Encyclopedia of Parkinson's Disease: Pathophysiology and Clinical Aspects

Volume II

Encyclopedia of Parkinson's Disease: Pathophysiology and Clinical Aspects
Volume II

Edited by **Kate White**

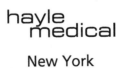

New York

Published by Hayle Medical,
30 West, 37th Street, Suite 612,
New York, NY 10018, USA
www.haylemedical.com

**Encyclopedia of Parkinson's Disease: Pathophysiology and
Clinical Aspects
Volume II**
Edited by Kate White

International Standard Book Number: 978-1-63241-190-7 (Hardback)

Printed in the United States of America.

Contents

Permissions

List of Contributors

Preface

The current book represents an elaborated study of the etiology and pathophysiology of Parkinson's disease, which is a complex neurological disorder. In this book, the ecological and biological agents which become the cause of Parkinson's disease have been described in detail. The book provides detailed description to readers about latest developments in several branches like neurotransmitters, inflammatory responses, oxidative pathways and biomarkers. Written by teachers of well reputed academic institutions the book highlights both primary and clinical approaches of Parkinson's disease. This book will be of great use for scientists and researchers. Also, neuroscience students and readers can gain ample knowledge from this book.

Various studies have approached the subject by analyzing it with a single perspective, but the present book provides diverse methodologies and techniques to address this field. This book contains theories and applications needed for understanding the subject from different perspectives. The aim is to keep the readers informed about the progresses in the field; therefore, the contributions were carefully examined to compile novel researches by specialists from across the globe.

Indeed, the job of the editor is the most crucial and challenging in compiling all chapters into a single book. In the end, I would extend my sincere thanks to the chapter authors for their profound work. I am also thankful for the support provided by my family and colleagues during the compilation of this book.

Editor

1

Brain Mitochondrial Dysfunction and Complex I Syndrome in Parkinson´s Disease

Laura B. Valdez[1], Manuel J. Bandez[2], Ana Navarro[2] and Alberto Boveris[1]
[1]Laboratory of Free Radical Biology, School of Pharmacy and Biochemistry,
University of Buenos Aires,
[2]Department of Biochemistry and Molecular Biology, School of Medicine,
University of Cádiz,
[1]Argentina
[2]Spain

1. Introduction

1.1 Clinical characteristics of Parkinson's disease

Parkinson's disease (PD) is an old-age neurodegenerative disease with a small but significant genetic risk. The prevalence of PD is of 0.3% in the whole population, affecting more than 1% of the humans over 60 years of age (de Lau & Breteler, 2006). Parkinson´s disease is characterized by the progressive loss of dopamine due to degeneration of dopaminergic neurons in the *substancia nigra, striatum* body and brain cortex. In addition, α-synuclein-positive Lewy bodies in brainstem and neocortex are consistently found at autopsy (Forno, 1996; Jellinger & Mizuno, 2003). Therefore, in patients with PD, movements, sleep, autonomic functions and cognition become progressively impaired.

Complex factors contribute to the appearance of PD but with a constant mitochondrial involvement and a decreased capacity to produce energy (ATP) in the affected brain areas (Shapira, 1998; Shapira, 2008). Mitochondrial dysfunction in the human frontal cortex is to be considered a factor contributing to impaired cognition in PD.

2. Environmental aspects and experimental models

Both environmental chemicals and genetic susceptibility are thought to contribute to the etiology of sporadic PD (Nagatsu, 2002). Despite of familial PD was correlated with a series of genes mutations, the etiology of idiopathic PD, which accounts for more than 90% of PD, is still not fully understood. It is well documented that there is an epidemiological link between PD and individuals who lives and works in rural areas and who has been exposed to various herbicides and insecticides (Gorell et al. 1998; Ayala et al., 2007; Gomez et al., 2007).

Although the etiopathogenesis of PD is still elusive, *post mortem* studies support the involvement of oxidative stress in neurons with an increased production of superoxide radical (O_2^-) and hydrogen peroxide (H_2O_2) and of mitochondrial dysfunction, especially of complex I of mitochondrial respiratory chain (Shapira et al., 1989; Shapira et al., 1990a, 1990b; Gomez et al., 2007; Navarro & Boveris, 2009; Navarro et al., 2009).

The early hints about the central role of mitochondria in the pathogenesis of PD resulted from the observation that human exposure to 1-methyl-4-phenyl-1,2,3,6-tetrahydropyridine (MPTP), a contaminant in synthetic opiates, triggered an acute and permanent parkinsonism with death of dopamine neurons (Langston et al., 1983). It was found that the MPTP active metabolite is the 1-methyl-4-phenilpyridinium ion (MPP^+). This compound is accumulated in mitochondria and produces their toxicity by inhibiting mitochondrial complex I, the proton pumping NADH:ubiquinone oxidoreductase.

As was mentioned above, epidemiological research indicates that exposure to pesticides and welding elevates the risk of PD (Chade et al., 2006; Dhillon et al., 2008). Most of pesticides are inhibitors of mitochondrial complex I, which is the first and the most vulnerable complex in the series of membrane H^+ pumps of the mitochondrial respiratory chain (Wallace et al., 1997). The pesticide rotenone ((2R,6aS,12aS)-1,2,6,6a,12,12a-hexahydro-2-isopropenyl-8,9-dimethoxychromeno [3,4-b]furo(2,3-h)chromen-6-one) is a powerful inhibitor of mitochondrial complex I: in isolated beef heart and liver mitochondria, rotenone median inhibitory concentration (IC_{50}) is 0.05 nmol/mg protein with a Ki of 4 nM (Degli, 1998). When neuron cultures are exposed to rotenone, the cells increase the O_2^- production rate leading them to death (Ahmadi et al., 2003; Moon et al., 2005). Furthermore, dopaminergic neuronal cells exposed to rotenone reproduce many of the features of PD including α-synuclein inclusions bodies in rats (Betarber et al., 2000; Sherer et al., 2003).

The above mentioned inhibitors of complex I, rotenone and MPTP, are typically used in the experimental model of PD in laboratory animals.

3. Genetic aspects

Although most PD cases are sporadic, the discovery of genes linked to familial form of disease due to mutations in the SNCA (α-synuclein), PARK2, DJ-1, PINK1, and LRRK2 genes has provided important clues about the disease progress (Henchcliffe & Beal., 2008; Zheng et al., 2010). In the sporadic disease, α-synuclein and degenerating mitochondria are the major components of Lewy bodies, the hall mark cytoplasmic inclusions found in PD brains. Biochemical complex I deficiency is found in PD patients not only in *substancia nigra* but also in platelets (Henchcliffe & Beal, 2008).

Recently, Zheng and coworkers (2010) reported that decreases in expression of 10 gene sets are associated with PD, even in probable subclinical disease and in tissues, outside *substancia nigra*. These 10 gene sets encode proteins responsible for interconnected cellular processes: nuclear-encoded mitochondrial electron transfer, mitochondrial biogenesis, glucose oxidation, and glucose sensing (Zheng et al., 2010). The authors showed that bioenergetics genes responsive to the master regulation of PGC-1α, including genes for nuclear-encoded electron transfer carriers are under expressed in patients with PD and in incipient Lewy body diseases. Furthermore, co-activation by PGC-1α up-regulates nuclear subunits of mitochondrial respiratory chain complexes I, II, III, IV, and V and blocks dopamine neuron loss in cellular models of PD-linked α-synocleinopathy and rotenone toxicity. Moreover, genetic ablation of PGC-1α in mice markedly enhanced MPTP-induced dopamine neuron loss in the *substancia nigra* (St-Pierre et al., 2006).

4. Pathophysiological aspects

Physiological, clinical and genetic studies support the relationship between PD and energy metabolism in neurons, including mitochondrial electron transport carriers and cytosolic glucose utilization. *In vivo* and *ex vivo* experimental results have shown that PD is primarily associated to two interdependent situations of brain mitochondria: (a) mitochondrial dysfunction; and (b) mitochondrial oxidative damage. In addition, defective oxidative phosphorylation was reported in muscle, and increased level of 8-hydroxydeoxyguanosine was found in PD patients plasma (Henchcliffe & Beal, 2008).

4.1 Mitochondrial complex I and physiological production of superoxide, nitric oxide and peroxynitrite

Mitochondrial complex I (NADH-UQ reductase) catalyzes electron transfer from NADH to ubiquinone and it is the main molecular pathway to link the tricarboxylic acid cycle, the coenzyme NADH and the mitochondrial respiratory chain. Complex I is a supra-molecular protein complex composed of about 40 polypeptide subunits and contains FMN and iron-sulphur centers (Walker, 1992; Walker et al., 1992). Two complex I-linked UQ-pools have been detected (Raha & Robinson, 2000). Non-covalent hydrophobic bonds are essential in keeping together the whole structure of complex I; low concentrations of detergents, natural and synthetic steroids (Boveris & Stoppani, 1970) and hydrophobic pesticides, such as rotenone and pyridaben (Gomez et al., 2007), are effective in disrupting intra-complex I polypeptide hydrophobic bonds and in inhibiting complex I electron transfer activity.

Complex I produces significant amounts of O_2^- in physiological conditions (0.80-0.90 nmol O_2^-/min.mg protein) through the auto-oxidation reaction of flavin-semiquinone (FMNH$^\bullet$) with molecular oxygen. It is understood that the ubisemiquinone (UQH$^\bullet$) auto-oxidation contribution, in complex I, is negligible (Boveris & Cadenas, 2000; Turrens & Boveris, 1980). Superoxide anion production yields an O_2^- steady state concentration of 0.1-0.2 nM in the mitochondrial matrix (Boveris & Cadenas, 2000; Boveris et al., 2006; Valdez et al., 2006). The O_2^- production rate by complex I is increased by inhibition of electron transfer with rotenone (Boveris & Chance, 1973) or by complex I dysfunction (Hensley et al., 2000; Navarro et al., 2009; Navarro et al., 2011).

Both, nitric oxide (NO) and peroxynitrite (ONOO-) have been proposed as direct inhibitors of complex I. Mitochondrial NO production is carried out by the mitochondrial nitric oxide synthase (mtNOS), an isoenzyme of the NOS family located in mitochondrial inner membrane (Tatoyan & Giulivi, 1998; Giulivi et al., 1998). Nitric oxide is produced at a rate of 1.0-1.4 nmol NO/min.mg protein and kept at a steady state level of 200-350 nM in the mitochondrial matrix (Boveris et al., 2006; Valdez et al., 2006). Peroxynitrite is generated in the mitochondrial matrix through the diffusion controlled reaction (k = 1.9×10^{10} M^{-1} s^{-1}) between two free radicals: O_2^- and NO. This reaction contributes with 0.38 μM ONOO-/sec in the mitochondrial matrix or 0.92 nmol/min. mg protein (Valdez et al., 2000). In this approximation the contribution of cytosolic NO has not been considered. Peroxynitrite is normally reduced by the mitochondrial reductants NADH, UQH$_2$ and GSH and kept at intramitochondrial steady state level of 2-5 nM (Valdez et al., 2000). When the steady state concentration of ONOO- is enhanced up to 25-40 nM, tyrosine nitration, protein oxidation and damage to iron sulfur centers might takes place, leading to a sustained complex I inhibition and increased generation of O_2^- by complex I.

4.2 Brain mitochondrial dysfunction: Complex I syndrome

Several studies have shown a mitochondrial dysfunction and a reduced activity of mitochondrial complex I in *substantia nigra* (Schapira et al., 1990a; Schapira et al., 1990b; Schapira, 2008b) and in frontal cortex (Navarro et al., 2009; Navarro & Boveris, 2009) in PD patients.

Gomez et al. (2007) and Navarro et al. (2009) have shown that the *in vitro* treatment of rat brain mitochondria with rotenone (1-10 μM) inhibits complex I activity without changes in complexes II, III and IV activities. In addition, coupled mitochondria isolated from rat brain incubated with rotenone showed a dose-dependent decrease in respiratory control with malate and glutamate as substrates, without modifications in the O_2 consumption when succinate was used as substrate (Gomez et al., 2007; Navarro et al., 2009).

Rats treated with rotenone (2 mg/kg weight, i.p. and daily, during 30 to 60 days) showed a selective nigrostriatal dopaminergic degeneration similar to the one observed in PD. Respiration rates were assessed in 1 mm³ brain cortex cubes, a thickness that allows O_2 diffusion to the center of the cube avoiding anaerobic areas. Control samples had a respiratory rate of about 0.45 μmol O_2/min. g striatum (Table 1). Rotenone treated rats during 30 and 60 days decreased 17% and 35%, respectively, the striatal O_2 uptake.

Experimental condition	O_2 consumption (ng-at O/ min.g striatum)
Control	896 ± 8
30 days rotenone	$744 \pm 8*$
60 days rotenone	$582 \pm 5*$#

Table 1. **Striatal O_2 consumption in rotenone-treated rats during 30 and 60 days.** Respiratory rates were determined in 1 mm³ rat striatum cubes in air-saturated Krebs suspending medium at 30°C. The values are means ± SEM: n = 3 per group (15 rats each group in pools of 5 rats). *p<0.05, rotenone treated rats *vs.* control rats; #p<0.05, 60 days-rotenone treated rats *vs.* 30 days-rotenone treated rats.

The same phenomenon was observed in isolated striatal mitochondria. Mitochondrial state 3 respiration decreased by about 13% and 30% after 30 and 60 days of rotenone treatment, with malate-glutamate as complex I substrate. Due to the fact that no changes were observed in state 4 respiration, the respiratory control also declined (Table 2). When succinate was used as complex II substrate, a slight impairment in state 3 respiration (20%) was observed after 60 days of rotenone administration.

The respiratory deficiency was further examined by assaying the activity of mitochondrial respiratory complexes. Table 3 shows that complex I activity decreased after 30 and 60 days of rotenone administration by 17% and 57%, respectively; complex IV activity declined 23% after 60 days of treatment; and complex II activity was not modified showing, once more, the highest and selective susceptibility of complex I to the oxidative, nitrosative and/or nitrative damage associated with rotenone treatment. The pattern observed for the decline of complex I activity in striatal mitochondria was also observed in the reduction of biochemical mtNOS (27% and 62%, in 30 and 60 days rotenone-treated rats) (Table 3) and functional mtNOS activities (29% and 71%), in accordance to the reported physical and functional interaction between complex I and mtNOS (Franco et al, 2006; Valdez & Boveris, 2007; Navarro et al., 2010).

Experimental conditions	Oxygen consumption (ng-at O/min. mg protein)		
	Control	Rotenone	
		30 days	60 days
Substrate: malate-glutamate			
State 4	42 ± 3	40 ± 3	38 ± 3
State 3	166 ± 9	144 ± 8*	116 ± 7*#
Respiratory control	3.9 ± 0.3	3.6 ± 0.3*	3.1 ± 0.4*
Substrate: succinate			
State 4	60 ± 4	58 ± 4	52 ± 4
State 3	240 ± 14	220 ± 11	192 ± 9*#
Respiratory control	4.0 ± 0.3	3.7 ± 0.3	3.7 ± 0.3

Table 2. **Striatum mitochondrial O_2 uptake of rotenone-treated rats during 30 and 60 days.** The values are means ± SEM: n = 3 per group (15 rats each in pools of 5 rats). *$p<0.05$, rotenone treated rats *vs.* control rats; # $p<0.05$, 60 days-rotenone treated rats *vs.* 30 days-rotenone treated rats.

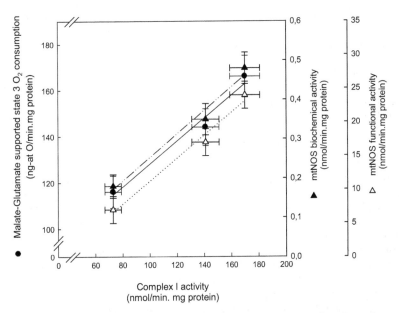

Fig. 1. Linear correlations between mitochondrial complex I activity and malate-glutamate supported state 3 respiration (•) ($r^2 = 0.97$) and between mitochondrial complex I activity and mtNOS biochemical (▲) ($r^2 = 0.98$) and functional activities (Δ) ($r^2 = 0.98$).

Linear correlations (Fig. 1) were obtained between mitochondrial complex I activity and either malate-glutamate supported state 3 O_2 uptake ($r^2 = 0.97$) or mtNOS biochemical ($r^2 = 0.98$) and functional activities ($r^2 = 0.98$), indicating that the pattern observed for the decline of complex I activity is associated to the reduction of mtNOS activity and to the impairment of striatum mitochondrial respiration.

Experimental condition	Complex I (nmol. min⁻¹. mg protein⁻¹)	Complex II (nmol. min⁻¹. mg protein⁻¹)	Complex IV (min⁻¹. mg protein⁻¹)	mtNOS (nmol. min⁻¹. mg protein⁻¹)
Control	170 ± 11	119 ± 9	75 ± 8	0.48 ± 0.04
30 days rotenone	$141 \pm 10*$	117 ± 9	61 ± 5	$0.35 \pm 0.04*$
60 days rotenone	$73 \pm 6*\#$	115 ± 9	$58 \pm 5*$	$0.18 \pm 0.03*\#$

Table 3. **Striatum mitochondrial enzymatic activities of rotenone-treated rats during 30 and 60 days.** The values are means ± SEM: n = 3 per group (15 rats each in pools of 5 rats). *p<0.05, rotenone treated rats *vs.* control rats; #p<0.05, 60 days-rotenone treated rats *vs.* 30 days-rotenone treated rats.

The experimental quantitative evidence shows a range of 35% to 73% of a decline of complex I activity in brain mitochondria in aging and in neurodegenerative diseases. A value of about 50% is considered a limit of a tolerable functional impairment in terms of energy production that is compatible with the physiological function. For instance, complex I is inactivated by 36% in aged rat whole brain mitochondria (Navarro & Boveris, 2007), by 73% in aged rat hippocampal mitochondria (Navarro et al., 2008), by 57% in rat striatal mitochondria in experimental parkinsonism (Table 3 and Fig. 1), and by 43% in cortex mitochondria of human PD patients (Navarro et al., 2010). The data included in Tables 1 and 2 and in Fig. 1 allow to making some quantitative considerations respect to the basal respiration of striatal tissue under no neurological stimulus (in physiological conditions the striatal route is constantly activated). Taking into account the striatal O_2 consumption in control rats of 896 ng-at O/min. g tissue, a mitochondrial content of 12 mg protein/g striatum, and the mitochondrial respirations (in ng-at O/min. mg protein) in state 3 of 166 (malate-glutamate) and of 240 (succinate) and in state 4 of 42 and 60 (respectively), the fraction of mitochondria in state 3 and in state 4 can be calculated (Boveris & Boveris, 2007):

$$\text{Tissue } O_2 \text{ consumption (ng-at O/min x g tissue)} =$$
$$\text{mg protein/g tissue x } [(a \text{ x state 3 } O_2 \text{ uptake}) + (1 - a) \text{ x (state 4 } O_2 \text{ uptake})]$$

The state 4 and state 3 mitochondrial O_2 consumption were calculated considering the detected O_2 uptake rates (Table 2) and the substrate supply in physiological conditions: [(3 x rate with malate-glutamate) + (rate with succinate)]/4. Therefore, striatal mitochondria are in the tissue about 20% in state 3 and about 80% in state 4. Under conditions of increased ATP demand, striatum mitochondria will be able to increase ATP synthesis up to 5 times by switching mitochondria from the resting state 4 to the active state 3. At variance, in experimental parkinsonism, after 60 days of rotenone treatment, mitochondria are 8% in state 3 and 92% in state 4, showing that in parkinsonism, striatal mitochondria are severely limited in their capacity to respond to ATP demands.

Moreover, similar mitochondrial complex I dysfunctions were reported in skeletal muscle and platelets of PD patients (Mann et al., 1992). This condition of complex I impairment is likely to be of pathogenic importance because intoxication of experimental animals with inhibitors of complex I (rotenone, MPTP, MPP⁺) (Bougria et al., 1995; Gomez et al., 2007) reproduces the clinical symptoms of PD in human subjects.

4.3 Brain mitochondrial oxidative damage
The mtNOS and complex I functional association in brain has been linked to the development of neurodegenerative diseases (Navarro et al., 2010). As it has been early

proposed (Hensley et al., 2000), changes in complex I proteins are certainly an explanation for the increase in O_2^- and H_2O_2 production rates. Rat treated with rotenone during 30 and 60 days increased the O_2^- production rates by about 13% and 37%, respectively (Table 4). This enhancement is in agreement with an increased generation of phospholipids oxidation and protein oxidation products in striatal mitochondria (Fig. 2 A and B).

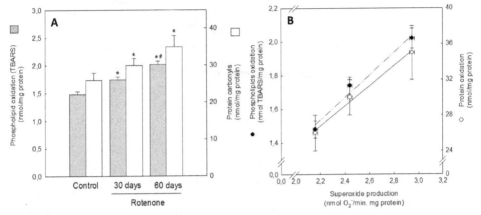

Fig. 2. **A**. Protein carbonyls and phospholipid oxidation products in striatal mitochondria of rotenone-treated rats. The values are means ± SEM: n=3 per group (15 rats each in pools of 5 rats). *p < 0.05, rotenone treated rats *vs.* control rats; #p<0.05, 60 days-rotenone treated rats *vs.* 30 days-rotenone treated rats. **B**. Linear correlations between O_2^- production rate and either phospholipid oxidation (•) ($r^2 = 0.98$) or protein oxidation (o) ($r^2 = 0.99$) products.

Navarro and co-workers (2009) have shown a marked impairments of tissue and malate-glutamate supported state 3 mitochondrial respiration and of complex I activity, associated with an oxidative damage, in frozen samples of frontal cortex (area 8) in PD patients in comparison to age-matched healthy controls (Navarro et al., 2009). Thus, human cortex mitochondrial dysfunction in PD is now added to the classical recognition of mitochondrial dysfunction in *substantia nigra*, which was early considered as specifically sensitive brain area in PD (Schapira et al., 1990a).

Experimental condition	O_2^- production (nmol/min. mg protein)
Control	2.16 ± 0.02
30 days rotenone	2.44 ± 0.02*
60 days rotenone	2.95 ± 0.02*#

Table 4. **Striatum mitochondrial superoxide anion production of rotenone-treated rats during 30 and 60 days.** The values are means ± SEM: n = 3 per group (15 rats each in pools of 5 rats). *p<0.05, rotenone treated rats *vs.* control rats; #p<0.05, 60 days-rotenone treated rats *vs.* 30 days-rotenone treated rats.

Mitochondrial complex I is particularly sensitive in terms of inhibition and inactivation to oxidants, oxygen free radicals and reactive nitrogen species. The mitochondrial dysfunction is currently described as "complex I syndrome", that includes decreased tissue O_2 uptake, decreased malate/glutamate-supported mitochondrial respiration, reduced complex I (NADH-dehydrogenase) activity, increased phospholipid and protein oxidation products, increased protein nitration products, and increased O_2^- and H_2O_2 production rates (Boveris et al., 2010). Interestingly, high doses of vitamin E are able to restore to normal the age-dependent complex I syndrome in hippocampus and brain cortex (Navarro et al., 2010).This "complex I syndrome" has been observed in PD and in other neurodegenerative diseases (Schapira et al., 1990a; Schapira et al., 1990b; Cooper et al., 1992; Schapira, 2008; Carreras et al., 2004; Navarro & Boveris, 2007; Navarro et al., 2009), as well as in aging (Boveris& Navarro, 2008) and in ischemia-reperfusion (Gonzalez-Flecha et al., 1993; Valdez et al., 2011).

The molecular mechanisms responsible for complex I syndrome are likely accounted for a series of processes and reactions that lead synergistically to complex I inactivation. The involved processes and reactions are, in the first place, the lipid peroxidation process and the reactions of the reactive free radical intermediates (mainly ROO$^•$) with complex I. In the second place, the reactions of the aldehydes produced in the lipid peroxidation process (4-HO-nonenal and malonaldehyde) with amino groups of the polypeptide chain of the complex I proteins. In the third place, nitration of complex I proteins following to the increased formation of ONOO-, the chemical species produced by the intramitochondrial reaction of NO and O_2^-at the vicinity of NADH-dehydrogenase active center (Turrens & Boveris, 1980). The three mentioned processes provide synergistically pathways leading to complex I inactivation. Interestingly, complex I inactivation is accompanied by increased auto-oxidation and O_2^- production rate and subsequently an enlarged generation of H_2O_2 (Hensley et al., 2000; Navarro et al., 2011). It is understood that the reactions that inactivate complex I, mediated by free radicals (ROO$^•$), aldehydes and ONOO-, change the native non-covalent intermolecular forces bonding and synergistically promote covalent cross linking with protein inactivation (Liu et al., 2003).

5. Conclusions

Parkinson's disease is characterized by persistent, coordinated, nuclear-encoded cellular energy defects to which nigral dopamine neurons are intrinsically more susceptible than others cells. Complex I dysfunction in PD may be a biochemically detectable "tip of the iceberg" of a deeper molecular defect comprising the entire nuclear-encoded electron transfer chain. Under expression of PGC-1α-controlled genes involved in cellular energetic might represent a common link for these diverse manifestations of defects in mitochondrial biogenesis, and abnormal glucose utilization. One of the basic postulates of the mitochondrial theory of aging and neurodegenerative diseases is that there is a significant reduction in the capacity for ATP production in the brain and other organs of old mammals. The concept of a decrease in the effectiveness of the mitochondrial process of energy transduction (or oxidative phosphorylation) is expressed as an under function of "the mitochondrial redox-energy axis" (Yap et al., 2010). Although mitochondrial complexes, complex I (Valdez et al., 2004; Boveris & Navarro, 2008; Navarro et al., 2009), complex IV (Valdez et al., 2004; Boveris & Navarro, 2008), and complex V (Lam et al., 2009), are considered the main targets in neurodegeneration and aging, there are also cytosolic enzymes whose activities are simultaneously decreased, such as succinyl-CoA-transferase (Lam et al. 2009) and as 6-phosphofructo-2-kinase (Herrero-Mendez et al., 2009). The cytosolic-mitochondrial interaction is certainly affected and there is recognition of a depressed glucose metabolism as the earliest and consistent abnormality in neurodegenerative diseases (Yap et al., 2009).

6. Acknowledgments

This work was supported by research grants from the University of Buenos Aires (B005), Agencia Nacional de Promoción Científica y Tecnológica (PICT 38326, PICT 1138), and Consejo Nacional de Investigaciones Científicas y Técnicas (PIP 688) in Argentina; and from Ministerio de Ciencia e Innovación (SAF2008-03690) and Plan Andaluz de Investigación 2007-2008 (CTS-194) in Spain.

7. References

Ahmadi, FA.,Linseman, DA., Grammatopoulos, TN., Jones, SM.,Bouchard, RJ., Freed, CR., Heidenreich, KA. &Zawada, WM. (2003). The pesticide rotenone induces caspase-3-mediatedapoptosis in ventral mesencephalic dopaminergic neurons. *J. Neurochem* 87: 914–921.

Ayala, A., Venero, JL., Cano, J. & Machado, A. (2007) Mitochondrial toxins and neurodegenerative diseases. *Front Biosci* 12: 986-1007

Betarbet, R., Sherer, TB., MacKenzie, G., Garcia-Osuna, M., Panov, AV. & Greenamyre, JT. (2000) Chronic systemic pesticide exposure reproduces features of Parkinson's disease. *Nat Neurosci* 3: 1301-1306

Bougria, M., Vitorica, J., Cano, J. & Machado, A. (1995) Implication of dopamine transporter system on 1-methyl-4-phenylpyridinium and rotenone effect in striatal synaptosomes. *Eur J Pharmacol* 291: 407-415

Boveris, A. & Cadenas, E. (2000) Mitochondrial production of hydrogen peroxide regulation by nitric oxide and the role of ubisemiquinone. *IUBMB Life* 50: 245-250.

Boveris, A. & Chance, B. (1973) The mitochondrial generation of hydrogen peroxide. *Biochem J.* 134: 617-630

Boveris, A. & Navarro, A. (2008) Brain mitochondrial dysfunction in aging. *IUBMB Life* 60: 308-314

Boveris, A. & Stoppani, AOM. (1970) Inhibition of electron and energy transfer in mitochondria by 19-nor-ethynyltestosterone acetate. *Arch Biochem Biophys* 141: 641-655

Boveris, A., Carreras, MC. & Poderoso, JJ. (2010) The regulation of cell energetics and mitochondrial signaling by nitric oxide. In: *Nitric oxide: Biology and Pathobiology*, Ignarro, L., pp. 441-482, Elsevier Academic Press Inc, London, UK.

Boveris, A., Valdez, LB., Zaobornyj, T. & Bustamante, J. (2006) Mitochondrial metabolic states regulate nitric oxide and hydrogen peroxide diffusion to the cytosol. *Biochim Biophys Acta* 1757: 535-542

Boveris, DL. & Boveris, A. (2007) Oxygen delivery to the tissues and mitochondrial respiration. *Front Biosci.* 12: 1014-1023

Carreras, MC., Franco, MC., Peralta, JG. & Poderoso, JJ. (2004) Nitric oxide, complex I, and the modulation of mitochondrial reactive species in biology and disease. *Mol Aspects Med* 25: 125-139

Chade, AR., Kasten, M. & Tanner, CM. (2006) Nongenetic causes of Parkinson's disease. *J Neural Transm Suppl* 70: 147-151

Cooper, JM., Mann, VM., Krige, D. & Schapira, AH. (1992) Human mitochondrial complex I dysfunction. *Biochim Biophys Acta* 1101: 198-120

de Lau, LM. & Breteler, MM. (2006) Epidemiology of Parkinson's disease. *Lancet Neurol* 5: 525-535

Degli, EM. (1998) Inhibitors of NADH-ubiquinone reductase: an overview. *Biochim Biophys Acta* 1364: 222-235

Dhillon, AS., Tarbutton, GL., Levin, JL., Plotkin, GM., Lowry, LK.,Nalbone, JT. & Shepherd, S. (2008) Pesticide/environmental exposures and Parkinson's disease in East Texas. *J Agromedicine* 13: 37-48

Forno, LS. (1996) Neuropathology of Parkinson's disease. *J Neuropathol Exp Neurol* 55: 259-272

Franco, MC., Arciuch, VG., Peralta, JG., Galli, S., Levisman, D., Lopez, LM., Romorini, L., Poderoso, JJ. & Carreras, MC. (2006) Hypothyroid Phenotype is contributed by mitochondrial complex I inactivation due to translocated neuronal nitric-oxide synthase. *J Biol Chem* 281: 4779-4786

Giulivi, C., Poderoso, JJ. & Boveris, A. (1998) Production of nitric oxide by mitochondria. *J. Biol Chem* 273: 11038-11043

Gomez, C., Bandez, MJ. & Navarro, A (2007) Pesticides and impairment of mitochondrial function in relation with the parkinsonian syndrome. *Front Biosci* 12: 1079-1093

González-Flecha, B., Cutrin, JC. & Boveris, A. (1993) Time course and mechanism of oxidative stress and tissue damage in rat liver subjected to in vivo ischemia-reperfusion. *J Clin Invest* 91: 456-464

Gorell, JM., Johnson, CC., Rybicki, BA., Peterson, EL. & Richardson, RJ. (1998) The risk of Parkinson's disease with exposure to pesticides, farming, well water, and rural living. *Neurology* 50: 1346-1350

Henchcliffe, C. & Beal, MF. (2008) Mitochondrial biology and oxidative stress in Parkinson disease pathogenesis. *Nat Clin Pract Neurol* 4: 600-609

Hensley, K., Kotake, Y., Sang, H., Pye, Q., Wallis, G., Kolker, L., Tabatabaie, T., Stewart, C., Konishi, Y., Nakae, D. & Floyd, R. (2000) Dietary choline restriction causes complex I dysfunction and increased H_2O_2 generation in liver mitochondria. *Carcinogenesis* 21: 983-989

Herrero-Mendez, A., Almeida, A., Fernández, E., Maestre, C., Moncada, S. & Bolaños, JP. (2009) The bioenergetic and antioxidant status of neurons is controlled by continuous degradation of a key glycolytic enzyme by APC/C-Cdh1. *Nat Cell Biol.* 11: 747-752

Jellinger, KA. & Mizuno, Y. (2003) Parkinson's disease. In: *Neurodegeneration: The molecular pathology of dementia and movement disorders*, Dickson, D., pp. 159-187, Neuropath Press

Lam, PY., Yin, F., Hamilton, RT., Boveris, A., Cadenas, E. (2009) Elevated neuronal nitric oxide synthase expression during ageing and mitochondrial energy production. *Free Radic Res* 43: 431-439

Langston, JW., Ballard, JW., Tetrud, JW. & Irwin, I. (1983) Chronic parkinsonism in human due to a product of meperidine-analog synthesis. *Science* 219: 979-980

Liu, Q., Raina, AK., Smith, MA., Sayre, LM. & Perry, G. (2003) Hydroxynonenal, toxic carbonyls, and Alzheimer disease. *Mol Aspects Med* 24: 305-313

Mann, VM., Cooper, JM., Krige, D., Daniel, SE., Schapira, AH. & Marsden, CD. (1992) Brain, skeletal muscle and platelet homogenate mitochondrial function in Parkinson's disease. *Brain* 115: 333-342

Mizuno, Y., Ohta, S., Tanaka, M., Takamiya, S., Suzuki, K., Sato, T., Oya, H., Ozawa, T. & Kagawa, Y. (1989) *Biochem Biophys Res Commun* 163: 1450-1455

Moon, Y., Lee, KH., Park, JH., Geum, D. & Kim, K. (2005). Mitochondrial membrane depolarization and the selective death of dopaminergic neurons by rotenone: protective effect of coenzyme Q10. *J. Neurochem.* 93: 1199–1208.

Nagatsu, T. (2002) Amine-related neurotoxins in Parkinson's disease: past, present, and future. *Neurotoxicol Teratol* 24: 565-569

Navarro, A. & Boveris, A. (2007) The mitochondrial energy transduction system and the aging process. *Am J Physiol Cell Physiol* 292: C670-686

Navarro, A. & Boveris, A. (2008) Mitochondrial nitric oxide synthase, mitochondrial brain dysfunction in aging, and mitochondria-targeted antioxidants. *Adv Drug Deliv Rev* 60: 1534-1544

Navarro, A. & Boveris, A. (2009) Brain mitochondrial dysfunction and oxidative damage in Parkinson's disease. *J Bioenerg Biomembr* 41: 517-521

Navarro, A., Bández, MJ., Gómez, C., Repetto, MG. &Boveris, A. (2010) Effects of rotenone and pyridaben on complex I electron transfer and on mitochondrial nitric oxide synthase functional activity. *J Bioenerg Biomembr* 42: 405-412

Navarro, A., Bandez, MJ., Lopez-Cepero, JM., Gómez, C. &Boveris, A. (2011) High doses of vitamin E improve mitochondrial dysfunction in rat hippocampus and frontal cortex upon aging. *Am J Physiol Regul Integr Comp Physiol* 300: R827-834

Navarro, A., Boveris, A., Bández, MJ., Sánchez-Pino, MJ., Gómez, C., Muntané, G. & Ferrer, I. (2009) Human brain cortex: mitochondrial oxidative damage and adaptive response in Parkinson disease and in dementia with Lewy bodies. *Free Rad Biol Med* 46: 1574-1580

Navarro, A., López-Cepero, JM., Bández, MJ., Sánchez-Pino, MJ., Gómez, C., Cadenas, E. & Boveris, A. (2008) Hippocampal mitochondrial dysfunction in rat aging. *Am J Physiol Regul Integr Comp Physiol* 294: R501-509

Persichini, T., Mazzone, V., Polticelli, F., Moreno, S., Venturini, G., Clementi, E. & Colasanti, M. (2005) Mitochondrial type I nitric oxide synthase physically interacts with cytochrome oxidase. *Neuroscience Lett* 384: 254-259

Raha, S. & Robinson, BH. (2000) Mitochondria, oxygen free radicals, disease and ageing. *Trends Biochem Sci* 25: 502-508.

Schapira, AH. (2008a) Mitochondria in the aetiology and pathogenesis of Parkinson's disease. *Lancet Neurol* 7: 97-109

Schapira, AH. (2008b) Mitochondrial dysfunction in neurodegenerative diseases. *Neurochem Res* 33: 2502-2509

Schapira, AH., Cooper, JM., Dexter, D., Clark, JB., Jenner, P. & Marsden, CD. (1990a) Mitochondrial complex I deficiency in Parkinson's disease. *J Neurochem* 54: 823-827

Schapira, AH., Cooper, JM., Dexter, D., Jenner, P., Clark, JB. & Marsden, CD. (1989) Mitochondrial complex I deficiency in Parkinson's disease. *Lancet* 1: 1269

Schapira, AH., Mann, VM., Cooper, JM., Dexter, D., Daniel, SE., Jenner, P., Clark, JB. & Marsden, CD. (1990b) Anatomic and disease specificity of NADH CoQ1 reductase (complex I) deficiency in Parkinson's disease. *J Neurochem* 55: 2142-2145.

Shapira, AH. (1998) Mitochondrial dysfunction in neurodegenerative disorders. *Biochim Biophys Acta* 1366: 225-233

Sherer, TB., Betarbet, R., Testa, CM., Seo, BB., Richardson, JR., Kim, JH., Miller, GW., Yagi, T., Matsuno-Yagi, A. & Greenamyre JT. (2003) Mechanism of toxicity in rotenone models of Parkinson's disease. *J Neurosci* 23: 10756-10764

St-Pierre, J., Drori, S., Uldry, M., Silvaggi, JM., Rhee, J., Jäger, S., Handschin, C., Zheng, K., Lin, J., Yang, W., Simon, DK., Bachoo, R., Spiegelman, BM. (2006) Suppression of reactive oxygen species and neurodegeneration by the PGC-1 transcriptional coactivators. *Cell* 127: 397-408.

Tatoyan, A. & Giulivi, G. (1998) Purification and characterization of a nitric-oxide synthase from rat liver mitochondria. *J Biol Chem* 273: 11044-11048

Turrens, JF. & Boveris, A. (1980) Generation of superoxide anion by the NADH dehydrogenase of bovine heart mitochondria. *Biochem J* 191: 421-427

Valdez, LB. & Boveris, A. (2007) Mitochondrial nitric oxide synthase, a voltage-dependent enzyme, is responsible for nitric oxide diffusion to cytosol. *Front Biosci* 12:1210-1219

Valdez, LB., Alvarez, S., LoresArnaiz, S., Schöpfer, F., Carreras, MC.,Poderoso, JJ. & Boveris A. (2000) Reactions of peroxynitrite in the mitochondrial matrix. *Free Rad Biol Med* 29: 349-356

Valdez, LB., Zaobornyj, T. & Boveris, A. (2006) Mitochondrial metabolic states and membrane potential modulate mtNOS activity. *Biochim Biophys Acta* 1757: 166-172

Valdez, LB., Zaobornyj, T., Alvarez, S., Bustamante, J., Costa, LE. & Boveris, A. (2004) Heart mitochondrial nitric oxide synthase. Effects of hypoxia and aging. *Mol Aspects Med* 25: 49-59

Valdez, LB., Zaobornyj, T., Bombicino, SS., Iglesias, DE. & Boveris, A. (2011) Regulation of heart mitochondrial nitric oxide synthase (mtNOS) by oxygen. In *Mitochondrial Pathophysiology*, Cadenas, S. & Palau, F. In press. Transworld Research Network, Kerala, India.

Walker, JE. (1992) The NADH:ubiquinoneoxidoreductase (complex I) of respiratory chains. *Q Rev Biophys* 25: 253-324

Walker, JE., Arizmendi, JM., Dupuis, A., Fearnley, IM., Finel, M., Medd, SM., Pilkington, SJ., Runswick, MJ. & Skehel, JM. (1992) Sequences of 20 subunits of NADH:ubiquinoneoxidoreductase from bovine heart mitochondria. Application of a novel strategy for sequencing proteins using the polymerase chain reaction. *J Mol Biol* 226: 1051-1072

Wallace, KB., Eells, JT., Madeira, VM., Cortopassi, G. & Jones, DP. (1997) Mitochondria-mediated cell injury. Symposium overview. *Fundam Appl Toxicol* 38: 23-37

Yap, LP., Garcia. JV., Han, DS. & Cadenas, E. (2011) Role of nitric oxide-mediated glutathionylation in neuronal function: potential regulation of energy utilization. *Biochem J* 428: 85–93

Zheng, B., Liao Z., Locascio, JJ., Lesniak, KA., Roderick, SS., Watt, ML., Eklund, AC., Zhang-James, Y., Kim, PD., Hauser, MA., Grünblatt, E., Moran, LB., Mandel, SA., Riederer, P., Mille,r RM., Federoff, HJ., Wüllner, U., Papapetropoulos, S., Youdim, MB., Cantuti-Castelvetri, I., Young, AB., Vance, JM., Davis, RL., Hedreen, JC., Adler, CH., Beach, TG., Graeber, MB., Middleton, FA., Rochet, JC., Scherzer, CR. (2010) Global PD Gene Expression (GPEX) Consortium. PGC-1α, a potential therapeutic target for early intervention in Parkinson's disease. *Sci Transl Med* 2: 52ra73

2

Oxidative DNA Damage and the Level of Biothiols, and L-Dopa Therapy in Parkinson's Disease

Dorszewska Jolanta and Kozubski Wojciech

Poznan University of Medical Sciences, Laboratory of Neurobiology Department of Neurology, Chair and Department of Neurology, Poland

1. Introduction

Parkinson's disease (PD) is a chronic and progressive neurological disorder characterized by resting tremor, rigidity, and bradykinesia, affecting at least 1% of individuals above the age of 65 years. Parkinson's disease is a result of degeneration of the dopamine-producing neurons of the *substantia nigra*. Available therapies in PD will only improve the symptoms but not halt progression of disease. The most effective treatment for PD patients is therapy with L-3,4-dihydroxy-phenylalanine (L-dopa) (Olanow, 2008). As indicated in literature reports, L-dopa therapy leads to motor fluctuations and disabling involuntary movements called L-dopa-induced dyskinesia (Carta et al., 2006; Obeso et al., 2008). Literature reports indicate also that long-term administration of L-dopa in PD patients may not only alter arginine (Arg) levels but may also lead to increased concentrations of homocysteine (Hcy), the factor responsible for development of atherosclerosis and dysfunction of nigral endothelial cells (Muller et al., 1999). Methylenetetrahydrofolate reductase (MTHFR) represents enzyme involved in remethylation of Hcy to methionine (Met). The C667T transition in *MTHFR* results in Ala>Val substitution in position 226 and, as a consequence, in 50 % decrease in the enzyme activity, and thus in an increased concentration of Hcy (Frosst et al., 1995). The study of Yasui et al. (2000) indicated that the TT genotype might be linked to pathogenesis of PD, particularly when the level of folates is low. Moreover, L-dopa metabolism via O-methylation by catechol-O-methyl-transferase (COMT) using S-adenosyl-L-methionine (SAM) leads to increase Hcy levels, hyper-Hcy (O'Suilleabhain et al., 2004a). A percentage 10-30% of PD patients exhibits hyper-Hcy. Hyper-Hcy in PD has been associated with affective and cognitive impairment, dementia, dyskinesia, and vascular disease (O'Suilleabhain et al., 2004b; Rogers et al., 2003; Zoccolella et al., 2006, 2009).

The exact mechanism of development and progression of PD pathology is not clear. It is known, that a complex interplay of multiple environmental and genetic factors has been involved in pathogenesis of PD and it is possibly that PD represents rather a syndrome but not a single disorder. Moreover, is likely that in pathogenesis of PD there are several mechanisms involved, such as: oxidative stress, mitochondrial dysfunction, DNA damage, protein aggregation, neuroinflammation, excitotoxicity, apoptosis and loss of trophic factors. The most probably is that all factors are represented targets for PD therapy.

2. 8-Oxo-2'-deoxyguanosine and L-dopa treatment in Parkinson's disease

Oxidative stress and excitotoxicity seems to play a pivotal role in pathogenesis of few major neurodegenerative diseases e.g. Alzheimer's disease (AD) and PD. The study of Jenner (2003) indicates that oxidative stress in the brain of PD patients may leads to formed reactive forms of oxygen (RFO). In the course of PD, RFO activate processes leading to the damage of DNA, proteins and lipids, and to a low level of antioxidants (Blake et al., 1997; Kikuchi et al., 2002). Moreover, in the patients suffering from PD, dopamine level-controlled deposition of ubiquitin- and α-synuclein-positive inclusion bodies (Lewy's bodies) takes place in the cytoplasm of dopaminergic neurons (Spillantini et al., 1997). Deposition of pathological proteins in brains of patients affected by the neurodegenerative diseases, result in pronounced neurotoxic effects on the central nervous system (CNS). In PD, augmented expression of α-synuclein may intensify oxidative stress (Hsu et al., 2000). Bergman et al. (1998) demonstrated that in the PD patients, dopaminergic neurons undergo oxidative damage of the compact portion of *substantia nigra* and dopamine levels decrease in putamen, a region of caudate nucleus. Moreover, ferrous ions released from damaged *substantia nigra* may provide an important substrate for oxidative reactions and for production of RFO (Jenner, 2003).

In PD, oxidative stress follows accumulation of the degradation products in the gray matter compact part of mesencephalon, and is accompanied not only by a high level of ferrous ions, and by decreased level of glutathione, malfunction of the respiratory chain complex I (Jenner, 2003; Schapira et al., 1990; Sian et al., 1994), and excessive oxidation processes, especially in patients treated with L-dopa (Spencer et al., 1994).

L-Dopa after oral intake undergoes metabolism, including oxidative metabolism of dopamine, and auto-oxidation, and is transported across the blood-brain barrier. Only less than 5% of an oral dose of L-dopa after took delivered to the brain. Remain plasmatic levels of L-dopa undergoes peripheral oxidative metabolism and may generate ROS. Likely peripheral oxidation status in PD might be affected by L-dopa therapy (Cornetta et al., 2009).

Some studies (e.g. Cornetta et al., 2009) suggest a toxic effect of L-dopa on neuronal cell *in vitro*, while *in vivo* studies in animal models are contradictory. However, in patients with PD some authors indicated on positive correlation between oxidative stress and L-dopa therapy (Florczak et al., 2008; Migliore at al., 2002), but there are also negative correlation between oxidative stress and L-dopa dosage in peripheral blood lymphocytes (in nine patients with PD et paper of Cornetta et al., 2009; Prigione et al., 2006).

As indicated by literature reports, interaction of reactive oxygen with nucleic acids leads to oxidation of guanine and formation of 8-oxo-2'-deoxyguanosine (8-oxo2dG). Oxidative modification of guanine at C8 position may take place either in nucleic acids or free cellular nucleosides and nucleotides, ready to be incorporated to newly synthesized DNA chains. Incorporation of the modified nucleotide to DNA may results in mutations due to pairing of 8-oxoguanosine with cytosine and adenosine. In the course of pairing with adenosine, 8-oxoguanosine induces GC→AT transversions (Hirano, 2008). 8-Oxoguanina or its nucleoside, 8-oxo2dG there are though to represent markers of oxidative DNA damage.

Augmented levels of 8-oxo2dG were demonstrated in brain and in lymphocytes of patients with PD (Alam et al., 1997; Dorszewska et al., 2007; Florczak et al., 2008; Kikuchi et al., 2002; Zhang et al., 1999). This indicates a gradual increase of nucleic acid damage during development of this disease, and high level of oxidized guanine in DNA is considered a risk factor for senescence and neurodegenerative diseases (e.g. PD).

The contribution of L-dopa therapy to oxidative damage and apoptosis in peripheral cells in PD patients is not clear, and is still debated.

2.1 Influence of L-dopa treatment on the level of 8-oxo-2dG in peripheral blood lymphocytes of Parkinson's disease patients

The aim of the study was to estimate the degree of oxidative damage to DNA (marker: 8-oxo2dG) in PD patients before and during treatment with L-Dopa, and in controls.

2.1.1 Patients

The studies were conducted on 98 patients with PD, including 37 women and 61 men aging 34-81 years (mean age: 60.8 ± 10.7 years). Among the patients with PD, 27 patients (9 women and 18 men) awaited L-dopa treatment (patients' age: 34-79 years) and the remaining 71 individuals, 28 women and 43 men (patients' age: 35-81 years) were treated with L-dopa preparations in daily doses (up to 5 years treatment to 500 mg/day, 5-10 year treatment 500-800 mg/day, and over 10 year treatment 800-1500 mg/day).

Control group included 50 individuals, 34 women and 16 men, 22-76 years of age (mean age: 44.6 ± 16.2 years).

Patients with PD were diagnosed using the criteria of UK Parkinson's Disease Society Brain Bank (Litvan et al., 2003), however stage of disease according to the scale of Hoehn and Yahr.

None of the control subjects had verifiable symptoms of dementia or any other neurological disorders and smoking, and drinking habits.

A Local Ethical Committee approved the study and the written consent of all patients or their caregivers was obtained.

2.1.2 Determination of 8-oxo2dG

Isolation of DNA. DNA was isolated from peripheral blood lymphocytes by fivefold centrifugation in a lytic buffer, containing 155 mM NH_4Cl, 10 mM $KHCO_3$, 0.1 mM Na_2EDTA, pH 7.4, in the presence of buffer containing 75 mM NaCl, 9 mM Na_2EDTA , pH 8.0, and sodium dodecyl sulfate and proteinase K (Sigma, St. Louis, MO). Subsequently, NaCl was added, the lysate was centrifuged, and DNA present in the upper layer was precipitated with 98% ethanol.

Enzymatic hydrolysis of DNA to nucleosides. DNA was hydrolyzed to nucleosides using P_1 nuclease (Sigma), for 2 h at 37ºC in 10 mM NaOAc, pH 4.5. The solution was buffered with 100 mM Tris-HCl, pH 7.5. Subsequently, the DNA was hydrolyzed with alkaline phosphatase (1U/μl; Roche, Germany) for 1 h at 37 ºC and the obtained nucleosides mixture was applied to high-pressure liquid chromatography system with both electrochemical and UV detection (HPLC/EC/UV).

Estimation of 8-oxo2dG. To determine 8-oxo2dG level, the nucleosides mixture was applied to the HPLC/UV system (P580A; Dionex, Germany) coupled to an electrochemical detector (CoulArray 5600; ESA, USA). Nucleosides were separated in a Termo Hypersil BDS C18 (250 x 4.6 x 5μm) column (Germany). The system was controlled, and the data were collected and processed using Chromeleon software (Dionex, Germany). The results were expressed as a ratio of oxidized nucleosides in the form of 8-oxo2dG to unmodified 2'dG (Olsen et al., 1999).

2.1.3 Results

In the patients with PD (Table 1), the levels of 8-oxo2dG in peripheral blood lymphocytes were significantly increased ($p<0.05$), as compared to the controls.

Parameter	Controls (22-76 years)	Patients with PD (34-81 years)
8-oxo2dG	13.7 ± 7.6	$21.8 \pm 17.8^*$

Table 1. Levels of DNA oxidative damage (8-oxo2dG/dG x 10^{-5}) in the PD patients and in control group. Results are expressed as a means ± SD. The nonparametric of Mann-Whitney test for unlinked variables was used. Differences significant at $^*p<0.05$, as compared to the controls.

In the PD patients (Table 2) disease progress from stage I to IV (according to the scale of Hoehn and Yahr) resulted in higher level of 8-oxo2dG in DNA ($p<0.05$) also observed between stages I and III, and a tendency to further decrease in stage IV.

Parameter	Stage I (35-79 years)	Stage II (34-81 years)	Stage III (46-81 years)	Stage IV (56-78 years)
8-oxo2dG	17.4 ± 16.9	20.5 ± 14.2	25.2 ± 22.7	$23.2 \pm 12.8^*$

Table 2. Levels of oxidative DNA damage (8-oxo2dG/dG x 10^{-5}), as related to the stage of the PD according to the scale of Hoehn and Yahr. Results are expressed as means ± SD. The nonparametric of Mann-Whitney test for unlinked variables was used. Differences significant at $^*p<0.05$, between stages I and IV of PD.

Pharmacotherapy with L-dopa (Table 3) affected the level of 8-oxo2dG ($p<0.01$), as compared to the healthy controls.

Parameter	Controls (22-76 years)	Patients with PD L-dopa (-) (34-79 years)	Patients with PD L-dopa (+) (35-81 years)
8-oxo2dG	13.7 ± 7.6	19.3 ± 17.3	$22.6 \pm 18.0^{**}$

Table 3. Levels of oxidative DNA damage (8-oxo2dG/dG x 10^{-5}), as related to pharmacotherapy with L-dopa (+) in the patients with PD. Results are expressed as means ± SD. The nonparametric of Mann-Whitney test for unlinked variables was used. Differences significant at $^{**}p<0.01$, as compared to the controls.

Our results indicated that, L-dopa can modify the level of oxidative DNA damage (8-oxo2dG) in the peripheral blood cells of PD patients. On the other hand, it is interesting that in PD a significant increase in DNA damage has been observed in the IVth stage of the disease development (according to Hoehn and Yahr), even so 8-oxo2dG levels are increased between the stages I and III of the disease evolution. It seems that in PD the reason for increasing levels of oxidative process altered nucleic acids is thought to involve overproduction of free radicals as well as decreased levels of enzymatic and non-enzymatic antioxidants and less effective repair mechanisms. In AD patients have been found to contain lowered activity of specific 8-oxoguanine glycosylase 1, OGG1, and more oxidative DNA damage which might induce of apoptosis (Dorszewska et al., 2005, 2009a, 2010).

It seems that analysis of the level of oxidative stress (8-oxo2dG) may be represented targets for diagnosis of PD and therapy in future.

2.2 Influence of L-dopa treatment on the level of apoptotic factors in peripheral blood lymphocytes of Parkinson's disease patients

At the neuropathological studies, PD is mainly characterized by neuronal intracellular inclusions named Lewy's bodies with α-synuclein. These inclusions are now known to be comprised of filamentous polymers of α-synuclein, which may generate oxidative stress in the brain of PD patients. It could results from several mechanisms, such as depletion of antioxidants, defects in mitochondrial electron transport, neurotoxin exposure, and excessive oxidation of dopamine in the patients given L-dopa. Conway et al. (2001) showed that dopamine or L-dopa inhibits the fibrillization of α-synuclein filaments by stabilization of their structure.

However Alves Da Costa et al. (2002) showed that α-synuclein drastically lowered caspase-3 activity and p53 protein expression, and transcriptional activity, proteins controlled the apoptotic cascade. Blandini et al. (2004), Dorszewska et al. (2009b) and Iwashita (2004) showed that, apoptotic proteins such as: Bcl-2 family proteins and PARP are involved in the pathogenesis of PD as well.

The aim of the study was to estimate the levels of p53, and PARP proteins, and 85 kDa fragment, and two Bcl-2 family proteins: Bcl-2 and Bax in peripheral lymphocytes of patients with PD and in control group. The attention was also paid to L-dopa pharmacotherapy in PD.

2.2.1 Patients

The studies were conducted on 45 patients with PD, among their 22 patients, including 9 women and 13 men, aging 41-79 years (mean age: 58.0±10.7 years) awaited L-dopa treatment and 23 patients, including 11 women and 12 men aging 45-81 years (mean age: 68.0±8.6 years) were treated with L-dopa preparations in daily doses (up to 5 years treatment to 500 mg/day, 5-10 year treatment 500-800 mg/day, and over 10 year treatment 800-1500 mg/day).

The control group included 27 individuals, 19 women and 8 men, 35-73 years of age (mean age: 54.0±10.7 years).

Patients with PD were diagnosed using the criteria of UK Parkinson's Disease Society Brain Bank (Litvan et al., 2003), however stage of disease according to the scale of Hoehn and Yahr.

None of the control subjects had verifiable symptoms of dementia or any other neurological disorders and smoking, and drinking habits.

A Local Ethical Committee approved the study and the written consent of all patients or their caregivers was obtained.

2.2.2 Estimation of p53, Bax, Bcl-2, PARP proteins and 85-kDa subunit

Isolation of proteins. Blood was gradiated onto gradisol L at a 1:1 ratio and centrifuged, followed by collection of the interphase which was then rinsed in PBS buffer (0.9% NaCl in phosphate buffer) and centrifuged. The obtained lymphocyte precipitate was rinsed with radioimmunoprotein assay (RIPA) buffer (50 mM Tris-HCl, pH 7.2, 150 mM NaCl, 1% IGEPAL CA-630, 0.05% SDS, and 1% sodium deoxycholate), supplemented with a protease inhibitor cocktail (Sigma) and homogenized in a mixture of RIPA with protease inhibitor cocktail (16:1) and 0.5 µl PSMF (Sigma) in isopropanol (10 mg/100 µl), centrifuged, and the obtained supernatant underwent further analysis (Ohnishi et al., 1996).

Western Blot. The Bax and Bcl-2 proteins were analyzed in 12% and p53, and PARP proteins were analyzed in 7.5% polyacrylamide gel. Equivalent amounts of protein (30 µg protein/lane) were loaded to the wells. The gel-separated proteins were electrotransferred to nitrocellulose filter in a semidry Western Blot analysis apparatus (Apelex, France). To estimate the levels of the PARP protein, the filters were exposed first to an anti-PARP monoclonal antibody (G-2-10, IgG, 0.05 ml, Sigma, USA), diluted 1:2000, while the p53, Bax, Bcl-2 proteins were identified using anti-p53 (IgG-2a, 200 µg/1.0 ml; Santa Cruz, USA), anti-Bax (IgG-2b, 200 µg/1.0 ml; Santa Cruz, USA) and anti-Bcl-2 (IgG-1, 200 µg/1.0 ml; Santa Cruz, USA) mouse monoclonal antibody, respectively, diluted 1:500.

Subsequently, individual sheets of nitrocellulose filter were incubated with the second antibody, goad antimouse IgG-HRP (200 µg/0.5 ml; Santa Cruz, USA) at a dilution of 1:2000. To stain immunoreactive bands, peroxidase BMB was added (BM blue POD substrate precipitation; Roche, Germany). The surface area of the immunoreactive bands was registered using a densitometer (GS-710; Bio-Rad, Hercules, CA) in the Quantity One System.

2.2.3 Results

The studies disclosed significant decreased levels of apoptotic proteins (p53, Bax:Bcl-2, PARP, $p < 0.01$; Bax, Bcl-2, $p < 0.001$) in PD as compared to the controls (Table 4). Decreased level of apoptotic proteins in PD patients probably was result influence of α–synuclein on lower p53 protein expression and caspase-3 activity.

Parameter	Controls 35-73 years of age	PD patients 41-81 years of age
p53	0.52 ± 0.37	0.25 ± 0.14**
Bax	0.60 ± 0.50	0.13 ± 0.07***
Bcl-2	1.20 ± 0.77	0.15 ± 0.08***
Bax/Bcl-2	1.46 ± 3.77	1.13 ± 0.83**
PARP	2.12 ± 0.83	1.61 ± 1.12**
85-kDa	0.42 ± 0.80	0.41 ± 0.31

Table 4. Level of p53, Bax, Bcl-2, PARP proteins and of 85-kDa protein subunit in peripheral blood lymphocytes in PD patients and in the control group. Apoptotic proteins represent % of area of immunoreactivity bonds. Results are expressed as a means ± SD. The nonparametric test of Mann-Whitney was used. Differences significant at **$p < 0.01$; ***$p < 0.001$ as compared to the controls.

Simultaneously, in PD patients treated with L-dopa preparations (Table 5) levels of p53, Bax, Bcl-2 proteins increased unsignificant as compared with untreatment patients. In the PD patients treated with L-dopa significant increased only the levels of PARP protein ($p < 0.001$ as compared to patients not treated with L-dopa) and 85-kDa fragment ($p < 0.01$ as compared to patients untreated with L-dopa).

Parameter	Controls 35-73 years of age	PD patients L-dopa (-) 41-79 years of age	PD patients L-dopa (+) 45-81 years of age
p53	0.52 ± 0.37	0.19 ± 0.11**	0.30 ± 0.15
Bax	0.60 ± 0.50	0.12 ± 0.06***	0.14 ± 0.08***
Bcl-2	1.20 ± 0.77	0.15 ± 0.06***	0.16 ± 0.10***
Bax/Bcl-2	1.46 ± 3.77	1.00 ± 0.64	1.26 ± 0.97*
PARP	2.12 ± 0.83	0.82 ± 0.36***	2.36 ± 1.08(***)
85-kDa	0.42 ± 0.80	0.22 ± 0.13	0.58 ± 0.32***(**)

Table 5. Level of p53, Bax, Bcl-2, PARP proteins and of 85-kDa protein subunit in peripheral blood lymphocytes in PD patients untreatment L-dopa (-) and treatment L-dopa (+), and in the control group. Apoptotic proteins represent % of area of immunoreactivity bonds. Results are expressed as a means ± SD. The nonparametric test of Kruskal-Wallis was used. Differences significant at *p<0.05; **p<0.01; ***p<0.001 as compared to the controls, and (**)p<0.01; (***)p<0.001 between PD patients untreatment L-dopa (-) and treatment L-dopa (+).

However, (Table 6) long-term (more than 5 years) therapy of L-dopa in PD patients probably leads to apoptosis, because elevated levels of Bax:Bcl-2 ratio (p<0.05 as compared to the controls) and 85-kDa fragment (p<0.05 as compared to the controls).

Parameter	Controls	PD patients L-dopa < 5 years	PD patients L-dopa > 5 years
p53	0.52 ± 0.37	0.30 ± 0.13	0.30 ± 0.16
Bax	0.60 ± 0.50	0.14 ± 0.09**	0.15 ± 0.08***
Bcl-2	1.20 ± 0.77	0.19 ± 0.08*	0.15 ± 0.11***
Bax/Bcl-2	1.46 ± 3.77	0.85 ± 0.69	1.40 ± 1.03*
PARP	2.12 ± 0.83	2.03 ± 1.00	2.48± 1.12
85-kDa	0.42 ± 0.80	0.44 ± 0.20	0.64 ± 0.35**

Table 6. Level of p53, Bax, Bcl-2, PARP proteins and of 85-kDa protein subunit in peripheral blood lymphocytes in PD patients treatment L-dopa less and more than 5 years, and in the control group. Apoptotic proteins represent % of area of immunoreactivity bonds. Results are expressed as a means ± SD. The nonparametric test of Kruskal-Wallis was used. Differences significant at *p<0.05; **p<0.01; ***p<0.001 as compared to the controls.

It seems that pharmacological treatment of PD patients with L-dopa has a major role in modulating of levels in lymphocytes of some apoptotic proteins, important for this process. Further investigation is thus requisite to analysis expression and mutations of genes encoding proteins important for effective repair and/or apoptosis in PD patients treatment with L-dopa.

3. Homocysteine and asymmetric dimethylarginine and L-dopa treatment in Parkinson's disease

Elevated Hcy level is a risk factor for vascular diseases, cognitive impairment and dementia, and neurodegenerative diseases (e.g. PD). It is also known that vascular dementia and cognitive impairment worsen the prognosis of PD patients, and it is important to minimize the risk of their occurrence as much as possible. Gorell et al. (1994) indicated that patients with PD have shown an increased risk for cardiovascular disease and stroke. In PD not only Hcy, but also cysteine (Cys), product of Hcy metabolism may promote pathological alterations such as: atherosclerosis and thrombogenesis (Muller, 2008).

3.1 Metabolism of biothiols

In the body, Hcy is a point of intersection of two main metabolic pathways: transsulfuration and remethylation. Under physiological conditions, around 50% of Hcy is catabolized by transsulfuration and undergoes transformation to cystathionine and then to Cys. The remaining 50% of Hcy undergoes methylation to Met (Fig. 1).

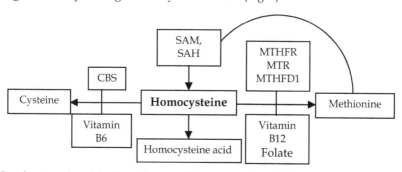

Fig. 1. Synthesis and metabolic pathways of homocysteine, CBS- cystationine β-synthase, MTHFR- 5,10-methylenetetrahydrofolate reductase, MTR- methionine synthase, MTHFD1- methylenetetrahydrofolate dehydrogenase/ methenyltetrahydrofolate cyclohydrolase/formyltetrahydrofolate synthetase, SAH- S-adenosylhomocysteine, SAM- S-adenosylmethionine.

Methionine is supplied with food and its transformation to Hcy involves several steps. At the first step, Met is transformed to SAM and is then demethylated to SAH (S-adenosylhomocysteine) and hydrolyzed to Hcy. SAM is the main donor of methyl groups in many reactions. A decreased content of SAM was demonstrated in the course of PD (Cheng et al., 1997).

The level of Hcy undergoes control, depending upon concentration of its metabolites: Cys and Met. In the case of Met deficit and low concentration of SAM, most Hcy undergoes remethylation to Met, catalyzed by methionine synthase (MTR). MTR is a vitamin B12-dependent enzyme responsible for transfer of methyl groups from N-methyltetrahydrofolate to Hcy, leading to formation of Met (Jarrett et al., 1996). Mutations in the MTR gene are responsible for decreased methylcobalamine level, and result in homocysteinuria, hyperhomocysteinemia and hypomethioninemia (Watkins et al., 2002). The tri-functional enzyme, methylenetetrahydrofolate dehydrogenase/ methenyltetrahydrofolate cyclohydrolase/formyltetrahydrofolate synthetase (MTHFD1) represents another enzyme linked to transformation of Hcy to Met. Homozygotes of both *MTHFR* and *MTHFD1* are at risk of cardiovascular diseases connected with elevated levels of Hcy, or folate level-related hypoplasia of neural tube (Hol et al., 1998). However, in the literature, less numerous data are available on the involvement of MTHFD1 in the pathogenesis of degenerative diseases (Dorszewska et al., 2007).

Under normal conditions, in the presence of a positive Met balance, most of Hcy undergoes transsulfuration catalyzed by cystathionine β-synthetase (CBS), which requires derivative of vitamin B6, pyridoxal phosphate.
Homocysteine or it oxidative product, homocysteine acid are thought to exhibit its pro-oxidative activity most probably through its direct interaction with NMDA receptors (it represents an agonist of NMDA receptor). Agnati et al. (2005) have shown that Hcy may pass the blood/brain barrier and that level of plasma Hcy corresponds to Hcy concentration in the brain.

3.2 Influence of L-dopa treatment on the plasma level of biothiols in Parkinson's disease

In PD, the high Hcy concentration may augment risk of the disease through its direct toxic effect on dopaminergic neurons. Studies *in vitro* on human dopaminergic neurons have documented a significant increase in neurotoxicity accompanying high Hcy levels (Duan et al., 2002). In parallel, elevated Hcy levels in PD have been shown to carry potential for deterioration of cognitive and motoric functions, for depression and elevated risk to develop vascular diseases (Kuhn et al., 1998).
Reports of the literature (Florczak et al., 2008; Miller et al., 2003) indicate that plasma Hcy levels in PD have been affected also by pharmacotherapy with L-dopa. It is indicated that in PD patients who are initiating L-dopa therapy, Hcy elevates within six weeks to a few months after L-dopa initiation (O'Suilleabhain et al., 2004a). Study Florczak et al., 2008 indicated that the sulfuric amino acids were also affected by duration of the L-dopa pharmacotherapy. The most exposed to neurotoxic effects of Hcy have seemed to be the patients during the first 5 years L-dopa treatment while its continued administration has resulted in stably elevated Hcy level. The study of Miller et al. (1997) indicates that L-dopa may induce elevated levels of Hcy during its methylation to 3-O-methyldopa (3-OMD) with involvement of COMT (catechol O-methyltransferase) both in peripheral blood leukocytes and in nigrostriatal neurons. In the course of the reaction, COMT in presence of magnesium ions induces in parallel transition of SAM to SAH and further hydrolysis of SAH to Hcy (Fig. 2).
Elevated level of Hcy in *substantia nigra* of PD patients has been demonstrated already after 3 months of L-dopa treatment (Yasui et al., 2003). Long-term administration of L-dopa is thought to promote benign vascular lesions in patients with PD and may result in the patients in cognitive disturbances or dementia, particular at late stages of treatment with the preparation (Muller et al., 1999). On the other hand, COMT has a broad detoxification potential in human. Two compounds are currently available, entacapone peripheral and tolcapone central blocking of COMT. COMT inhibition is also under suspicion to prevent motor complications and seems that has beneficial effect on the L-dopa-related hyper-Hcy as well (Muller, 2009a; Nevrly et al., 2010). Some animal studies shown that COMT inhibition can eliminate L-dopa-induced hyper-Hcy but not all previous studies confirm it.
Study Dorszewska et al. (2007) have shown that augmented plasma levels of Hcy in PD possibly could have developed due to altered processes of Hcy remethylation to Met and transsulfuration to Cys. Simultaneuosly, in the PD patients a decreased concentration of Met has been observed, paralleled by elevated levels of Cys and lowered ratio of Met and Cys to Hcy. The demonstrated at present decrease in Met to Hcy ratio may be linked to transformation of Hcy to thiolactone in endothelial cells. According to one of more recent hypothesis, sulfonic sulfur of thiol compounds may be involved in development of Hcy-induced arteriosclerotic lesions (Toohey, 2001). At the same time, the demonstrated at

present increased plasma Cys level in PD may result from intensified release of the amino acid from proteins, due to substitution by the circulating Hcy or due to diminished transformation of Cys to glutathione, important for maintenance of redox homeostasis in the body.

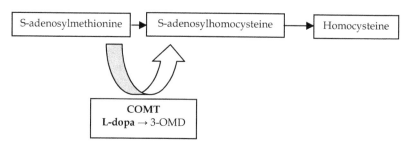

Fig. 2. COMT-mediated O-methylation of L-dopa, which results in formation of 3-methyldopa product, COMT- catecholamine-O-methyltrasferase, 3-OMD- 3-O-methyldopa.

In the literature there are studies of plasma Cys concentrations in PD patients (Dorszewska et al., 2007; Muller & Kuhn, 2009b) but there are no reported about relation between L-dope treatment and Cys status.

3.2.1 Patients

The studies were conducted on 98 patients with PD, including 37 women and 61 men aging 34-81 years (mean age: 60.8±10.7 years). Among the patients with PD, 27 patients (9 women and 18 men) awaited L-dopa treatment (patients' age: 34-79 years) and the remaining 71 individuals, 28 women and 43 men (patients' age: 35-81 years) were treated with L-dopa preparations in daily doses (up to 5 years treatment to 500 mg/day, 5-10 year treatment 500-800 mg/day, and over 10 year treatment 800-1500 mg/day).

Control group included 50 individuals, 34 women and 16 men, 22-76 years of age (mean age: 44.6±16.2 years).

Patients with PD were diagnosed using the criteria of UK Parkinson's Disease Society Brain Bank (Litvan et al., 2003), however stage of disease according to the scale of Hoehn and Yahr.

None of the control subjects had verifiable symptoms of dementia or any other neurological disorders and smoking, and drinking habits.

A Local Ethical Committee approved the study and the written consent of all patients or their caregivers was obtained.

3.2.2 Analysis of Cys concentrations

Preparation of samples. The analyzed plasma thiol compounds (Cys, Sigma, USA) were diluted with water at 2:1 ratio and reduced using 1% TCEP (Tris-(2-carboxyethyl)-phosphin-hydrochloride; Applichem, Germany) at 1:9 ratio. Subsequently, the sample was deproteinized using 1M $HClO_4$ (at 2:1 ratio) and applied to the HPLC/EC system.

Determination of thiol concentration. The samples were fed to the HPLC system (P580A; Dionex, Germany) coupled to an electrochemical detector (CoulArray 5600; ESA, USA). The analysis was performed in Termo Hypersil BDS C18 column (250 x 4.6 x 5μm) (Germany) in isocratic conditions, using the mobile phase of 0.15 M phosphate buffer, pH 2.8 supplemented with 8-10% acetonitrile for estimation of Cys (Accinni et al., 2000).

The system was controlled, and the data were collected and processed using Chromeleon software (Dionex, Germany).

3.2.3 Results
Pharmacotherapy with L-dopa of PD patients (Tables 7 and 8) leads to increase of the concentrations of metabolic product of Hcy, Cys ($p < 0.01$) as compared to the controls, in the patients treated ($p < 0.05$) as well as untreated ($p < 0.01$) with L-dopa. Consequently, the ratio of Cys/Hcy in PD patients decreased, as compared to the controls ($p < 0.05$) and to the untreated patients ($p < 0.01$) as compared to treated PD patients with L-dopa.

Parameter	Controls (22-76 years)	Patients with PD (34-81 years)
Cys	220.7 ± 46.6	250.6 ± 49.6**
Cys/Hcy	19.3 ± 6.7	16.3 ± 6.5*

Table 7. Cysteine (µM) concentrations in the patients with PD and in control group. Results are expressed as a means ± SD. The nonparametric test of Mann-Whitney was used. Differences significant at *$p < 0.05$, **$p < 0.01$ as compared to the controls.

Parameter	Controls (22-76 years)	Patients with PD L-dopa (-) (34-79 years)	Patients with PD L-dopa (+) (35-81 years)
Cys	220.7 ± 46.6	263.6 ± 42.9**	244.7 ± 51.9*
Cys/Hcy	19.3 ± 6.7	20.7 ± 6.9	14.4 ± 5.4**(**)

Table 8. Cysteine (µM) concentrations as related to pharmacotherapy with L-dopa (+) in the patients with PD. Results are expressed as means ± SD. The nonparametric test of Mann-Whitney was used. Differences significant at *$p < 0.05$, **$p < 0.01$ as compared to the controls. Differences significant at (**)$p < 0.01$, as compared to patients not treated with L-dopa (-).

Muller & Kohn (2009) indicated that only PD patients with an elevated level of Hcy above 15 µM showed an increase of Cys plasma level and elevated concentration of both risk factors (Hcy, Cys) may intervene in the neurodegenerative process. Present study indication that especially PD patients before L-dopa treatment showed increased level of Cys and L-dopa treatment only little decreased higher level of Cys. Increased plasma Cys level in PD may result from intensified release of the amino acid from proteins, due to substitution by the circulating Hcy or due to diminished transformation of Cys to glutathione, important for maintenance of redox homeostasis in the body. In culture of human hepatocytes 50% Cys has been demonstrated to transform into GSH (Mosharov et al., 2000). It seems also that intensity of dementive disease in particular disturbs transsulfuration of Hcy and leads to decreased levels of the agent (Cys), which provides the natural antioxidant, GSH. Homocysteine as well as Cys may serve as biomarkers for severity or progression of PD.

3.3 Influence of L-dopa treatment on the plasma level of Hcy and ADMA in Parkinson's disease patients
In the body Hcy is metabolized along two metabolic pathways, by the way of trassulfution and remethylation, involvement of SAM and SAH (Fig. 1). SAM is thought to provide the principal donor of methyl groups in numerous metabolic reactions, leading to formation of

methyl derivatives. One of the products of SAM methylation is thought to be asymmetric dimethylarginine (ADMA) (Gary & Clarke, 1998).

ADMA is an endogenous inhibitor of nitrogen oxide synthase (NOS) (Vallace et al., 1992). It arises from Arg contained in body proteins and may undergo hydrolysis to L-citruline and dimethylamine with involvement of dimethylaminohydrolase (DDAH). Homocysteine is thought to inhibit activity of DDAH (Stuhlinger et al., 2001) and might promote accumulation of ADMA that leads to a decreased production of nitrogen oxide (NO) and L-citruline from Arg with participation of NOS (Fig. 3).

NO plays an important role in control of vascular tone, in neurotransmission and in body protective mechanisms as well as in memory processes. Literature reports indicate that in PD the augmented activity of glia results in increased production of NO (McGeer et al., 1988).

ADMA is regarded to act as a risk factor for vascular diseases (Yoo & Lee, 2001). Its elevated levels were demonstrated in patients with hypercholesterolemia, hypertension, chronic heart failure and in atherosclerotic processes and during physiological aging (Kielstein et al., 2003). Role of ADMA in pathogenesis of PD is less known. Until now, in PD the levels on non-methylated substrate in biosynthesis of ADMA were examined only, and the elevated levels of Arg in cerebrospinal fluid were shown in PD patients with the decrease after L-dopa administration (Qureshi et al., 1995). Literature reports indicate also that long-term administration of L-dopa in PD patients may not only lead to increased concentrations of Hcy but may also alter Arg levels (Muller et al., 1999).

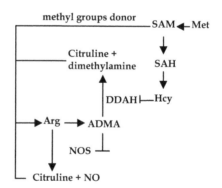

Fig. 3. The roles of methionine, homocysteine and arginine in metabolism of asymmetric dimethylarginine, Hcy- homocysteine, Met- methionine, ADMA- asymmetric dimethylarginine, Arg- arginine, NO- nitric oxide, NOS- NO synthase, DDAH-dimethylarginine dimethylaminohydrolase, SAM- S-adenosylmethionine, SAH- S-adenosylhomocysteine.

The present study was aimed at the estimation of plasma levels of Hcy and ADMA together with Met and Arg in patients with PD. The attention was also paid to developmental stages of the analyzed degenerative diseases and to L-dopa pharmacotherapy in PD.

3.3.1 Patients

The studies were conducted on 47 patients with PD, including 21 women and 26 men aging 41-86 years (mean age: 63.0±11.1 years). Among the patients with PD, 13 patients (3 women and 10 men) awaited L-dopa treatment (patients' age: 41-78 years) and the remaining 34 individuals, 18 women and 16 men (patients' age: 46-86 years) were treated with L-dopa preparations in daily doses (up to 5 years treatment to 500 mg/day, 5-10 year treatment 500-800 mg/day, and over 10 year treatment 800-1500 mg/day).

The control group included 35 individuals, 20 women and 15 men, 22-76 years of age (mean age: 45.1±16.0 years).

Patients with PD, on the other hand, were diagnosed using the criteria of UK Parkinson's Disease Society Brain Bank (Litvan et al., 2003). The stage of evolution of Parkinson's disease was defined according to the scale of Hoehn and Yahr. The tested patients represented stages I to IV of the disease evolution.

None of the control subjects had verifiable symptoms of dementia or any other neurological disorders.

A Local Ethical Committee approved the study and the written consent of all patients or their caregivers was obtained.

3.3.2 Analysis of Hcy and Met concentrations

Preparation of samples. The analyzed plasma thiol compounds (Hcy, Fluka Germany; Met, Sigma, USA) were diluted with water at 2:1 ratio and reduced using 1% TCEP (Tris-(2-carboxyethyl)-phosphin-hydrochloride; Applichem, Germany) at 1:9 ratio. Subsequently, the sample was deproteinized using 1M $HClO_4$ (at 2:1 ratio) and applied to the HPLC/EC system.

Determination of thiol concentration. The samples were fed to the HPLC system (P580A; Dionex, Germany) coupled to an electrochemical detector (CoulArray 5600; ESA, USA). The analysis was performed in Termo Hypersil BDS C18 column (250 x 4.6 x 5μm) (Germany) in isocratic conditions, using the mobile phase of 0.15 M phosphate buffer, pH 2.9, supplemented with 12.5-17% acetonitrile for estimation of Hcy and Met and 0.15 M phosphate buffer (Accinni et al., 2000).

The system was controlled and the data were collected and processed using Chromeleon software (Dionex, Germany).

3.3.3 Analysis of Arg and ADMA concentrations

Preparation of samples and derivatization. Plasma and the standard, containing solution of Arg and ADMA (Sigma, USA) were diluted with water at the ratio of 1.5:1.0 and, then, they were deproteinised using 8M $HCLO_4$ at the ratio of 5:1. Directly before HPLC analysis the samples were subjected to derivatization in a solution containing 10 mg OPA per 100 μl methanol supplemented with 900 μl 0.4 M borate buffer (pH 8.5) and 5μl 2-mercaptoethanol at the ratio of 1:1 (Pi et al., 2000).

Analysis of Arg and ADMA. The samples were fed to the HPLC system (P580A; Dionex, Germany) coupled to a fluorescence detector (RF2000; Dionex, Germany). The analysis was performed in a Termo Hypersil BDS C18 column (250 x 4.6 x 5μm) (Germany) in an isocratic conditions using 0.1 M phosphate buffer, pH 6.75 with 25 % methanol as the mobile phase. Arg and its methylated metabolites were measured fluorimetrically at excitation and emission wavelengths of 340 nm and 455nm, respectively.

The system was controlled and the data were collected and processed using Chromeleon software (Dionex, Germany).

3.3.4 Results

The study indicated that in patients with the diagnosed PD (Table 9) the augmented export of Hcy to plasma, (p<0.001 as compared to the controls), was accompanied by increased levels of circulating ADMA in analyzed neurodegenerative disease ($p<0.001$ as compared to the controls). In parallel, in the patients lower levels were observed of both Met ($p<0.01$ as compared to the controls), and Arg ($p<0.05$ as compared to the controls) expressed also by the lowered Met/Hcy and Arg/ADMA ratio ($p<0.001$ as compared to the controls).

Parameter	Controls (22-76 years)	Patients with PD (41-86 years)
Hcy	13.0 ± 4.3	$20.1 \pm 14.1^{***}$
Met	24.0 ± 6.9	$18.7 \pm 8.6^{**}$
Met/Hcy	2.1 ± 0.9	$1.2 \pm 0.8^{***}$
Arg	79.7 ± 24.4	$68.4 \pm 21.9^{*}$
ADMA	2.0 ± 1.0	$3.8 \pm 1.9^{***}$
Arg/ADMA	55.3 ± 40.5	$25.8 \pm 20.9^{***}$

Table 9. Homocysteine (μM), methionine (μM), asymmetric dimethylarginine (μM) and arginine (μM) concentrations in the patients with PD and in control group. Results are expressed as a means $\pm$ SD. The nonparametric test of Mann-Whitney was used. Differences significant at $^{*}p<0.05$, $^{**}p<0.01$, $^{***}p<0.001$, as compared to the controls.

Moreover, in the patients with PD (Fig. 4) development of the degenerative disease resulted in increased levels the risk factor for vascular diseases (Hcy), particularly pronounced in IVth stage of PD development ($p<0.05$ between Ist and IVth stage and between IInd and IVth stage of PD evolution). On the other hand, the Hcy remethylation product demonstrated a decreasing tendency only in the stage III of the disease, as compared to stage I of PD. In parallel, levels of the other analyzed risk factor of vascular diseases (ADMA) manifested higher correlation with concentration of its precursor. In parallel to the development of PD from stage I to stage IV of the disease evolution augmented levels of ADMA were accompanied by a decrease in the level of Arg (as compared to the Ist stage of PD). Also at the IInd stage of the degenerative disease evolution the highest levels of Met and ADMA and practically unaltered levels of Arg were accompanied by the lowest value of Arg/ADMA ratio ($p<0.01$ between stages I and II of PD evolution). In the IVth stage of PD development, however, both Met/Hcy ratio and Arg/ADMA ratio behaved in a similar manner demonstrating practically the lowest level ($p<0.05$, as compared to the Ist stage of the disease development).

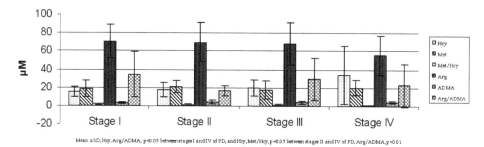

Mean $\pm$ SD; Hcy, Arg/ADMA, p<0.05 between stages I and IV of PD, and Hcy, Met/Hcy, p<0.05 between stages II and IV of PD; Arg/ADMA, p<0.01 between stages I and II of PD

Fig. 4. Hcy, Met, Arg and ADMA concentrations as related to the stage of the PD according to the scale of Hoehn and Yahr.

Pharmacotherapy with L-dopa preparations was demonstrated also to increase levels of both factors of vascular disease risk (Table 10), Hcy (p<0.001 as compared to the controls and p<0.05 as compared to patients not treated with L-dopa) and ADMA (p<0.001 as compared to the controls), although levels of ADMA increased also as a result of development of the degenerative disease (p<0.01 as compared to the controls). In parallel, in patients treated with L-dopa preparations levels of Met decreased (p<0.001 as compared to the controls) and so did concentrations of Arg (p<0.05 as compared to the controls and to L-dopa untreated patients), Met/Hcy ratios (p<0.001 as compared to the controls and p<0.05 as compared to patients not treated with L-dopa) and Arg/ADMA ratios (p<0.001, only as compared to the controls).

Parameter	Controls (22-76 years)	Patients with PD L-dopa (-) (41-78 years)	Patients with PD L-dopa (+) (46-86 years)
Hcy	13.0 ± 4.3	15.1 ± 5.1	22.0 ± 15.9***(*)
Met	24.0 ± 6.9	21.0 ± 7.8	17.8 ± 8.8***
Met/Hcy	2.1 ± 0.9	1.6 ± 1.0*	1.0 ± 0.6***(*)
Arg	79.7 ± 24.4	77.5 ± 19.7	64.4 ± 22.0*(*)
ADMA	2.0 ± 1.0	3.3 ± 1.1**	4.1 ± 2.1***
Arg/ADMA	55.3 ± 40.5	22.8 ± 7.8***	26.7 ± 23.6***

Table 10. Homocysteine (μM), methionine (μM), asymmetric dimethylarginine (μM) and arginine (μM) concentrations as related to pharmacotherapy with L-dopa (+) in the patients with PD. The nonparametric test of Mann-Whitney was used. Results are expressed as means ± SD. Differences significant at *p<0.05, **p<0.01, ***p<0.001, as compared to the controls. Differences significant at (*)p<0.05, as compared to patients not treated with L-dopa (-).

Present study indicated that ADMA may be involved in pathogenesis of PD. In development of PD the principal role is thought to be played by peroxinitrates (Padovan-Neto et al., 2009). This seems consistent with the demonstrated in present study ADMA level not elevated till the IInd stage of the disease development and the lower level of Arg, particularly accentuated in the IVth stage of PD evolution. Thus, a probability exists for involvement of reactive NO derivatives in induction of toxic damage to *substantia nigra* in PD.

In present study we have observed particularly in PD patients an evident decrease in Arg/ADMA ratio. The lowered ratio in blood is thought (Matsuoka et al., 1997) to be linked to development of hypercholesterolemia, congestive heart failure, arterial occlusive disease, heart failure and hypertension.

The levels of ADMA in PD have probably been affected also by pharmacotherapy with L-dopa. Both in the studies of Qureshi et al. (1995), and in present study decreased levels of Arg have been shown in patients treated with the drug. In the study of Qureshi et al. (1995) pharmacotherapy with L-dopa has been shown to generate nitrites, agents of neurotoxic activity, but in present studies seem that ADMA has not been shown to participate in their generation. Increased NO levels in PD have seemed to result rather from elevated activity of the glutaminergic system and altered neuronal metabolism.

It seems that ADMA may be regarded to represent a risk factor for PD and may be involved in pathogenesis of this neurodegenerative disease. Present results indicate also that developing neurodegenerative diseases are accompanied by disturbed metabolism of Hcy and ADMA and administration of L-arginine, in line with vitamins B6, B12 and folates, to PD patients may offer a modern therapy in this neurodegenerative disease.

4. Polymorphisms of *MTHFR*, *MTR*, *MTHFD1* and the level of biothiols in Parkinson's disease

The enzyme MTHFR plays a key role in regulating of Hcy metabolism. The study of Yasui et al. (2000) indicated that the TT *MTHFR* C677T genotype might also be linked to pathogenesis of PD, particularly when the level of folates is low. However, Fong et al. (2011) indicated on synergistic effects of polymorphisms in the folate metabolic pathway genes in PD not only C677T *MTHFR*, but also A2756G of *MTR* and A1049G, C1783T of *MTRR* (methionine synthase reductase). Yuan et al. (2009) showed on synergism between Hcy elevation after L-dopa administration in PD patients and *MTHFR*, CT and TT (C677T) genotypes. The study of Dorszewska et al. (2007) indicated that the genotypes TT (C677T), CC (A1298C) and AA (G1793A) of *MTHFR* have been the least frequent in patients with neurodegenerative disorders and their incidence has been slightly increased in the degenerative diseases (e.g. PD). In study of Dorszewska et al. (2007) also indicated that in PD patients Hcy has reached higher levels only in patients with CT genotype of *MTHFR* C677T. It seems that, particularly in persons with CT genotype of the C677T polymorphism of *MTHFR*, processes of Hcy transsulfuration to Cys become disturbed. Moreover, in PD the most pronounced alterations in Hcy levels in cases of A1298C polymorphism of *MTHFR* have been manifested in both genotypes AA and AC, even if this has not been expressed by the increased in parallel levels of oxidized guanine in DNA.

The enzyme of MTR is responsible for transfer of methyl groups from methyltetrahyrofolate to Hcy with involvement of methylcobalamin as the cofactor. The AG genotype of the A2756G polymorphism of *MTR* is probably linked to augmented levels of Hcy (Dorszewska et al., 2007). The increase of Hcy concentrations most probably results from lowered activity of MTR, induced by excessive oxidation of cobalamin (McCaddon et al. 2002) due to a more pronounced oxidative stress in degenerative syndromes. In parallel, the studies of Matsuo et al. (2001) indicate that *MTR* AG leads also to hypomethylation of DNA and to inactivation of several genes (low levels of SAM).

It seems also that the polymorphism G1958A of the gene coding for MTHFD1 enzyme may be involved in pathogenesis of PD, and heterozygote as well as homozygote (GA, AA) are thought to be responsible for increased levels of Hcy (Dorszewska et al., 2007). MTHFD1 represents another folate-dependent enzyme, which catalyzes transformation of tetrahydrofolate to 10-formyl, 5,10-methenyl and 5,10-methylene derivatives. 10-Formyltetrahydrofolate and 5,10-methylenetetrahydrofolate are regarded to serve as donors of methyl groups in DNA biosynthesis. The study of Dorszewska et al. (2007) also indicated that significant differences of the levels of Cys/Hcy, *MTHFD1* GA (G1958) were between AD and PD groups. The results indicate that only polymorphisms of folate-dependent enzyme *MTHFD1* have pointed to significant differences in intensity of turnover of circulating thiols between both neurodegenerative diseases, AD and PD.

Some studies confirmed that the C677T *MTHFR* polymorphism should consider as a genetic risk factor in patients who are going to take L-dopa preparations and folates and vitamins B (6, 12) supplementation may be given to the treated PD patients.

5. Influence of L-dopa treatment duration on the level of oxidative damage to DNA and thiols compounds concentration in patients with Parkinson's disease

The discussion about value of the L-dopa treatment in PD concerning on: toxicity, biochemical effects, clinical motor complications, especially after long-term its administrations (Belcastro et al., 2010; Muller, 2009a). Long-term treatment with L-dopa in PD patients may be promotes Hcy levels increase. Moreover, only PD patients with hyper-Hcy (Hcy above 15 µM) may have disturbed metabolism Hcy to Cys. As showed, hyper-Hcy in PD patients has been correlated with duration of disease and L-dopa dose.

5.1 Patients (see point 2.1.1)
5.2 Analysis of Hcy and Met (see point 3.3.2), and Cys (see point 3.2.2) concentrations, and 8-oxo2dG level (see point 2.1.2)
5.3 Results

During the initial five years and within the following 10 years of treatment with L-dopa (Table 11), the levels of 8-oxo2dG were augmented ($p<0.05$, as compared to the controls). Similarly to 8-oxo2dG, the levels of Hcy were highest after the initial five years of L-dopa administration ($p<0.05$, as compared to the controls). Subsequent treatment for another five to ten years resulted in the elevated levels of Hcy ($p<0.01$, as compared to the controls) which were even more significant if the treatment was extended over ten years ($p<0.001$, as compared to the controls). Moreover, the initial five years of L-dopa treatment were accompanied by relatively low levels of Met ($p<0.05$, as compared to the controls) and a slight increase in concentration of Cys. After ten years of treatment, similar levels of Hcy and Met were detected (Met, $p<0.01$), as compared to the controls, and Cys, ($p<0.05$), as compared to the group treated for five to ten years.

Parameter	Controls (22-76 years)	Patients with PD		
		up to 5 year treatment (34-78 years)	5-10 year treatment (46-81 years)	over 10 year treatment (46-81 years)
8-oxo2dG	13.7 ± 7.6	21.5 ± 15.1*	17.5 ± 11.1	27.8 ± 23.0*
Hcy	12.6 ± 4.3	28.5 ± 33.6*	19.7 ± 9.0**	18.3 ± 6.9***
Met	24.2 ± 6.7	19.2 ± 6.2*	20.4 ± 9.1	18.2 ± 8.2**
Met/Hcy	2.2 ± 0.9	1.1 ± 0.5**	1.2 ± 0.6**	1.1 ± 0.5***
Cys	220.7 ± 46.6	232.3 ± 52.5	267.9 ± 47.1**	238.2 ± 53.3(*)
Cys/Hcy	19.3 ± 6.7	12.8 ± 5.3*	15.4 ± 5.1	14.4 ± 5.8**

Table 11. Levels of oxidative DNA damage (8-oxo2dG/dG x 10⁻⁵), and homocysteine (µM), methionine (µM) and cysteine (µM) concentrations as related to duration of L-dopa administration to patients with PD. Results are expressed as means ± SD. Differences significant at *$p<0.05$, **$p<0.01$, ***$p<0.001$, as compared to the controls. Differences significant at (*)$p<0.05$ between patients treated with L-dopa for 5-10 year and those treated for over 10 year.

As shown by the literature (Spencer et al., 1995) and by our studies, the elevated level of oxidized guanine in DNA (8-oxo2dG) in PD reflects also pharmacotherapy with L-dopa preparations. In present study, levels of 8-oxo2dG in the patients treated with L-dopa preparations have reflected duration of administration of the drug. Patients have seemed most exposed to oxidative stress, resulting from L-dopa administration, during the first 5 years of treatment with the preparation and following long-term (over 10 years) its administration. According to Spencer et al. (1995), the augmented oxidative stress in patients treated with L-dopa might have resulted from lowered levels of antioxidants (GSH), disturbed mitochondrial transport and from excessive oxidation of dopamine.

Reports of the literature (Miller et al., 2003) and present results indicate that plasma Hcy levels in PD have been affected also by pharmacotherapy with L-dopa. In present study levels of the sulfuric amino acid were also affected by duration of the pharmacotherapy. The most exposed to neurotoxic effects of Hcy have seemed to be the patients during the first 5 years L-dopa treatment while its continued administration has resulted in stably elevated Hcy level, it seems that all time are disturbed metabolism of Hcy to Met and Cys.

Treatment with L-dopa preparations seems to be a potential risk factor for vascular diseases in PD patients. According to Lamberti et al. (2005), administration of vitamin B12 and of folates decreases plasma level of Hcy particularly in patients with PD during treatment with L-dopa preparations and in this way prevents against intensification of vascular lesions and dementia in the patients.

6. Conclusion

In conclusion, L-dopa metabolism after administration in PD patients is an important component for Hcy elevation and for increase toxicity in peripheral blood lymphocytes. Therapy of L-dopa leads to increases of the level factors inducing in oxidative stress and apoptosis as well as changes concentrations of risk factors of vascular diseases such as: Hcy, Cys and ADMA especially after long-term therapy. Analysis of the level of 8-oxo2dG, Hcy, Cys and ADMA may be a new biomarkers of severity and progression of PD.

It seems that for elevated levels of biothiols in PD, is not only important genotype MTHFR, TT (C677T) but also CC (A1298C), AA (G1793A), and MTHFD1, AA (G1958A) and MTR, GG (A2756G), which have a tendency for increased frequency in PD patients. In PD, there are more significant differences of the levels of biothiols in patients with one of genotype: Hcy [MTHFR: CT (C677T) and GG (G1793A); MTR, AG (A2756G)], Met [MTR, AA (A2756G)], Cys [MTR, AG (A2756G)], and Met/Hcy [MTHFR: CC, CT (C677T) and AA (A1298C), and GG (G1793A); MTHFD1 AA (G1958A); MTR AA (A2756G)]. Moreover only polymorphisms of folate-dependent enzyme MTHFD1 have pointed to significant differences in intensity of turnover of circulating biothiols between both neurodegenerative diseases: AD, and PD, which differ in the localization of neurotoxic lesions in the CNS.

Therefore in PD, monitoring of thiols compound levels in particular Hcy, is recommended. In the patients with PD administration of vitamins B6, B12, folates may cause a decrease in Hcy level, due to increased efficiency of remethylation and transsulfuration processes.

7. References

Accinni, R., Bartesaghi, S., De Leo, G., Cursano, C.F., Achilli, G., Loaldi, A., Cellerino, C., & Parodi, O. (2000). Screening of homocysteine from newborn blood spots by high-performance liquid chromatography with coulometric array detection. *Journal of Chromatography A*, Vol.896, No.1-2, (Obctober 2000), pp. 183-189, ISSN 0021-9673

Agnati, L.F., Genedani, S., Rasio, G., Galantucci, M., Saltini, S., Filaferro, M., Franco, R., Mora, F., Ferre, S., & Fuxe, K. (2005). Studies on homocysteine plasma levels in Alzheimer's patients. Relevance for neurodegeneration. *Journal of Neural Transmission*, Vol.112, No.1, (January 2005), pp. 163-169, ISSN 0300-9564

Alam, Z.I., Jenner, A., Daniel, S.E., Lees, A.J., Cairns, N., Marsden, C.D., Jenner, P., & Halliwell, B. (1997). Oxidative DNA damage in the parkinsonian brain: an apparent selective increase in 8-hydroxyguanine levels in substantia nigra. *Journal of Neurochemistry*, Vol.69, No.3, (September 1997), pp. 1196-1203, ISSN 0022-3042

Alves Da Costa, C.A., Paitel, E., Vincent, B., & Checler, F. (2002). α-Synuclein lowers p53-dependent apoptotic response of neural cells. Abolishment by 6-hydroxydopamine and implication for Parkinson's disease. *Journal of Biological Chemistry*, Vol.277, No.52, (December 2002), pp. 50980-50984, ISSN 0021-9258

Belcastro, V., Pierguidi, L., Castrioto A., Menichetti, C., Gorgone, G., Ientile, F., Pisani F., Rossi, A. Calabresi P., & Tambasco N. (2010). Hyperhomocysteinemia recurrence in levodopa-treated Parkinson's disease patients. *European Journal of Neurology*, Vol.17, No.5, (May 2010), pp. 661-665, ISSN 1351-5101

Blake, C.I., Spitz, E., Leehey, M., Hoffer, B.J., & Boyson, S.J. (1997). Platelet mitochondrial respiratory chain function in Parkinson's disease. *Movement Disorders*, Vol.12, No.1, (January 1997), pp. 3-8, ISSN 0885-3185

Blandini, F., Cosentino, M., Mangiagalli, A., Marino, F., Samuele, A., Rasini, E., Fancellu, R., Tassorelli, C., Pacchetti, C., Martignoni, E., Riboldazzi, G., Calandrella, D., Lecchini, S., Frigo, G., & Nappi, G. (2004). Modifications of apoptosis-related protein levels in lymphocytes of patients with Parkinson's disease. The effect of dopaminergic treatment. *Journal of Neural Transmission*, Vol.111, No.8, (August 2004), pp. 1017-1030, ISSN 0300-9564

Bergman, H., Feingold, A., Nini, A., Raz, A., Slovin, H., Abeles, M., & Vaadia, E. (1998). Physiological aspects of information processing in the basal ganglia of normal and parkinsonian primates. *Trends in Neurosciences*, Vol.21, No.1, (January 1998), pp. 32-38, ISSN 0166-2236

Carta, M., Lindgren, H.S., Lundblad, M., Stancampiano, R., Fadda, F., & Cenci, M.A. (2006). Role of striatal L-DOPA in the production of dyskinesia in 6-hydroxydopamine lesioned rats. *Journal of Neurochemistry*, Vol.96, No.6, (March 2006), pp. 1718-1727, ISSN 0022-3042

Cheng, H., Gomes-Trolin, C., Aquilonius, S.M., Steinberg, A., Lofberg, C., Ekblom, J., & Oreland, L. (1997). Levels of L-methionine S-adenosyltransferase activity in erythrocytes and concentrations of S-adenosylmethionine and S-adenosylhomocysteine in whole blood of patients with Parkinson's disease. *Experimental Neurology*, Vol.145, No.2 Pt 1, (January 1997), pp. 580-585, ISSN 0014-4886

Conway, K.A., Rochet, J.C., Bieganski, R.M., & Lansbury, P.T.Jr. (2001). Kinetic stabilization of the alpha-synuclein protofibril by a dopamine-alpha-synuclein adduct. *Science*, Vol.249, No.5545, (November 2001), pp. 1346-1349, ISSN 0036-8075

Cornetta, T., Palma, S., Aprile, I., Padua, L., Tonali, P., Testa, A., & Cozzi, R. (2009). Levodopa therapy reduces DNA damage in peripheral blood cells of patients with Parkinson's disease. *Cell Biology & Toxicology*, Vol.25, No.4, (August 2009), pp. 321-330, ISSN 0742-2091

Dorszewska, J., Florczak, J., Rózycka, A., Jaroszewska-Kolecka, J., Trzeciak, W.H., & Kozubski, W. (2005). Polymorphisms of the CHRNA4 gene encoding the alpha4 subunit of nicotinic acetylcholine receptor as related to the oxidative DNA damage and the level of apoptotic proteins in lymphocytes of the patients with Alzheimer's disease. *DNA & Cell Biology*, Vol.24, No.12, (December 2005), pp. 786-794, ISDN 1044-5498

Dorszewska, J., Florczak, J., Rozycka, A., Kempisty B., Jaroszewska-Kolecka, J., Chojnicka K., Trzeciak,W.H., & Kozubski, W. (2007). Oxidative DNA damage and level of thiols as related to polymorphisms of MTHFR, MTR, MTHFD1 in Alzheimer's and Parkinson's diseases. *Acta Neurobiologiae Experimentalis*, Vol.67, No.2, (2007), pp. 113-129, ISSN 0065-1400

Dorszewska, J., Kempisty, B., Jaroszewska-Kolecka, J., Rozycka, A., Florczak, J., Lianeri, M., Jagodzinski, P.P., & Kozubski, W. (2009a). Expression and polymorphisms of gene 8-oxoguanine glycosylase 1 and the level of oxidative DNA damage in peripheral blood lymphocytes of patients with Alzheimer's disease. *DNA & Cell Biology*, Vol.28, No.11, (November 2009), pp. 579-588, ISSN 1044-5498

Dorszewska, J., Florczak, J., & Kozubski, W. (2009b). Level of oxidative DNA damage and expression of apoptotic proteins in patients with Parkinson's disease treatment with L-dopa. *Parkinsonism & Related Disorders*, 15, Suppl. 2, 111, ISSN 1353-8020, Abstracts of the XVIII WFN World Congress on Parkinson's Disease and Related Disorders. Miami Beach, FL, USA, December 13-16, 2009

Dorszewska, J., Dezor, M., Florczak, J., Kozubski, W. (2010). Expression of 8-oxoguanine DNA glycosylase 1 (OGG1) and the level of p53 and TNF-alpha proteins in peripheral lymphocytes in patients with Alzheimer's disease. *Alzheimer's Dementia*, 6, 4, P3186, Supp. 1, ISSN 1552-5260, Alzheimer's Association International Conference on Alzheimer's disease. Honolulu, Hawaii, USA, July 10-15, 2010

Duan, W., Ladenheim, B., Cutler, R.G., Kruman, I.I., Cadet, J.L., & Mattson, M.P. (2002). Dietary folate deficiency and elevated homocysteine levels endanger dopaminergic neurons in models of Parkinson's disease. *Journal of Neurochemistry*, Vol.80, No.1, (January 2002), pp. 101-110, ISSN 0022-3042

Florczak, J., Dorszewska, J., & Kozubski, W. (2008). Influence of L-dopa treatment duration on the level of oxidative damage to DNA and thiol compound concentration in patients with Parkinson's disease. *Neurologia i Neurochirurgia Polska*, Vol.42, No.1, Suppl. 1, (in Polish), pp. S36-S44, ISSN 0028-3843

Fong, C.S., Shyu, H.Y., Shieh, J.C., Fu, Y.P., Chin, T.Y., Wang, H.W., & Cheng C.W. (2011). Association of MTHFR, MTR, and MTRR polymorphisms with Parkinson's disease among ethnic Chinese in Taiwan. *Clinica Chimica Acta*, Vol.412, No.3-4, (January 2011), pp. 332-338, ISSN 0009-8981

Frosst, P., Blom, H.J., Milos, R., Goyette, P., Sheppard, C.A., Matthews, R.G., Boers, G.J., den Heijer, M., Kluijtmans, L.A., van den Heuvel, L.P., & Rozen, R. (1995). A candidate genetic risk factor for vascular disease: a common mutation in methylenetetrahydrofolate reductase. *Nature Genetics*, Vol.10, No.1, (May 1995), pp. 111-113, ISSN 1061-4036

Gary, J.D., & Clarke, S. (1998). RNA and protein interactions modulated by protein arginine methylation. *Progress in Nucleic Acid Research & Molecular Biology*, Vol.61, pp. 65-131, ISSN 0079-6603

Gorell, J.M., Johnson, C.C., & Rybicki, B.A. (1994). Parkinson's disease and its comorbid disorders: an analysis of Michigan mortality data, 1970 to 1990. *Neurology*, Vol.44, No.10, (October 1994), pp. 1865-1868, ISSN 0028-3878

Hirano, T. (2008). Repair system of 7, 8-dihydro-8-oxoguanine as a defense line against carcinogenesis. *Journal of Radiation Research*, Vol.49, No.4, (July 2008), pp. 329-340, ISSN 0449-3060

Hol, F.A., van der Put, N.M., Geurds, M.P., Heil, S.G., Trijbels, F.J., Hamel, B.C., Mariman, E.C., & Blom, H.J. (1998). Molecular genetic analysis of the gene encoding the trifunctional enzyme MTHFD (methylenetetrahydrofolate-dehydrogenase, ethenyltetrahydrofolate-cyclohydrolase, formyltetrahydrofolate synthetase) in patients with neural tube defects. *Clinical Genetics*, Vol.53, No.2, (February 1998), pp. 119-125, ISSN 1178-704X

Hsu, L.J., Sagara, Y., Arroyo, A., Rockenstein, E., Sisk, A., Mallory, M., Wong, J., Takenouchi, T., Hashimoto, M., & Masliah, E. (2000). alpha-synuclein promotes mitochondrial deficit and oxidative stress. *American Journal of Pathology*, Vol.157, No.2, (August 2000), pp. 401-410, ISSN 0002-9440

Iwashita, A., Yamazaki, S., Mihara, K., Hattori, K., Yamamoto, H., Ishida, J., Matsuoka, N., & Mutoh, S. (2004). Neuroprotective effects of a novel poly(ADP-ribose) polymerase-1 inhibitor, 2-{3-[4-(4-chlorophenyl)-1-piperazinyl]propyl}-4(3H)-quinazolinone (FR255595), in an in vitro model of cell death and in mouse 1-methyl-4-phenyl-1,2,3,6-tetrahydropyridine model of Parkinson's disease. *Journal of Pharmacology and Experimental Therapeutics*, Vol.309, No.3, (June 2004), pp. 1067-1078, ISSN 0022-3565

Jarrett, J.T., Amaratunga, M., Drennan, C.L., Scholten, J.D., Sands, R.H., Ludwig, M.L., & Matthews, R.G. (1996). Mutations in the B12-binding region of methionine synthase: how the protein controls methylcobalamin reactivity. *Biochemistry*, Vol.35, No.7, (February 1996), pp. 2464-2475, ISSN 0006-2979

Jenner, P. (2003). Oxidative stress in Parkinson's disease. *Annals Neurology*, Vol.53, pp. S26-S38, ISSN 0364-5134

Kielstein, J.T., Bode-Boger, S.M., Frolich, J.C., Ritz, E., Haller, & H., Fliser, D. (2003). Asymmetric dimethylarginine, blood pressure, and renal perfusion in elderly subjects. *Circulation*, Vol.107, No.14, (April 2003), pp. 1891-1895, ISSN 0009-7322

Kikuchi, A., Takeda, A., Onodera, H., Kimpara, T., Hisanaga, K., Sato, N., Nunomura, A., Castellani, R.J., Perry, G., Smith, M.A., & Itoyama, Y. (2002). Systemic increase of oxidative nucleic acid damage in Parkinson's disease and multiple system atrophy. *Neurobiology of Disease*, Vol.9, No.2, (March 2002), pp. 244-248, ISSN 0969-9961

Kuhn, W., Roebroek, R., Blom, H., van Oppenraaij, D., Przuntek, H., Kretschmer, A., Buttner, T., Woitalla, D., & Muller, T. 1998). Elevated plasma levels of homocysteine in Parkinson's disease. *European Neurology*, Vol.40, No.4, (November 1998), pp. 225-227, ISSN 0014-3022

Lamberti, P., Zoccolella, S., Armenise, E., Lamberti, S.V., Fraddosio, A., de Mari, M., Iliceto, G., & Livrea, P. (2005). Hyperhomocysteinamia in L-dopa treated Parkinson's disease patients: effect of cobalamin and folate dministration. *European Journal of Neurology*, Vol.12, No.5, (May 2005), pp. 365-368, ISSN 1351-5101

Litvan, I., Bhatia, K.P., Burn, D.J., Goetz, C.G., Lang, A.E., McKeith, I., Quinn, N., Sethi, K.D., Shults, C., & Wenning, G.K. (2003). Movement Disorders Society Scientific Issues Committee report: SIC Task Force appraisal of clinical diagnostic criteria for Parkinsonian disorders. *Movement Disorders*, Vol.18, No.5, (May 2003), pp. 467-486, ISSN 0885-3185

Matsuo, K., Suzuki, R., Hamajima, N., Ogura, M., Kagami, Y., Taji, H., Kondoh, E., Maeda, S., Asakura, S., Kaba, S., Nakamura, S., Seto, M., Morishima, Y., & Tajima, K. (2001). Association between polymorphisms of folate- and methionine-metabolizing enzymes and susceptibility to malignant lymphoma. *Blood*, Vol.97, No.10, (May 2001), pp. 3205-3209, ISSN 0006-4971

Matsuoka, H., Itoh, S., Kimoto, M., Kohno, K., Tamai, O., Wada, Y., Yasukawa, H., Iwami, G., Okuda, S., & Imaizumi, T. (1997). Asymmetric dimetylarginine, an endogenous nitric oxide synthase inhibitor, in experimental hypertension. *Hypertension*, Vol.29, No.1 Pt 2, (January 1997), pp. 242-247, ISSN 0914-911X

McCaddon, A., Regland, B., Hudson, P., & Davies, G. (2002). Functional vitamin B(12) deficiency and Alzheimer disease. *Neurology*, Vol.58, No.9, (May 2002), pp. 1395-1399, ISSN 0028-3878

McGeer, P.L., Itagaki, S., Boyes, B.E., & McGeer, E.G. (1988). Reactive microglia are positive for HLA-DR in the substantia nigra of Parkinson's and Alzheimer's disease brains. *Neurology*, Vol.38, No.8, (August 1988), pp. 1285-1291, ISSN 0028-3878

Migliore, L., Petrozzi, L., Lucetti, C., Gambaccini, G., Bernardini, S., Scarpato, R., Trippi, F., Barale, R., Frenzilli, G., Rodilla, V., & Bonuccelli, U. (2002). Oxidative damage and cytogenetic analysis in leukocytes of Parkinson's disease patients. *Neurology*, Vol.58, No.12, (June 2002), pp. 1809-1815, ISSN 0028-3878

Miller, J.W., Shukitt-Hale, B., Villalobos-Molina, R., Nadeau, M.R., Selhub. J., & Joseph, J.A. (1997). Effect of L-Dopa and the catechol-O-methyltransferase inhibitor Ro 41-0960 on sulfur amino acid metabolites in rats. *Clinical Neuropharmacology*, Vol.20, No.1, (February 1997), pp. 55-66, ISSN 0362-5664

Miller, J.W., Selhub, J., Nadeau, M.R., Thomas, C.A., Feldman, R.G., & Wolf, P.A. (2003). Effect of L-dopa on plasma homocysteine in PD patients: relationship to B-vitamin status. *Neurology*, Vol.60, No.7, (April 2003), pp. 1125-1129, ISSN 0028-3878

Mosharov, E., Cranford, M.R., & Banerjee, R. (2000). The quantitatively important relation ship between homocysteine metabolism and glutathione synthesis by the transsulfuration pathway and its regulation by redox changes. *Biochemistry*, Vol.39, No.42, (October 2000), pp. 13005-13011, ISSN 0006-2979

Muller, T., Werne, B., Fowler, B., & Kuhn, W. (1999). Nigral endothelial dysfunction, homocysteine, and Parkinson's disease. *Lancet*, Vol.354, No.9173, (July 1999), pp. 126-127, ISSN 0140-6736

Muller, T. (2008). Role of homocysteine in the treatment of Parkinson's disease. *Expert Review of Neurotherapeutics*, Vol.8, No.6, (June 2008), pp. 957-967, ISSN 1473-7175

Muller, T. (2009a). Possible treatment concept for the levodopa-related hyperhomocystenemia. *Cardiovascular Psychiatry & Neurology*, (September 2009), pp. 1-5, ISSN 2090-0163

Muller, T. & Kuhn, W. (2009b). Cysteine elevation in levodopa-treated patients with Parkinson's disease. *Movement Disorders*, Vol.24, No.6, (April 2009), pp. 929-932, ISSN 0885-3185

Nevrly, M., Kanovsky, P., Vranova, H., Langova, K., & Hlustik, P. (2010). Effect of entacapone on plasma homocysteine levels in Parkinson's disease patients. *Neurological Sciences*, Vol.31, No.5, (October 2010), pp. 565-569, ISSN 1590-1874

Obeso, J.A., Rodriguez-Oroz, M.C., Benitez-Temino, B. Blesa, F.J., Guridi, J., Marin, C., & Rodriguez, M. (2008). Functional organization of the basal ganglia: therapeutic implications for Parkinson's disease. *Movement Disorders*, Vol.23, Suppl. 3, pp. S548-S559, ISSN 0885-3185

Ohnishi, T., Inoue, N., Matsumoto, H., Omatsu, T., Ohira, Y., & Nagaoka, S. (1996). Cellular content of p53 protein in rat skin after exposure to the space environment. *Journal of Applied Physics*, Vol.81, No.1, (July 1996), pp. 183-185, ISSN 0021-8979

Olanow, C.W. (2008). Levodopa/dopamine replacement strategies in Parkinson's disease: future directions. *Movement Disorders*, Vol.23, Suppl. 3, pp. S613-S622, ISSN 0885-3185

Olsen, A., Siboska, G.E., Clark, B.F., & Rattan, S.I. (1999). N[6]-Furfuryladenosine, kinetin, protects against Fenton reaction-mediated oxidative damage to DNA. *Biochemical Biophysical Research Communications*, Vol.265, No.2, (November 1999), pp. 499-502, ISSN 0006-291X

O'Suilleabhain, P.E., Bottiglieri, T., Dewey, R.B., Sharma, S., & Diaz-Arrastia, R. (2004a). Modest increase in plasma homocysteine follows levodopa initiation in Parkinson's disease. *Movement Disorders*, Vol.19, No.12, (December 2004), pp. 1403-1408, ISSN 0885-3185

O'Suilleabhain, P.E., Sung, V., Hernandez, C., Lacritz, L., Dewey, R.B.Jr., Bottiglieri, T., & Diaz-Arrastia, R. (2004b). Elevated plasma homocysteine level in patients with Parkinson disease: motor, affective, and cognitive associations. *Archives of Neurology*, Vol.61, No.6, (June 2004), pp. 865-868, ISSN 0003-9942

Padovan-Neto, F.E., Echeverry, M.B., Tumas, V., & Del-Bel, E.A. (2009). Nitric oxide synthase inhibition attenuates L-DOPA-induced dyskinesias in a rodent model of Parkinson's disease. *Neuroscience*, Vol.159, No.3, (March 2009), pp. 927-935, ISSN 0306-4522

Pi, J., Kumagai, Y., Sun, G., & Shimojo, N. (2000). Improved method for simultaneous determination of L-arginine and its mono- and dimethylated metabolites in biological samples by high-performance liquid chromatography. *Journal of Chromatography B: Biomedical Sciences & Applications*, Vol.742, No.1, (May 2000), pp. 199-203, ISSN 0378-4347

Prigione, A., Begni, B., Galbussera, A., Beretta, S., Brighina, L., Garofalo, R., Andreoni, S., Piolti, R., & Ferrarese C. (2006). Oxidative stress in peripheral blood mononuclear cells from patients with Parkinson's disease: negative correlation with levodopa dosage. *Neurobiology of Disease*, Vol.23, No.1, (July 2006), pp. 36-43, ISSN 0969-9961

Qureshi, G.A., Baig, S., Bednar, I., Sodersten, P., Forsberg, G., & Siden, A. (1995). Increased cerebrospinal fluid concentration of nitrite in Parkinson's disease. *Neuroreport*, Vol.6, No.12, (August 1995), pp. 1642-1644, ISSN 0959-4965

Rogers, J.D., Sanchez-Saffon, A., Frol, A.B., & Diaz-Arrastia, R. (2003). Elevated plasma homocysteine levels in patients treated with levodopa: association with vascular disease. *Archives of Neurology*, Vol.60, No.1, (January 2003), pp. 59-64, ISSN 0003-9942

Schapira, A.H., Cooper, J.M., Dexter, D., Clark, J.B., Jenner, P., & Marsden, C.D. (1990). Mitochondrial complex I deficiency in Parkinson's disease. *Journal of Neurochemistry*, Vol.53, No.3, (March 1990), pp. 823-827, ISSN 0022-3042

Sian, J., Dexter, D.T., Lees, A.J., Daniel, S., Agid, Y., Javoy-Agid, F., Jenner, P., & Marsden, C.D. (1994). Alterations in glutathione levels in Parkinson's disease and other neurodegenerative disorders affecting basal ganglia. *Annals of Neurology*, Vol.36, No.3, (September 1994), pp. 384-355, ISSN 0364-5134

Spencer, J.P., Jenner, A., Aruoma, O.I., Evans, P.J., Kaur, H., Dexter, D.T., Jenner, P., Lees, A.J., Marsden, D.C., & Halliwell, B. (1994). Intense oxidative DNA damage promoted by L-dopa and its metabolites. Implications for neurodegenerative disease. *FEBS Letters*, Vol.353, No.3, (October 1994), pp. 246-250, ISSN 0014-5793

Spencer, J.P., Jenner, P., & Halliwell, B. (1995). Superoxide-dependent depletion of reduced glutathione by L-DOPA and dopamine. Relevance to Parkinson's disease. *Neuroreport*, Vol.6, No.11, (July 1995), pp. 1480-1484, ISSN 0959-4965

Spillantini, M.G., Schmidt, M.L., Lee, V.M., Trojanowski, J.Q., Jakes, R., & Goedert, M. (1997). α-synuclein in Lewy bodies. *Nature*, Vol.388, No.6645, (August 1997), pp. 839-840, ISSN 0028-0836

Stuhlinger, M.C., Tsao, P.S., Her, J.H., Kimoto, M., Balint, R.F., & Cooke, J.P. (2001). Homocysteine impairs the nitric oxide synthase pathway: role of asymmetric dimethylarginine. *Circulation*, Vol.104, No.21, (November 20001), pp. 2569-2575, ISSN 0009-7322

Toohey, J.I. (2001). Possible involvement of sulfane sulfur in homocysteine-induced atherosclerosis. *Medical Hypotheses*, Vol.56, No.2, (February 2001), pp. 259-261, ISSN 0306-9877

Yasui, K., Kowa, H., Nakaso, K., Takeshima, T., & Nakashima, K. (2000). Plasma homocysteine and MTHFR C677T genotype in levodopa-treated patients with PD. *Neurology*, Vol.55, No.3, (August 2000), pp. 437-440, ISSN 0028-3878

Vallance, P., Leone, A., Calver, A., Collier, J., & Moncada, S. (1992). Accumulation of an endogenous inhibitor of nitric oxide synthesis in chronic renal failure. *Lancet*, Vol.339, No.8793, (March 1992), pp. 572-575, ISSN 0140-6736

Watkins, D., Ru, M., Hwang, H.Y., Kim, C.D., Murray, A., Philip, N.S., Kim, W., Legakis, H., Wai, T., Hilton, J.F., Ge, B., Dore, C., Hosack, A., Wilson, A., Gravel, R.A., Shane, B., Hudson, T.J., & Rosenblatt, D.S. (2002). Hyperhomocysteinemia due to methionine synthase deficiency, cblG: structure of the MTR gene, genotype diversity, and recognition of a common mutation, P1173L. *American Journal of Human Genetics*, Vol.71, No.1, (July 2003), pp. 143-153, ISSN 0002-9297

Yasui, K., Kowa, H., Nakaso, K., Takeshima, T., & Nakashima, K. (2000). Plasma homocysteine and MTHFR C677T genotype in levodopa-treated patients with PD. *Neurology*, Vol.55, No.3, (August 2000), pp. 437-440, ISSN 0028-3878

Yasui, K., Nakaso, K., Kowa, H., Takeshima, T., & Nakashima, K. (2003). Levodopa-induced hyperhomocysteinaemia in Parkinson's disease. *Acta Neurologica Scandinavica*, Vol.108, No.1, (July 2003), pp. 66-67, ISSN 0001-6314

Yoo, J.H. & Lee, S.C. (2001). Elevated levels of plasma homocysteine and asymmetric dimethylarginine in elderly patients with stroke. *Atherosclerosis*, Vol.158, No.2, (October 2001), pp. 425-430, ISSN 0021-9150

Yuan, R.Y., Sheu, J.J., Yu, J.M., Hu, C.J., Tseng, I.J., Ho, C.S., Yeh, C.Y., Hung, Y.L., & Chiang, T.R. (2009). Methylenetetrahydrofolate reductase polymorphisms and plasma homocysteine in levodopa-treated and non-treated Parkinson's disease patients. *Journal of Neurological Sciences*, Vol.287, No.1-2, (December 2009), pp. 64-68, ISSN 0022-510X

Zhang, J., Perry, G., Smith, M.A., Robertson, D., Olson, S.J., Graham, D.G., & Montine, T.J. (1999). Parkinson's disease is associated with oxidative damage to cytoplasmic DNA and RNA in substantia nigra neurons. *American Journal of Pathology*, Vol.154, No.5, (May 1999), pp. 1423-1429, ISSN 0002-9440

Zoccolella, S., Lamberti, P., Iliceto, G., Dell'Aquila, C., Diroma, C., Fraddosio, A., Lamberti, S.V., Armenise, E., Defazio, G., de Mari,.M., & Livrea, P. (2006). Elevated plasma homocysteine levels in L-dopa-treated Parkinson's disease patients with dyskinesias. *Clinical Chemistry and Laboratory Medicine*, Vol.44, No.7, pp. 863-866, ISSN 1434-6621

Zoccolella, S., Dell'Aquila, C., Abruzzese, G., Antonini, A., Bonuccelli, U., Canesi, M., Cristina, S., Marchese, R., Pacchetti, C., Zagaglia, R., Logroscino, G., Defazio, G., Lamberti, P., & Livrea, P. (2009). Hyperhomocysteinemia in levodopa-treated patients with Parkinson's disease dementia. *Movement Disorders*, Vol.24, No.7, (May 2009), pp. 1028-1033, ISSN 0885-3185

3

Inflammatory Responses and Regulation in Parkinson's Disease

Lynda J. Peterson and Patrick M. Flood
The University of North Carolina at Chapel Hill,
U.S.A.

1. Introduction

Parkinson's disease (PD) is a slow, progressive neurodegenerative disorder affecting an estimated 6 million people worldwide (Litteljohn, Mangano et al. 2011). The etiology of the disease is characterized by increasing loss over time of dopaminergic neurons (DA-neurons) in the substantia nigra (SN) as well as the depletion of dopamine in the striatum, which eventually leads to pathological and clinical symptoms (Jenner and Olanow 2006). PET imaging and post-mortem analyses of the brains of PD patients indicate that the appearance of symptoms, including tremor, bradykinesia, rigidity, slowness of movement, and postural instability (Jellinger 2001), generally are manifest once 60% of DA-neurons have died and a 70% threshold decrease in normal DA activity has been reached (Klockgether 2004; Litteljohn, Mangano et al. 2011). Epidemiological studies indicate that only about 10% of PD cases are early onset , i.e. prior to the age of 50 and occur mainly in familial clusters (Mizuno, Hattori et al. 2001). These cases have established genetic bases due to mutations in several recently identified genes, including parkin, leucine-rich repeat kinase 2 (LRRK2), α-synuclein, PINK-1, or DJ-1 (Polymeropoulos, Lavedan et al. 1997; Lucking, Durr et al. 2000; Abou-Sleiman, Healy et al. 2003; Farrer, Haugarvoll et al. 2006; Sun, Latourelle et al. 2006; Jiang, Wu et al. 2007; Weng, Chou et al. 2007; Bonifati, Wu-Chou et al. 2008). The majority of PD cases (approximately 90%) are late onset and idiopathic (Tanner 2003). Although the etiology of idiopathic PD is uncertain, this form of PD particularly affects the elderly, with average onset of clinical symptoms between 60 and 65 years of age (Litteljohn, Mangano et al. 2011). Idiopathic PD is thus age-associated, with approximately 1% of the population being affected by 65-70 year of age, increasing to 4-5% at 85 years (Fahn 2003; Tansey, McCoy et al. 2007). However, the causes of idiopathic non-familial PD are probably multifactorial, with some form of genetic predisposition, environmental insults and/or aging all likely to be important factors in disease initiation and progression (Nagatsu and Sawada 2006; Dickson 2007; Vilar, Coelho et al. 2007; Singh, Singh et al. 2008).

While the exact cause of chronic neurodegeneration of PD is not known, increasing evidence suggests that chronic inflammation is the fundamental process mediating the progressive nature of the neurodegeneration characteristic of PD (McGeer, Yasojima et al. 2001; Hirsch and Hunot 2009). In animal PD models, long-term inflammation induces progressive loss of DA neurons within the SN brain region (Gao, Jiang et al. 2002; Dauer and Przedborski 2003; Bartels and Leenders 2007). Neuroinflammation, which is characterized by activation of both the innate and adaptive immune response, has been demonstrated in PD patients by the preponderance of activated microglia within the SN, and the increased production in the CNS of inflammatory mediators, such as cytokines, chemokines, reactive oxygen species (ROS) and reactive nitrites (Cicchetti, Lapointe et al. 2005; Loeffler, Camp et al. 2006; Ghosh, Roy et al. 2007; Cicchetti, Drouin-Ouellet et al. 2009). Post mortem analyses of brains from PD patients provide clear evidence of large numbers of human leukocyte antigen (HLA-DR) and CD11b-positive microglia in the SN, the brain region in which the degeneration of DA neurons is most prominent (McGeer, Itagaki et al. 1988). Expression of the inflammatory markers MHC II, TNFα and cyclooxygenase (COX-2) is also higher in SN tissue of patients with PD than in comparable tissue from unaffected controls (McGeer, Itagaki et al. 1988; Boka, Anglade et al. 1994; Knott, Stern et al. 2000). Additionally, levels of proinflammatory mediators, including TNFα, IL-1β, IL-6, (ROS), and eicosanoids, are all elevated in the SN, striatum, cerebrospinal fluid (CSF) and/or peripheral blood mononuclear cells (PBMC) of PD patients (McGeer, Itagaki et al. 1988; Qureshi, Baig et al. 1995; Mogi, Harada et al. 1996; Nagatsu, Mogi et al. 2000; Imamura, Hishikawa et al. 2003; Teismann and Schulz 2004; Nagatsu and Sawada 2006; Sawada, Imamura et al. 2006; Hirsch and Hunot 2009; Pisani, Moschella et al. 2010). Nitric oxide (NO) free radicals are also elevated in PD as indicated by increased nitrite (an indicator for NO) present in the CSF, as well as increased expression of inducible nitric oxide synthase (iNOS) within the SN of PD patients (Qureshi, Baig et al. 1995). Oxidative damage measured by the presence of nucleoside oxidation product 8-hydroxyguanosine, is approximately 16-fold higher in SN of PD patients and post-mortem analysis of the brains of PD patients also show evidence of the oxidation of lipids, DNA and proteins (Owen, Schapira et al. 1996; Spencer, Jenner et al. 1998; Halliwell 2006). Reduced levels of antioxidant glutathione (GSH) concomitant with increased concentrations of oxidized GSH, are found in the surviving SN neurons of PD patients compared to normal controls, indicating these neurons were undergoing increased oxidative stress (OS) at the time of death (Sofic, Lange et al. 1992; Pearce, Owen et al. 1997).

In addition to direct evidence for increased inflammatory activity within the CNS of patients with PD, other aspects of the etiology of PD suggest this is primarily an inflammatory disorder. For example, PD patients display decreased activity in mitochondrial complexes I and I/III (Krige, Carroll et al. 1992), and the inhibition of mitochondria respiratory complex-I after exposure to MPTP gives rise to PD-like pathologies in humans (Tetrud, Langston et al. 1989; Langston, Forno et al. 1999), primates, mice and rats (Yazdani, German et al. 2006; Jackson-Lewis and Przedborski 2007). This is because DA neurons appear to have an intrinsic sensitivity to complex I defects based on studies that demonstrate the selective neurotoxic effects of the pesticide rotenone on DA neurons only, despite the fact that rotenone inhibits complex I throughout the brain (Sherer, Betarbet et al. 2002). However, even direct inhibition of complex-I by MPTP in DA neurons results in neurodegeneration that is primarily inflammatory in nature (Ghosh, Roy et al. 2007; Qian, Gao et al. 2007; Qian and Flood 2008). Further evidence of the key role of inflammation in PD is seen in other features of the disease. For example, blood-brain-barrier (BBB) leakage has been found in positron-emission tomography (PET) images of the brains of PD patients (Kortekaas, Leenders et al. 2005), and is likely caused by increased inflammation in PD. In addition, increased angiogenesis also occurs in PD patients (Faucheux, Bonnet et al. 1999) , and in the SN of a monkey-model of PD (Barcia, Bautista et al. 2005). Increased expression of the angiogenic-stimulant vascular endothelial growth factor (VEGF) and its major receptor

VEGFR1, have been found post mortem in the SN of PD patients (Wada, Arai et al. 2006), and this is consistent with increased angiogenesis found in PD brains (Faucheux, Bonnet et al. 1999). Excess VEGF induces increased macrophage migration mediated by VEGFR1 (Huusko, Merentie et al. 2009) and VEGF also induces BBB disruption in animal models after brain injury (Zhang, Zhang et al. 2000; Nguyen, Julien et al. 2002; Rite, Machado et al. 2007; Argaw, Gurfein et al. 2009) as well as in a rat model of PD (Rite, Machado et al. 2007). The VEGFR antagonist, Cyclo-VEGI, reduces inflammation and vascular leakiness, and is neuroprotective against excitotoxin-induced neurodegeneration in rats (Ryu and McLarnon 2008). This suggests dysregulated VEGF expression in the PD brain is also a key part of the neuroinflammatory response and increased edema in PD (Kirk and Karlik 2003; Suidan, Dickerson et al. 2010) (Nguyen, Julien et al. 2002; Nguyen, Tatlipinar et al. 2006; Zhang, Wang et al. 2006).

It is also worth noting that the innate immune cells of the brain, including microglia, become more reactive with age and that this might contribute to increased neuroinflammation in the elderly at some time point after activation of the peripheral immune response (Godbout and Johnson 2009). It has been suggested that prolonged exposure over a lifetime to inflammatory cytokines in the brain might eventually lead to various neurologic disorders (Godbout and Johnson 2009). This increased susceptibility to chronic inflammation in the elderly could contribute to the increased risk of PD associated with age. With growing elderly populations in many countries, PD is potentially an expanding public health problem. It is therefore critical that therapeutic interventions be identified and developed, that can halt and eventually reverse the neurodegeneration characteristic in PD. Treatments that focus on reducing chronic inflammation and pro-inflammatory microglial cell activation offer great promise for this sort of therapy. Therapies that foster microglia phenotypes which are non-inflammatory and supportive of neuroregeneration, could also prove beneficial in treating PD in the future.

In this chapter, we will discuss inflammatory mechanisms that play a crucial role in the progression of PD, and the therapeutic efficacy of using several anti-inflammatory compounds to treat progressive PD. We will also discuss the biology of microglial cells, including the cellular and molecular mechanisms that activate and regulate their inflammatory response, the evidence that implicates their different inflammatory mediators in the destruction of DA-neurons, and the efficacy of using different anti-inflammatory cytokines such as IL-10 and 1β, natural anti-inflammatory compounds such as *sinomenine*, *luteolin*, and *curcumin*, and the anti-inflammatory drugs morphinans and cyclosporine A, cell-based treatments such as Treg therapy, and specific anti-inflammatory therapies such as NF-κB inhibitors and β2-Adrenergic Receptor (β2AR) agonists. in halting or reversing the degenerative effects of inflammation within the SN. Finally, we will propose a model for PD as it relates to chronic inflammation, and discuss some possible future directions for the therapeutic treatment of PD.

2. Neuroinflammation in Parkinson's Disease

2.1 Microglia and chronic inflammation in neurodegeneration

Over two decades ago, high levels of activated microglia were discovered in the SN of PD patients (McGeer, Itagaki et al. 1988), first suggesting a connection between inflammation and PD. Since then, a wide range of inflammatory mediators produced by active microglia have been identified post mortem in PD tissue samples (Hirsch 2000; Orr, Rowe et al. 2002). The presence of activated microglia has also been verified in the SN of PD animal models (rodents and primates) (Akiyama and McGeer 1989; Barcia, Sanchez Bahillo et al. 2004; Gao, Miao et al. 2011). Studies using animal models of PD have begun to elucidate the inflammatory mechanisms that underlie the neurodegeneration of DA neurons and loss of DA production which are hallmarks of the disease. It has been found that intranigral injection of the pathogen product lipopolysaccharide (LPS) induces increased levels of CD11b+ and microglia and neutrophils in the SN of rats when compared to levels found in the cortex (Ji, Kronenberg et al. 2009). This same study also observed pronounced damage to endothelial cells and BBB permeability within the SN of the LPS-injected rats (Ji, Kronenberg et al. 2009). In this model, direct intranigral injection LPS or administration of the neurotoxin 1-methyl-4-phenyl-1,2,3,6-tetrahydropyridine (MPTP) induced PD-like symptoms accompanied by increased activation of microglia in the SN. Of particular significance is another finding that activated microglia and elevated levels of pro-inflammatory TNFα could be detected in the SN of monkeys from 1 to 14 years after an initial brief administration of MPTP (McGeer, Schwab et al. 2003; Barcia, Sanchez Bahillo et al. 2004; Barcia, de Pablos et al. 2005). These observations suggested that a brief insult to the brain by toxins could induce a chronic inflammatory state with concomitant progressive neurodegeneration. Additional support for sustained inflammation after insult is provided by an unfortunate human example of accidental exposure to MPTP in contaminated illegal street-drugs. Post-mortem evidence of activated microglia and degeneration in the SN of these human patients remained evident from 3 to 16 years after intravenous injection of the toxin (Langston, Forno et al. 1999).

Among the many inflammatory factors produced by microglia, superoxide is one of the major mediators of neurodegeneration. DA neurons are especially vulnerable to oxidative insults and this strongly supports the association of microglia activation with progressive PD (Block and Hong 2007). It is known that the normal midbrain region encompassing the SN contains nearly five times more microglia than other areas of the brain (Kim, Mohney et al. 2000). Understanding the progressive nature of microglia-mediated neurotoxicity, and the common mechanism of microglia activation by various diverse toxins or insults, thus has prime therapeutic importance for treating PD (Nguyen, Julien et al. 2002).

2.2 Inflammatory mechanisms and dopaminergic-neuron death

Several different animal models of PD have found that both systemic inflammation and direct dopaminergic neurotoxicity can initiate or exacerbate the neuroinflammation and neurodegeneration that are hallmarks of the disease. Injection of MPTP results in chronic neuroinflammation and progressive neurotoxicity in humans (Langston, Forno et al. 1999) and other primates (McGeer, Schwab et al. 2003). In the former case, an accidental intravenous injection of MPTP-contaminated street-drugs left several patients ill with progressive motor-dysfunction which was shown in post mortem analysis to be mediated by DA-neuron loss in the SN, very similar to what is observed following MPTP injection in both rodent and primate models of neurodegeneration (Langston, Forno et al. 1999; Qin, Wu et al. 2007). Similarly a single systemic injection of LPS in an rodent model results in significant loss (23%) of DA neurons in the SN beginning at 7-months post treatment, increasing to a 47% loss at 10-months post injection (Qin, Wu et al. 2007). This delayed, progressive loss of DA neurons in the SN recapitulates some of the hallmark characteristics of PD. This model is further supported as a model for PD by a clinical case report that a patient displayed PD-related symptoms after accidental peripheral exposure to LPS (Niehaus and Lange 2003). However, the underlying mechanism that advances the progressive nature of the disease remains unclear. It is known that systemically injected LPS cannot readily cross the blood-brain barrier, and studies have shown that pro-inflammatory cytokines, actually mediate the mechanism of systemic LPS-induced DA neurotoxicity (Qin, Wu et al. 2007). Interestingly, systemic administration of LPS enhances motor neuron degeneration in animal models of another neurodegenerative disease, amyotrophic lateral sclerosis (ALS), 6 months after LPS injection (Nguyen, D'Aigle et al. 2004), suggesting this may be a common etiology for a number of chronic neurodegenerative conditions. In addition, systemic exposure to LPS was also shown to significantly exacerbate neuronal-cell death associated with ischemic insult in neonatal rats (Lehnardt, Massillon et al. 2003). The effects of systemic inflammation on neuronal survival may depend upon several factors such as brain region affected, length of time to allow cumulative effects, age of exposure to the inflammagen, presence of systemic TNFα, and severity of the inflammatory stimulation.

It now appears that it is the inflammatory cytokines TNFα, IL-1β and IL-6 which play major roles in the etiology of PD both systemically and within the CNS. First, TNFα produced in the periphery after systemic LPS injection is transported across BBB to enter the brain through a TNFα-receptor dependent mechanism (Gutierrez, Banks et al. 1993; Pan and Kastin 2002; Qin, Wu et al. 2007). TNFα then initiates an inflammatory cascade by interacting with TNFα receptors on the microglia, leading to the activation of transcription factor NF-κB within microglial cells, and resulting in the production of additional TNFα and other pro-inflammatory factors, and thus creating a persistent and self-perpetuating neuroinflammatory response that drives delayed and progressive loss of DA neurons in the SN (Park and Bowers 2010). In addition, TNFα is one of the primary pro-inflammatory cytokines that promote overproduction of ROS (Fernandez-Checa, Kaplowitz et al. 1997), a key player in DA-neurodegeneration (Gao and Hong 2008) (Qian, Flood et al. 2011). Another pro-inflammatory cytokine, IL-1β, is also under transcriptional control of NF-κB and is consequently up-regulated in neuroinflammation. Direct injection of recombinant IL-1β into the brains of rats induces astrocytic expression of hypoxia inducible factor (HIF-1α) which contributes to the induction of oxidative stress (Argaw, Zhang et al. 2006). IL-1β also induces the HIF-1α-VEGF pathway that results in increased BBB permeability and increased angiogenesis (Argaw, Zhang et al. 2006; Argaw, Gurfein et al. 2009), which are all found to be increased in PD patients (Kortekaas, Leenders et al. 2005). Similarly, IL-6 expression is controlled by NF-κB (Lappas, Permezel et al. 2002) and is increased under a variety of inflammatory conditions (Van Snick 1990; Dendorfer 1996), including an MPTP-induced mouse model of PD (Kohutnicka, Lewandowska et al. 1998). IL-6 expression from activated microglia coincides in the SN with loss of TH+ DA neurons after MPTP injection but is absent from the SN in uninjected controls (Kohutnicka, Lewandowska et al. 1998). Neuronal levels of IL-6 are also increased by oxidative stress which is another mediator of microglia activation, neuroinflammation and degeneration (Lee, Cho et al. 2010; Naik and Dixit 2011; Negi, Kumar et al. 2011).

In addition to inflammatory cytokines, oxidative stress appears to play a crucial role in the DA-neurodegeneration seen in PD. Oxidative stress occurs because of intracellular accumulation of reactive oxygen and nitrogen species (ROS & RNS) and, along with mitochondrial dysfunction and inflammation, has been identified as central in the mechanism underlying the inflammatory pathogenesis of PD (Bartels and Leenders 2007; Monahan, Warren et al. 2008). Impaired mitochondrial function has been observed in PD (Schapira, Cooper et al. 1989; Schapira 1994; Jenner and Olanow 1996; Sherer, Betarbet et al. 2002; Keeney, Xie et al. 2006; Schapira 2006), in which mitochondria generate ROS as by-products of molecular oxygen consumption in the electron transport chain. Oxidative stress is hypothesized to initiate DA neuron loss in the SN (Jenner and Olanow 1998; Lin and Beal 2006). The brain is hypersensitive to oxidative damage in part due to the fact that oxygen consumption by brain cells constitutes 20% of total oxygen consumption in body. Brain tissue is also enriched in peroxidizable fatty acids and has low levels anti-oxidant defenses (catalase, SOD, glutathione, glutathione peroxidase) (Floyd 1999; Floyd 1999). Within the brain, the SN is amongst regions most vulnerable to oxidative insult. The SN is characterized by a pro-oxidative state, and has a high metabolic rate with high levels of the oxidizable species DA, DA-derived ROS, neuromelanin and other molecules that render the SN vulnerable to the possible effects of peroxynitrite and sulfite (Marshall, Reist et al. 1999). Oxidative stress is part of the pro-inflammatory response of microglia within the CNS, and it has been found that NADPH oxidase (PHOX), is the major superoxide-producing enzyme of microglia. It is a molecular complex of membrane-associated cytochrome b558 (composed of 2 subunits: gp91phox and p22phox) and the cytosolic components: p47phox, p67phox, p40phox, and a small GTPase rac2 (Groemping and Rittinger 2005). Upon activation, the cytosolic subunits translocate to the membrane and form a functional enzyme to generate superoxide. Therapy directed against the oxidative stress response has proved beneficial in treatment for PD (Smith and Zigmond 2003; Jackson-Lewis and Smeyne 2005). Anti-inflammatory agents that inhibit NADPH oxidase activity are neuroprotective (Liu and Hong 2003; Qian, Block et al. 2006; Qian, Gao et al. 2007), and reduced DA neurotoxicity induced by LPS or MPTP has been demonstrated in PHOX-/- compared to wild-type mice (Gao, Liu et al. 2003; Qin, Liu et al. 2004). Pharmacological inhibition of PHOX by the specific inhibitor diphenyliodonium (DPI), also shows potent DA-neuroprotection *in vitro* (Qian, Gao et al. 2007). PHOX activity also regulates production of pro-inflammatory cytokines, such as TNFα, by activated microglia *in vitro* following LPS stimulation (Qin, Liu et al. 2004). This suggests that PHOX not only mediates superoxide production, but also controls the levels of other pro-inflammatory neurotoxic factors produced by activated microglia. Cell signaling pathways that regulate PHOX activity are still being elucidated but it has been shown that a microglial adhesion molecule, the integrin MAC1 (macrophage antigen complex 1), is closely linked with PHOX and plays an important role in microglia-mediated neuroinflammation and neurotoxicity (Hu, Zhang et al. 2008). Microglial- cell expressed MAC1 is indispensable for the enhanced neurotoxicity induced by LPS, a-synuclein, or MPTP in neuron-glia mixed cell cultures (Pei, Pang et al. 2007; Zhang, Dallas et al. 2007; Hu, Zhang et al. 2008). Furthermore, MAC1-deficient mice show resistance to MPTP-induced DA neurotoxicity *in vivo*. NADPH oxidase-generated oxygen free radicals are also required for MAC1-mediated phagocytosis in neutrophils (Coxon, Rieu et al. 1996). Therefore, the dual activity between MAC1 and NADPH oxidase might be a central mechanism underlying the reactive microgliosis that mediates oxidative damage and consequent progressive neurodegeneration after microglia activation.

2.3 Peripheral inflammation, microglial-cell activation and neurodegeneration

Neuroinflammation is an important defense mechanism against pathogens and environmental toxins damaging the brain. Under normal conditions, the central nervous system (CNS) and the brain especially are considered to be immune privileged (Neuwelt and Clark 1978; Smith, DeGirolami et al. 1992; Lotan and Schwartz 1994). Any immune response is very highly regulated with a finely balanced anti-inflammatory environment within the CNS combined with vigilant immune surveillance by circulating immune cells and those that are resident in the CNS. Under pathological conditions, the brain mounts an aggressive, acute inflammatory response to invading pathogens, infection, trauma, stroke or any other threat to homeostasis. These perturbations trigger the activation of microglia, the brain resident macrophages (Ransohoff and Perry 2009), as well as local invasions of circulating immune cells and the production of ROS and RNS (Mosley, Benner et al. 2006; Tansey, McCoy et al. 2007; Whitton 2007). The resident microglia aid in functional regulation of other immune cells particularly the helper T-cells and dendritic cells (DC) which also play critical roles in the initiation and maintenance of any neuroinflammatory response to pathological threats. However, inflammation in the brain is a 'two-edged sword' (Wyss-Coray and Mucke 2002) because if the tight regulation of the inflammatory process breaks down in any manner, the inflammatory response can switch from being beneficial to highly detrimental to brain function. In acute situations short-lived inflammatory mechanisms limit injury and promote healing (Wyss-Coray and Mucke 2002; McGeer and McGeer 2004). Microglia are the critical elements in an acute neuroinflammatory response that minimize tissue damage, restore tissue to homeostasis and promote would healing processes. Conversely, when inflammation is chronically sustained at high levels, this can lead to brain-tissue damage with concomitant initiation and progression of neuroinflammatory diseases such as PD.

While microglial cells are the major immunocompetent cells in the CNS and are important mediators in the pathogenesis of PD (Herrera, Tomas-Camardiel et al. 2005; Smeyne, Jiao et al. 2005; Zhou, Wang et al. 2005), up-regulation of humoral response and other peripheral immune components has been identified in both idiopathic and genetic cases of PD (Orr, Rowe et al. 2005). Elevated levels of IL-1β, TNFα, IL-6 have been described in post mortem tissue from PD patients (Mogi, Harada et al. 1994; Mogi, Harada et al. 1994; Mogi, Harada et al. 1996), and PD patients show higher levels of IL-1β, TNFα, Il-1, CD4+ and CD8+ cells in serum and CSF (Dobbs, Charlett et al. 1999; Bas, Calopa et al. 2001; Hisanaga, Asagi et al. 2001; Reale, Greig et al. 2009). CD8+ T cells have also been found associated with degenerating SN neurons (McGeer, Itagaki et al. 1988), and classical complement components have been isolated in the Lewy bodies that form in the SN of PD patients (Yamada, McGeer et al. 1992). Significantly, compromised BBB integrity has also been observed in PD patients (Kortekaas, Leenders et al. 2005), indicating that factors in peripheral inflammation have ready access to the brain and may also be involved in the neurodegenerative process probably via an effect on the activation of microglia. Complement proteins normally circulate in the blood in an inactive state, but in response to pathogenic threat, these proteins become activated in cascades of events that precipitate destruction and removal of the threat. Importantly for PD, studies have shown that complement factors C1q and mannose-binding lectins (MBL), participate in microglial cell activation and could be important in pathogenesis of neurodegeneration (Yamada, McGeer et al. 1992; Webster, Galvan et al. 2001; Whitton 2007). The importance of the classical complement pathway in PD has been established (Yamada, McGeer et al. 1992; Yamada, Chong et al. 1993), and MBL infiltration into the brain accompanies degeneration of TH+ neurons in MPTP-injected mice up to 28 days post MPTP administration in an animal model of PD (Chao, He et al. 2009). In the latter study, clear evidence of BBB breakdown was also documented, providing further evidence that peripheral immunity probably participates in the activation of microglia and consequent DA-neuron destruction.

Normally, immune surveillance protects the healthy brain from pathogen assault and damage. Memory T-cell surveillance of the CNS is first regulated via migration from the blood into the cerebral spinal fluid (CSF) through the choroid plexus barrier (Engelhardt and Ransohoff 2005), while the recruitment and infiltration of immune cells into brain tissue occurs through the post-capillary venules into the perivascular space that surrounds microvascular endothelial cells (MVEC) which are joined together by tight-junctions that form the blood-brain-barrier (Carrithers, Visintin et al. 2000; Pachter, de Vries et al. 2003). MVEC in the brain closely interact with astrocytes, pericytes, perivascular microglia and neuronal cells such as DA-producing neurons to form the neurovascular unit. Thus, at these crucial checkpoints the specific microenvironment within the CNS tissues determines whether the immune cells survive to mount antigen-specific inflammatory response or if they will be eliminated. CD4+ T cells play a critical role in the initiation and maintenance of any immune response in the CNS including the brain, but to survive in this normally anti-inflammatory environment, they need additional stimulatory signals. Generally, CD4+ must be activated in the peripheral lymphoid system prior to migration into the CNS. Activated CD4+Th cells differentiate into distinct effector subsets that express unique suites of cytokines that perform different immunoregulatory functions. For example Th1 and Th2 produce predominantly INF-γ and IL-4 respectively which have differential effects on the activation state of microglia amongst other disparate outcomes (Appel, Beers et al. 2009)

T cells express many sensor receptors with which they assess the microenvironment milieu. CD+4 interact with other immune cells such as antigen presenting cells (APC) that take-up, process and present antigens via the major histocompatibility complex molecules (MHC). MHCII is expressed mainly in cells of the lymphoid system such as T cells, B cells, macrophages, and DC (Matarese, De Rosa et al. 2008). Under non-inflammatory conditions, cells of the CNS express low levels of MCH and in the absence of histocompatibility molecules the survival or further differentiation of activated T cells is low. Constitutively expressed mediators also help prevent differentiation of Th cells, and conversely promote development of Tregs. For example, the neuropeptide Vasoactive Intestinal Peptide (VIP) up-regulates Treg function which has an inhibitory effect on microglia and macrophages (Delgado, Chorny et al. 2005; Fernandez-Martin, Gonzalez-Rey et al. 2006). Additionally, anti-inflammatory cytokines secreted by astrocytes and glial cells, such as IL-10 and TGFβ1, induce differentiation of Tregs (Chen and Wahl 2003). However, during inflammation TGFβ1 works with IL-6 or IL-21 to induce differentiation of pro-inflammatory IL-17-producing T cells (Th17) indicating the distinction between anti-inflammatory and pro-inflammatory is not always straight forward. In an animal model of PD, the DA-neuron neurodegenerative effects of MPTP administration were Th17-cell mediated, and the induction of Tregs by VIP attenuated this effect (Reynolds, Banerjee et al. 2007; Reynolds, Stone et al. 2010). However, as it has also been shown that TGFβ1/IL-6 increases production of IL-10 as well as IL-17, this IL-10 is then capable of suppressing the degenerative effects mediated by Th17 cells (McGeachy, Bak-Jensen et al. 2007).

3. Efficacy of anti-inflammatory agents halting or reversing degeneration

Mounting evidence indicates that numerous types of inflammatory mediators such as TNFα, prostaglandin (PGE2), NO, free radicals, and other products of activated immune cells can also play a role in the DA-neuron degeneration in several models of PD (Gao, Jiang et al. 2002; Dauer and Przedborski 2003; Bartels and Leenders 2007). Treatment using anti-inflammatory agents directed at a number of different pro-inflammatory targets could potentially halt, slow or even reverse PD disease progression. For example, steroidal anti-inflammatory drugs (SAIDS) such as dexamethasone have been used to stimulate neuroprotection against MPTP or LPS-induced toxicity (Kurkowska-Jastrzebska, Wronska et al. 1999; Castano, Herrera et al. 2002; Kurkowska-Jastrzebska, Litwin et al. 2004). In addition, non-steroidal anti-inflammatory drugs (NSAIDS), e.g. aspirin and ibuprofen, can reduce inflammation by inhibition of COX activity (Sairam, Saravanan et al. 2003)(Sairam et al. 2003). A prospective study found a significantly lower risk of developing PD in users of ibuprofen compared to non-users, and that the efficacy of taking ibuprofen was dose-dependently related to the number of weekly tablets of the drug taken (Gao, Chen et al. 2011). Microglial cell inhibitors such as minocycline have also shown neuroprotective characteristics in PD animal models (Du, Ma et al. 2001; Wu, Jackson-Lewis et al. 2002). Recently, strategies that directly inactivate the activation of the pro-inflammatory transcription factor NF-κB (Ghosh, Roy et al. 2007; Zhang, Qian et al. 2010), and/or activate the peroxisome proliferator-activated receptor-c (PPARc) (Bernardo, Ajmone-Cat et al. 2005), have produced beneficial modulation of inflammatory responses. Other strategies, including inhibition of ion channels in microglial cells (Thomas, Chartrand et al. 2007) can also be effective treatments aimed at halting progressive PD in an animal model of the disease. We will focus on five relatively new approaches in anti-inflammatory therapy for PD: (1) the use of exogenous anti-inflammatory cytokines IL-10 or TGFβ1, (2) the use of cell-based therapies such as regulatory T cells (Tregs), which are the major source of IL-10 or TGFβ1 in the resolution of neuroinflammation; (3) the use of morphinan-related compounds; (4) the targeting of NF-κB, the major transcriptional regulator of inflammation, and (5) the administration of beta2-adrenergic receptor (β2AR) agonists.

3.1 Therapies using anti-inflammatory cytokines: IL-10 and TGFβ

When acute inflammation is not resolved, i.e. the agent or event that originated the inflammatory response has not been eliminated, chronic inflammation can become entrenched and lead to neuroinflammation and degeneration. Normally, endogenous anti-inflammatory cytokines provide a negative-feedback mechanism which controls the continued activation of immune cells from potentially pathological effects (Moore, Lahiri et al. 2001; Strle, Zhou et al. 2001). Therefore, replacing or elevating the level of these anti-inflammatory regulators could be a therapeutic means to halt the chronic, pathological aspects of inflammation. IL10 and TGFβ1 are two major anti-inflammatory cytokines that are normally produced by Treg cells. Studies using exogenously supplied IL10 and TGFβ1 have shown potent effects in reducing neurotoxicity induced by either LPS or MPTP in PD models. In an *in vitro* model of PD, application of IL-10 to a mixed glial cell-neuron cell culture abrogated the degeneration of the neuron cells induced by either LPS or MPTP (Qian, Block et al. 2006). This inhibitory effect of IL10 was mediated through its inhibition of the production of TNFα, nitric oxide, and extracellular superoxide in the microglia cells within the mixed cell culture (Qian, Block et al. 2006). These *in vitro* effects of IL-10 are confirmed by *in vivo* results from a 6-OHDA rat model of PD. In this model, sustained administration of IL10 via a viral-vector, significantly protected DA-neuron from death and ameliorated behavioral deficits induced by intra-striatal delivery of 6-OHDA (Johnston, Su et al. 2008).

Several *in vitro* studies have shown that TGFβ1 can also protect neurons from cell death induced by oxidative stress (Prehn and Krieglstein 1994), glutamate excitotoxicity (Zhu, Yang et al. 2002), or chemical-induced hypoxia (Ruocco, Nicole et al. 1999). TGFβ1 suppresses the progression of neurodegeneration *in vivo* in an EAE model of MS (Szczepanik, Tutaj et al. 2005). Additionally, recombinant TGFβ1, intracerebrally delivered by a viral-vector, protects against brain injury induced by ischemia (Unsicker and Krieglstein 2002), excitotoxic-induced death (Ruocco, Nicole et al. 1999), and oxidative stress (Henrich-Noack, Prehn et al. 1996). Although exogenous TGFβ1 has thus been strongly suggested as a neuroprotective treatment, the molecular mechanisms underlying its neuroprotection have not been clearly elucidated. Recent evidence indicates that the neuroprotective effects of both IL10 and TGFβ1 are mainly due to their inhibition of ROS production in microglia during initial activation or in reactive microgliosis (Qian, Block et al. 2006; Qian, Wei et al. 2008). In mixed glial cell-neuronal cell cultures, application of TGFβ1 blocked neuron cell death through the inhibition of PHOX activity in cultures exposed to either LPS or MPTP. TGFβ1 prevented the ERK-dependent phosphorylation on p47phox in the microglial cells and blocked translocation and assembly of the PHOX molecular complex to the plasma membrane. Inhibition of PHOX activation consequently reduced oxidase activities induced by LPS (Qian, Wei et al. 2008). While the complete *in vivo* roles of IL10 and TGFβ1 in the regulation of chronic CNS inflammation in PD remain to be determined, both may provide promising basis for therapeutic use in PD treatments.

3.2 Morphinan-based anti-inflammatory therapeutics

Dextromethorphan (DM) is a well established drug that is used as the active ingredient in many cough suppressants. Over twenty years ago, it was recognized that DM and the metabolite dextrorphan (DX) could have anti-seizure effects in models of convulsive disorders such as epilepsy (Tortella, Ferkany et al. 1988). Dextrorphan was also shown to antagonize the *in vitro* excitation of spinal neurons by application of N-methyl-D-aspartate (NMDA), a glutamate receptor ligand (Church, Lodge et al. 1985). In addition, DX was found to block cortical neuron injury induced by NMDA or by glutamate (Choi 1987; Choi, Maulucci-Gedde et al. 1987; Choi, Peters et al. 1987; Koh and Choi 1987). Because NMDA receptors were known to mediate hypoxic injury in neuronal cell cultures, it was suggested that morphinan drugs, especially DX and DM, might be potential therapeutic treatments for brain injury from hypoxia of ischemia (Goldberg, Weiss et al. 1987). Additionally, since the loss of DA-neuron in PD leads to the secondary effect of hyperactive glutamatergic function, it was postulated that DM and DX might also be useful as adjunct therapies in treating PD (Albin, Young et al. 1989; Greenamyre and O'Brien 1991).

Several studies using PD animal models or *in vitro* cell cultures have shown that dextromethorphan and its metabolites are neuroprotective due to their anti-inflammatory properties and inhibitory function towards microglia activation (Liu, Qin et al. 2003; Zhang, Wang et al. 2004; Zhang, Qin et al. 2005). In the first of these studies, DM treatment protected DA-neurons from LPS-induced neuron death in mixed glial-neuronal cell cultures (Liu, Qin et al. 2003). Furthermore, the neuroprotective effects of DM were mediated through inhibiting microglial cell activation (Liu, Qin et al. 2003). Similarly, DM inhibited microglia activation and was neuroprotective when administered daily to mice that had been injected with MPTP (Zhang, Wang et al. 2004). Another metabolite of DM, 3-hydroxymorphinan (3-HM), was shown to have the greatest potency (of several tested methorphinans) for attenuating the loss of DA-neurons in the SN, as well as restoring motor functions in an MPTP-injection mouse-model of PD (Zhang, Qin et al. 2005). 3-HM also protected neuronal cells in mixed glial-neuronal cells cultures by reducing MPTP-induced microgliosis and decreasing the production of ROS. In addition to this neuroprotective property, 3-HM was also found to have neurotrophic effects. The neurotrophic effects of 3-HM were mediated by induction of increased expression of neurotrophic factors, including GDNF, EGF, NTF and TGFβ1, by astroglial cells in mixed cultures with neuronal cells (Zhang, Wang et al. 2004; Zhang, Shin et al. 2006). In another study using mixed neuron-glia cultures, both l-morphine and it synthetic steroenantiomer, d-morphine, reduced LPS or MPTP-induced DA-neuron death with similar efficacy (Qian, Tan et al. 2007). These results indicated that morphine exerts anti-inflammatory effects either by inhibition of direct microglial cell activation via LPS or through attenuating reactive microgliosis induced by MPTP. A naturally occurring d-morphinan, sinomenine, also has neuroprotective effects and will be discussed below (Qian, Xu et al. 2007).

While DM and other morphinan compounds appear to have strong neuroprotective properties in animal model systems of PD, early human trials using DM to treat PD patients were contradictory. While one study found daily high doses of DM could improve some motor-behavioral deficits in PD patients (Bonuccelli, Del Dotto et al. 1992), another similar trial using the same dose regimen reported no beneficial effects on PD motor-associated symptoms (Montastruc, Fabre et al. 1994). Significantly, more recent double-blind trials have confirmed that DM can improve motor function in PD patients, especially the dyskinesia associated with long-term levadopa treatment (Verhagen Metman, Blanchet et al. 1998; Verhagen Metman, Del Dotto et al. 1998). It has been suggested that the uncertainty over the true effects of DM might be due to the relatively rapid metabolism of DM *in vivo* (Werling, Lauterbach et al. 2007). Although, DX and other DM metabolites have shown similar neuroprotective properties in preclinical studies, only DM seems to function through multiple mechanisms rather than simply blocking activity of the NMDA-receptor (Werling, Lauterbach et al. 2007). In situ DM concentrations can be increased if given in conjunction with a low dose of the drug quinidine which retards metabolism of DM and leads to increased DM concentrations in plasma, resulting in greater bioavailability (Pope, Khalil et al. 2004). Clearly, DM presents an attractive potential for use in combinatorial treatment for at least ameliorating the motor deficits characteristic of PD and possibly for attenuating the activation of microglia and chronic inflammation also prominent in PD.

3.3 Sinomenine, luteolin and curcumin as treatments for Parkinson's disease

Several natural compounds isolated from plants, including sinomenine, luteolin and curcumin, are also being investigated for their ability to attenuate inflammation and provide neuroprotection against the loss of DA neurons. Although these three agents belong to different families of organic compounds, they have all shown anti-oxidant, anti-inflammatory and neuroprotective qualities *in vitro* cell-culture models of neurodegenerative diseases including PD. The first of these is sinomenine, a morphinan related alkaloid compound purified from a medicinal plant (Sinomenine acutum) that has been traditionally used to treat inflammatory disorders (Liu, Resch et al. 1994; Liu, Buchner et al. 1996). In a study using rat midbrain mixed glial cell-neuron cell cultures, sinomenine protected the neuronal cells from both LPS and MPP+ induced cell death (Qian, Xu et al. 2007). Sinomenine protected neurons by reducing release of extracelluar ROS and inhibiting PHOX/p47 from translocation to the plasma membrane where the complex becomes activated. These effects were mediated by inhibition of microglial cells since sinomenine failed to protect neuronal-cell enriched cultures which lacked microglia from MPP+ induced damage and death (Qian, Xu et al. 2007).

Another plant extract, the flavonoid luteolin, has also been used for its anti-oxidant and anti-inflammatory properties. Luteolin was demonstrated to have neuroprotective effects by inhibiting oxidative stress-induced cell death in the DA-producing SH-SY5Y cell line (Kang, Lee et al. 2004). In mixed glial-neuron midbrain cell cultures from rats, luteolin attenuated the loss of TH+ DA-neurons after addition of increasing concentrations of LPS. The protective effect of luteolin in these experiments was shown to be mediated through the inhibition of microglial cell activation, and reduced production of TNFα, NO and ROS (Chen, Jin et al. 2008). Similarly, curcumin, the active anti-inflammatory isolate from turmeric (Curcuma longa), is known to have anti-inflammatory neuroprotective effects in CNS disorders. In an experimental allergic encephalomyelitis (EAE) mouse model of MS, curcumin inhibited EAE development by attenuating microglia activation and IL-12 production as well as Th1 cell differentiation (Natarajan and Bright 2002). Curcumin also has shown protective effects against LPS-induced DA neuron cell death in mixed rat neuron-glial cell cultures which were mediated by inhibition of the production of proinflammatory factors in microglia (Yang, Zhang et al. 2008). Taken together, the neuroprotective results from these three natural plant products suggest an interesting possibility for PD therapeutics. Since these and other similar plant-based isolates can cross the BBB and have anti-inflammatory as well as anti-oxidant properties, they may provide new directions for adjunct therapy.

4. Anti-inflammatory cell-based strategy for Parkinson's disease therapy: Regulatory T-cells

An anti-inflammatory strategy currently being studied as a cell-based therapy in PD involves the therapeutic introduction of Treg cells. It is now believed that Tregs suppress immune reactivity through multiple mechanisms, such as release of IL-10 and TGFβ, induction of apoptotic tolerance, and suppression of metabolic functions in effector immune cells such as microglia and effector T-cells. As the primary source IL10 and TGF1β *in vivo*, Tregs have been shown to be the major cells which regulate the inflammatory response in a number of disorders through their effects on the innate and adaptive immune responses that have escaped normal pathways of control. Recent studies using models of neurodegeneration demonstrated that induction of an anti-inflammatory Treg response inhibited microglial activation, and promoted neuronal survival (Reynolds, Banerjee et al. 2007; Liu, Gong et al. 2009; Reynolds, Stone et al. 2009). In another report, adoptively transferred Treg cells attenuated a Th17-mediated inflammatory response in mice that had been injected with MPTP and concomitantly vaccinated with nitrated (N) α-synuclein. In this model, injection of N-α-synuclein elicited an adaptive immune response in conjunction with the MPTP-induced neurotoxicity both of which were ameliorated by the transfer of natural or VIP-induced Treg cells in these mice (Reynolds, Stone et al. 2010). Tregs have also been shown to promote neurotrophic factor production from astrocytes (Reynolds, Banerjee et al. 2007; Reynolds, Stone et al. 2010), indicating their potential for neuroregeneration of DA neurons.

Strategies that use Th2 cells are also being employed. Th2 cells inhibit microglial cell activation through the production of IL4 and IL10, and stimulate the production of GDNF by astrocytes, thereby providing neuroprotection against MPTP-induced neuronal death (Benner, Mosley et al. 2004). Copaxone, a peptide-based therapy approved for patients with MS, is thought to promote the development of Th2 cells which function to decrease CNS inflammation through the release of anti-inflammatory cytokines and neurotrophic factors (Kipnis and Schwartz 2002; Angelov, Waibel et al. 2003; Benner, Mosley et al. 2004; Schwartz 2004). Copaxone-induced T-cells also have neuroprotective effects in animal models of ALS and PD (Angelov, Waibel et al. 2003; Benner, Mosley et al. 2004). However, because the interactions amongst regulatory T cells, glial cells, neurons and other infiltrating leukocytes within the SN is incredibly complex and not well understood, further studies to elucidate the regulatory pathways involved are necessary to develop Th2-cell based therapies for PD patients.

5. Specific anti-inflammatory therapies

5.1 Therapies targeting pro-inflammatory transcription factor NF-κB

Many of the inflammatory mediators involved in inflammation and DA-neurodegeneration in PD are expressed in microglial cells and their regulation is primarily mediated by the transcription factor NF-κB. NF-κB was first described in 1986 as a transcription factor which is essential for the expression of mouse kappa light chain genes (Sen and Baltimore 1986; Sen and Baltimore 1986). It has since been shown that NF-κB functions to control gene expression of many of pro-inflammatory mediators (Tsoulfas and Geller 2001). Inflammatory cytokines such as TNFα and IL-1α and β, bacterial products such as lipopolysaccharide (LPS), and products of cellular damage strongly activate inflammatory responses through the activation of NF-κB. NF-κB subsequently plays an essential positive-feedback role in the inflammatory response through regulation of genes encoding inflammatory cytokines IL-1β, TNFα, and IL-12/23, as well as chemokines IL-8, MIP-1α, and MCP-1(Xia, Pauza et al. 1997; Roebuck 1999; Roebuck, Carpenter et al. 1999). NF-κB also mediates nitric oxide production (iNOS), expression of NADPH oxidase subunits p47 and p67 (Gauss, Nelson-Overton et al. 2007; Lawrence 2009), and adhesion molecules ICAM-1, VCAM, and E-selectin (Chen and Manning 1995; Tak and Firestein 2001). Activation of NF-κB is a key event in many chronic inflammatory diseases such as cardiovascular disease (Van der Heiden, Cuhlmann et al.), tissue reperfusion injury (Latanich and Toledo-Pereyra 2009), experimental autoimmune encephalomyelitis (EAE) (Vandenbroeck, Alloza et al. 2004), rheumatoid arthritis (Criswell 2010), and inflammatory bowel disease (IBD) (Atreya, Atreya et al. 2008). A large number of the therapeutic agents for treating human inflammatory conditions, including sulfasalazine, 5-aminosalicylates, and corticosteroids, as well as some natural anti-inflammatory compounds such as IL-10, TGFβ1, β2AR agonists, glutamate, and curcumin, may owe their anti-inflammatory effects to inhibition of NF-κB (Lawrence and Fong ; Wang, Boddapati et al. ; Pereira and Oakley 2008; Lawrence 2009). These anti-inflammatory agents are potent inhibitors of microglial activation, and are neuroprotective to DA neurons *in vitro* and *in vivo*. Clearly, NF-κB activity presents a key target to ameliorate chronic inflammation in humans. Therapeutic strategies to inhibit NF-κB activity in microglial cells may lead to more effective treatments for PD (Zhang, Qian et al. 2010; Flood, Qian et al. 2011).

The NF-κB family consists of dimeric transcription factors which include five members: c-Rel, RelA (p65), RelB, NF-κB1 (p50/p105), and NF-κB2 (p52/p100) (Flood, Qian et al. 2011). There are two major activation pathways: (1) the classical or canonical pathway, and (2) the alternate or noncanonical pathway. While the non-canonical pathway does not appear to play a major role in the activation of inflammation, the classical pathway is thought to regulate the production of most pro-inflammatory mediators and is characterized by activation of a dimer of Rel proteins p50 and p65. In the inactive state this Rel dimer is complexed within the cytosol to the inhibitory protein IκBα complex (Lawrence 2009). The classical NF-κB pathway is initiated upon phosphorylation, ubiquitination, and subsequent proteasome-dependent degradation of IκBα. The phosphorylation of IκBα on serine residues is mediated by IκB kinase (IKK), which is a molecular complex of three proteins consisting of a heterodimer of the two catalytic subunits IKKα and IKKβ, along with IKKγ (the NF-κB essential modulator, NEMO) (May, Marienfeld et al. 2002; Huxford and Ghosh 2009; Oeckinghaus and Ghosh 2009). Embryonic cells derived from genetic knock-out mice lacking IKKβ, IKKγ, or p65 are unresponsive to classical NF-κB inducers such as TNFα and IL-1β (Reuther-Madrid, Kashatus et al. 2002; Sizemore, Lerner et al. 2002; Sizemore, Agarwal et al. 2004). Activation of IKK in response to inflammatory mediators such as TNFα, IL-1β, and LPS, depends critically on the presence of the IKKγ (NEMO) subunit of the IKK complex (Rudolph, Yeh et al. 2000; May, Marienfeld et al. 2002), which results in the phosphorylation of the IκB by the kinase activity of IKKβ (Huxford and Ghosh 2009; Oeckinghaus and Ghosh 2009). An N-terminal region of NEMO associates with a hexapeptide sequence within the C-terminus of both IKKα and IKKβ (NEMO binding domain or NBD), and disruption or mutation of this NEMO-NBD interaction site on either IKKβ or IKKγ results in a loss of responsiveness of cells to pro-inflammatory signaling (Flood, Qian et al. 2011). Agents that block the activation of NF-κB are capable of inhibiting the two major inflammatory pathways in microglia—activation of oxidative stress and production of inflammatory mediators, including cytokines TNFα, IL-1β, IL-6, as well as chemokines associated with inflammation (Qian, Flood et al. 2010).

Selective IKKβ and IKKγ inhibitors that do not target IKKα or the non-canonical P100/p52 pathway, should be promising therapeutic agents for treating chronic inflammatory disorders including PD. Such specific NF-κB inhibitors have recently been used in murine models of PD to halt the progression of neurodegeneration induced by the neurotoxin MPTP (Ghosh, Roy et al. 2007), or by activation of CNS inflammation by the intracranial injection of LPS (Zhang, Qian et al. 2010). Pretreatment of animals with a peptide against the NEMO-binding domain (NBD peptide) prior to injection of MPTP into mice, significantly inhibits the activation of NF-κB within the midbrain region. This inhibition of NF-κB activation is accompanied by a concomitant reduction in inflammatory mediator mRNA expression within the SN, as well as the expression of microglial cell activation marker CD11b. Mice receiving the NBD peptide prior to MPTP injection also showed highly significant protection of the nigrostriatum from MPTP-induced neurodegeneration of the TH+ neurons and the loss of dopamine production, as well as improvement in their locomotor function compared with MPTP-injected mice given mutant peptide. More importantly, administration of NBD peptide 2 days after injection of MPTP showed substantial protection of TH+ neurons, suggesting that NBD peptide can be used therapeutically to slow down or halt the progression of DA-neurodegeneration in MPTP-treated animals (Ghosh, Roy et al. 2007). In addition, infrared analysis of the brains of NBD-treated animals determined that significant levels of the NBD peptide localized within the brain tissue, suggesting that the NBD peptide could cross the BBB and reach sites of neuroinflammation. The nature of the mechanism of NF-κB inhibition within the SN remains to be determined, but these data suggest NF-κB is a viable target for therapy for PD patients (Ghosh, Roy et al. 2007).

A second approach to inhibit inflammation has been to use small molecule inhibitors that specifically block function of IKKβ. One such specific inhibitor, called Compound A, is a small molecule inhibitor of the kinase activity of IKKβ but not IKKα. Compound A, also known as BAY-65-1942 (7-[2-(cyclopropylmethoxy)-6-hydroxyphenyl]-5-[(3S)-3-piperidinyl]-1,4-dihydro-2Hpyrido [2,3- d] [1,3]-oxazin-2-one hydrochloride), has been shown to specifically and effectively block the catalytic activity of IKKβ, inhibiting its ability to phosphorylate IκB and activate the cytosolic p50/p65 NF-κB heterodimers (Moss, Stansfield et al. 2007; Zhang, Qian et al. 2010). In one recent study, Zhang and colleagues (2010) used Compound A in an LPS-induced neurodegeneration model to inhibit the canonical NF-κB pathway and halt inflammation-induced DA-neurodegeneration. In this model, LPS was injected directly into one side of the midbrain of rats, leading to inflammation-induced degeneration of DA-neurons (Zhang, Qian et al. 2010). It was found that Compound A strongly inhibited the activation of NF-κB *in vitro* and *in vivo*, as well as the mRNA expression and subsequent release of pro-inflammatory mediators. Compound A also significantly inhibited LPS- and MPTP-induced DA-neurotoxicity *in vitro*, and this neuroprotective activity required the presence of microglial cells. Most importantly, administration of Compound A to animals injected intranigrally with LPS, attenuated LPS-induced DA neuronal loss and microglia activation within the SN ((Zhang, Qian et al. ; Zhang, Qian et al. 2010). These data provide strong evidence that NF-κB offers a promising potential therapeutic target to halt DA-neurodegeneration, and that much additional work needs to be performed to determine the optimal approach and agent best suited for the treatment of PD.

5.2 β2-AR agonists as PD therapeutics

A family of compounds that have recently been shown to potentially reduce inflammation and DA-neurodegeneration in animal models are the β2 adrenergic receptor agonists. The β2 adrenergic receptor (β2AR) is a G-protein coupled receptor (GPCR) which is known to regulate of smooth muscle function in the airway and vasculature. Interestingly, β2AR expression has also been identified on immune cells such as macrophages, microglia, T cells, and B cells, and signaling through this receptor can inhibit the inflammatory response of these cells (Koff, Fann et al. 1986; Severn, Rapson et al. 1992; van der Poll, Jansen et al. 1994; Sekut, Champion et al. 1995; Panina-Bordignon, Mazzeo et al. 1997; Farmer and Pugin 2000; Kin and Sanders 2006). Both short-acting and long-acting β2AR agonists have been used for pharmacological studies and clinical therapy, and results have indicated that they possess the ability to inhibit the inflammatory responses by immune cells. Several of these long-acting agonists such as salmeterol (Advair®) and formoterol (Symbicort®) are currently being used as anti-inflammatory therapeutics to treat asthma and chronic obstructive pulmonary disease (COPD) (Koto, Mak et al. 1996; Tashkin and Cooper 2004; McKeage and Keam 2009). However, potential use of β2AR agonists in neurodegenerative diseases in the CNS has not been well studied. Since most long-acting β2AR agonists are highly lipophilic and should readily cross the BBB, it is likely that these compounds could have an immunomodulatory effect on the progression of inflammation in PD patients by inhibiting the activation of microglia that normally express high levels of β2AR (Tanaka, Kashima et al. 2002).

When long-acting β2AR agonists were tested for DA-neuroprotective properties, it was found that the compounds can inhibit DA-neurodegeneration *in vitro,* even if used at extremely low doses. Furthermore, administration of the long-acting β2AR agonist salmeterol significantly protects DA neurons against LPS- and MPTP-induced cytotoxicity *in vivo* (Qian, Wu et al. 2011). Mechanistic studies using primary midbrain neuron-glia cultures demonstrated that salmeterol, as well as several other long-acting β2AR agonists, have potent neuroprotective effects through their inhibition of microglial inflammatory mediator production. These anti-inflammatory effects of salmeterol require the presence of β2AR, are mediated through the inhibition of both MAPK and NF-κB signaling pathways in activated microglia, and function independently of the canonical GPCR/cAMP/PKA signaling pathway. It was further determined that this inhibition is dependent on the expression of β-arrestin 2, which suggests a novel mechanism for the long-acting β2AR agonists in regulating CNS inflammatory conditions (Qian, Wu et al. 2011). Therefore, the high specific activity and effectiveness of β2AR agonists such as salmeterol at inhibiting inflammation and DA-neurodegeneration within the CNS in these animal models suggests they have potential for the treatment of chronic inflammatory disorders and in particular, Parkinson's disease.

6. Proposed model of neuroinflammation in PD

Inflammation associated with PD can be initiated in the brain by internal factors such as a brain injury, a genetic mutation or some other brain insult or dysfunction (Nagatsu and Sawada 2006; Tansey, McCoy et al. 2007; Hirsch and Hunot 2009; Qian, Flood et al. 2010)(Figure 1). These sorts of intracerebral inflammatory stimuli activate the microglia which then up-regulate production of inflammatory factors including inflammatory cytokines such as TNFα, IL-1β or IL-6, as well as NO and ROS (Nagatsu, Mogi et al. 2000; Nagatsu and Sawada 2006; Tansey, McCoy et al. 2007). These in turn stimulate a further inflammatory response which results in a self-perpetuating chronic inflammatory condition (Qian and Flood 2008; Qian, Flood et al. 2010). Alternatively, inflammation in the periphery might induce the initial inflammatory response within the brain. Normally, the microvascular endothelial cells that line the blood vessels in the brain are tightly joined to each other through cell-cell tight junctions, and thus form the blood-brain-barrier which excludes most substances or cells from entry into the brain (Zlokovic 2008). A chronic peripheral inflammatory response can work to disrupt the cell-cell junctions and the blood-brain barrier, allowing access of inflammatory factors and cells into the brain (Stamatovic, Keep et al. 2008; Zlokovic 2008). These can then activate microglia and initiate the perpetual round of pro-inflammatory factor production leading to chronic neuroinflammation. Once microglia are activated, from whatever the source of initial inflammatory stimulus, the microglial response increases secretion of inflammatory cytokines and release of NO (Qian and Flood 2008). Microglial activation also precipitates an enhanced respiratory burst and release of ROS (Colton and Gilbert 1987). These various inflammatory mediators can trigger cell death in neurons (Chao, Hu et al. 1992; Colton and Gilbert 1993; Taylor, Jones et al. 2005), including DA neurons which seem to be especially vulnerable. Dying neurons then stimulate an intensified inflammatory response as the brain attempts to restore stasis (Qian, Flood et al. 2010). Therapies aimed at halting neurodegeneration are increasingly based on intervention to top the chronic inflammatory response, including introduction of anti-inflammatory drugs, compounds, cytokines and Treg cells, which inherently release anti-inflammatory cytokines such as TGFβ1 and IL-10.

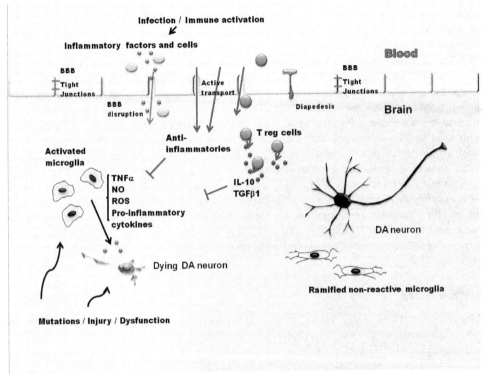

Fig. 1. Model relating chronic inflammation to dopaminergic (DA)-neuron death in Parkinson's Disease.

7. Future directions for PD therapy

Five relatively new approaches in anti-inflammatory therapy described above all show some promise for short-term or long-term therapeutics in PD. The use of exogenous anti-inflammatory cytokines such as IL10 or TGFβ1, has been shown to have potent effects in reducing neurotoxicity in both *in vitro* and in animal models of PD. However, although both cytokines are considered to be predominantly anti-inflammatory, they each can have pro-inflammatory effects in certain contexts. More thorough functional studies are needed for these anti-inflammatory cytokines, especially in the context of PD models before these might be readily used in human therapy. Particularly important factors include what form and what mode of delivery will optimize the anti-inflammatory effects of the cytokines as therapy and ameliorate any unintended negative effects. Cell-based therapies such as regulatory T cells (Tregs) offer great promise for long-term therapy in many degenerative disorders including PD. Both the use of T cells and stem cell transplantation focus on regeneration as well as intervening in neuronal death processes. However, some of the potential problems with these cell-transplant strategies are obvious since these are invasive therapies and as such carry the attendant problems associated with transplants in general as well as the specific consequences of introducing these cells into PD patients. Much remains to be determined before they become readily applicable for PD therapy. Anti-inflammatory therapies have already been developed in animal models of PD and are being used to a limited extent in human studies. The finding that the chronic use of certain NSAIDs seems to lower the risk of PD is promising for possibly reducing PD incidence. Additionally, NSAIDS (or SAIDS) might be used profitably in combinatorial therapy for PD, but the long-term use of these drugs already has well documented potential health problems. Careful determination of the potential risks to PD patients as compared to what benefits may be gained from long-term use of NSAIDS or SAIDS needs to be addressed. This is particularly important since these drugs might be well suited to combinatorial therapy in conjunction with existing PD treatments. Similarly, morphinan-based drugs, or other drugs already used for treatment of other diseases such as beta2-adrenergic receptor agonists, hold the most immediate potential for development as therapeutics to treat PD. The normal pharmacokinetics and safety profiles have already been established for some of these drugs such as salmeterol, and although preclinical studies indicate potential efficacy in PD, again the specific pharmacokinetics and safety for treating the neuroinflammation underlying PD must be determined. Orally available NF-kB inhibitors are equally attractive as PD therapies and are currently being studied in preclinical applications in a variety of diseases including PD.

8. References

Abou-Sleiman, P. M., D. G. Healy, et al. (2003). "The role of pathogenic DJ-1 mutations in Parkinson's disease." Ann Neurol 54(3): 283-6.

Akiyama, H. and P. L. McGeer (1989). "Microglial response to 6-hydroxydopamine-induced substantia nigra lesions." Brain Res 489(2): 247-53.

Albin, R. L., A. B. Young, et al. (1989). "The functional anatomy of basal ganglia disorders." Trends Neurosci 12(10): 366-75.

Angelov, D. N., S. Waibel, et al. (2003). "Therapeutic vaccine for acute and chronic motor neuron diseases: implications for amyotrophic lateral sclerosis." Proc Natl Acad Sci U S A 100(8): 4790-5.

Appel, S. H., D. R. Beers, et al. (2009). "T cell-microglial dialogue in Parkinson's disease and amyotrophic lateral sclerosis: are we listening?" Trends Immunol 31(1): 7-17.

Argaw, A. T., B. T. Gurfein, et al. (2009). "VEGF-mediated disruption of endothelial CLN-5 promotes blood-brain barrier breakdown." Proc Natl Acad Sci U S A 106(6): 1977-82.

Argaw, A. T., Y. Zhang, et al. (2006). "IL-1beta regulates blood-brain barrier permeability via reactivation of the hypoxia-angiogenesis program." J Immunol 177(8): 5574-84.

Atreya, I., R. Atreya, et al. (2008). "NF-kappaB in inflammatory bowel disease." J Intern Med 263(6): 591-6.

Barcia, C., V. Bautista, et al. (2005). "Changes in vascularization in substantia nigra pars compacta of monkeys rendered parkinsonian." J Neural Transm 112(9): 1237-48.

Barcia, C., V. de Pablos, et al. (2005). "Increased plasma levels of TNF-alpha but not of IL1-beta in MPTP-treated monkeys one year after the MPTP administration." Parkinsonism Relat Disord 11(7): 435-9.

Barcia, C., A. Sanchez Bahillo, et al. (2004). "Evidence of active microglia in substantia nigra pars compacta of parkinsonian monkeys 1 year after MPTP exposure." Glia 46(4): 402-9.

Bartels, A. L. and K. L. Leenders (2007). "Neuroinflammation in the pathophysiology of Parkinson's disease: evidence from animal models to human in vivo studies with [11C]-PK11195 PET." Mov Disord 22(13): 1852-6.

Bas, J., M. Calopa, et al. (2001). "Lymphocyte populations in Parkinson's disease and in rat models of parkinsonism." J Neuroimmunol 113(1): 146-52.

Benner, E. J., R. L. Mosley, et al. (2004). "Therapeutic immunization protects dopaminergic neurons in a mouse model of Parkinson's disease." Proc Natl Acad Sci U S A 101(25): 9435-40.

Bernardo, A., M. A. Ajmone-Cat, et al. (2005). "Nuclear receptor peroxisome proliferator-activated receptor-gamma is activated in rat microglial cells by the anti-inflammatory drug HCT1026, a derivative of flurbiprofen." J Neurochem 92(4): 895-903.

Block, M. L. and J. S. Hong (2007). "Chronic microglial activation and progressive dopaminergic neurotoxicity." Biochem Soc Trans 35(Pt 5): 1127-32.

Boka, G., P. Anglade, et al. (1994). "Immunocytochemical analysis of tumor necrosis factor and its receptors in Parkinson's disease." Neurosci Lett 172(1-2): 151-4.

Bonifati, V., Y. H. Wu-Chou, et al. (2008). "LRRK2 mutation analysis in Parkinson disease families with evidence of linkage to PARK8." Neurology 70(24): 2348; author reply 2348-9.

Bonuccelli, U., P. Del Dotto, et al. (1992). "Dextromethorphan and parkinsonism." Lancet 340(8810): 53.

Carrithers, M. D., I. Visintin, et al. (2000). "Differential adhesion molecule requirements for immune surveillance and inflammatory recruitment." Brain 123 (Pt 6): 1092-101.

Castano, A., A. J. Herrera, et al. (2002). "The degenerative effect of a single intranigral injection of LPS on the dopaminergic system is prevented by dexamethasone, and not mimicked by rh-TNF-alpha, IL-1beta and IFN-gamma." J Neurochem 81(1): 150-7.

Chao, C. C., S. Hu, et al. (1992). "Activated microglia mediate neuronal cell injury via a nitric oxide mechanism." J Immunol 149(8): 2736-41.

Chao, Y. X., B. P. He, et al. (2009). "Mesenchymal stem cell transplantation attenuates blood brain barrier damage and neuroinflammation and protects dopaminergic neurons against MPTP toxicity in the substantia nigra in a model of Parkinson's disease." J Neuroimmunol 216(1-2): 39-50.

Chen, C. C. and A. M. Manning (1995). "Transcriptional regulation of endothelial cell adhesion molecules: a dominant role for NF-kappa B." Agents Actions Suppl 47: 135-41.

Chen, H. Q., Z. Y. Jin, et al. (2008). "Luteolin protects dopaminergic neurons from inflammation-induced injury through inhibition of microglial activation." Neurosci Lett 448(2): 175-9.

Chen, W. and S. M. Wahl (2003). "TGF-beta: the missing link in CD4+CD25+ regulatory T cell-mediated immunosuppression." Cytokine Growth Factor Rev 14(2): 85-9.

Choi, D. W. (1987). "Dextrorphan and dextromethorphan attenuate glutamate neurotoxicity." Brain Res 403(2): 333-6.

Choi, D. W., M. Maulucci-Gedde, et al. (1987). "Glutamate neurotoxicity in cortical cell culture." J Neurosci 7(2): 357-68.

Choi, D. W., S. Peters, et al. (1987). "Dextrorphan and levorphanol selectively block N-methyl-D-aspartate receptor-mediated neurotoxicity on cortical neurons." J Pharmacol Exp Ther 242(2): 713-20.

Church, J., D. Lodge, et al. (1985). "Differential effects of dextrorphan and levorphanol on the excitation of rat spinal neurons by amino acids." Eur J Pharmacol 111(2): 185-90.

Cicchetti, F., J. Drouin-Ouellet, et al. (2009). "Environmental toxins and Parkinson's disease: what have we learned from pesticide-induced animal models?" Trends Pharmacol Sci 30(9): 475-83.

Cicchetti, F., N. Lapointe, et al. (2005). "Systemic exposure to paraquat and maneb models early Parkinson's disease in young adult rats." Neurobiol Dis 20(2): 360-71.

Colton, C. A. and D. L. Gilbert (1987). "Production of superoxide anions by a CNS macrophage, the microglia." FEBS Lett 223(2): 284-8.

Colton, C. A. and D. L. Gilbert (1993). "Microglia, an in vivo source of reactive oxygen species in the brain." Adv Neurol 59: 321-6.

Coxon, A., P. Rieu, et al. (1996). "A novel role for the beta 2 integrin CD11b/CD18 in neutrophil apoptosis: a homeostatic mechanism in inflammation." Immunity 5(6): 653-66.

Criswell, L. A. (2010). "Gene discovery in rheumatoid arthritis highlights the CD40/NF-kappaB signaling pathway in disease pathogenesis." Immunol Rev 233(1): 55-61.

Dauer, W. and S. Przedborski (2003). "Parkinson's disease: mechanisms and models." Neuron 39(6): 889-909.

Delgado, M., A. Chorny, et al. (2005). "Vasoactive intestinal peptide generates CD4+CD25+ regulatory T cells in vivo." J Leukoc Biol 78(6): 1327-38.

Dendorfer, U. (1996). "Molecular biology of cytokines." Artif Organs 20(5): 437-44.

Dickson, D. W. (2007). "Linking selective vulnerability to cell death mechanisms in Parkinson's disease." Am J Pathol 170(1): 16-9.

Dobbs, R. J., A. Charlett, et al. (1999). "Association of circulating TNF-alpha and IL-6 with ageing and parkinsonism." Acta Neurol Scand 100(1): 34-41.

Du, Y., Z. Ma, et al. (2001). "Minocycline prevents nigrostriatal dopaminergic neurodegeneration in the MPTP model of Parkinson's disease." Proc Natl Acad Sci U S A 98(25): 14669-74.

Engelhardt, B. and R. M. Ransohoff (2005). "The ins and outs of T-lymphocyte trafficking to the CNS: anatomical sites and molecular mechanisms." Trends Immunol 26(9): 485-95.

Fahn, S. (2003). "Description of Parkinson's disease as a clinical syndrome." Ann N Y Acad Sci 991: 1-14.

Farmer, P. and J. Pugin (2000). "beta-adrenergic agonists exert their "anti-inflammatory" effects in monocytic cells through the IkappaB/NF-kappaB pathway." Am J Physiol Lung Cell Mol Physiol 279(4): L675-82.

Farrer, M. J., K. Haugarvoll, et al. (2006). "Genomewide association, Parkinson disease, and PARK10." Am J Hum Genet 78(6): 1084-8; author reply 1092-4.

Faucheux, B. A., A. M. Bonnet, et al. (1999). "Blood vessels change in the mesencephalon of patients with Parkinson's disease." Lancet 353(9157): 981-2.

Fernandez-Checa, J. C., N. Kaplowitz, et al. (1997). "GSH transport in mitochondria: defense against TNF-induced oxidative stress and alcohol-induced defect." Am J Physiol 273(1 Pt 1): G7-17.

Fernandez-Martin, A., E. Gonzalez-Rey, et al. (2006). "Vasoactive intestinal peptide induces regulatory T cells during experimental autoimmune encephalomyelitis." Eur J Immunol 36(2): 318-26.

Flood, P. M., L. Qian, et al. (2011). "Transcriptional Factor NF-kB as a Target for Therapy in Parkinson's Disease." Inflammation and Parkinson's Disease, SAGE-Hindawi, pub. in press.

Floyd, R. A. (1999). "Antioxidants, oxidative stress, and degenerative neurological disorders." Proc Soc Exp Biol Med 222(3): 236-45.

Floyd, R. A. (1999). "Neuroinflammatory processes are important in neurodegenerative diseases: an hypothesis to explain the increased formation of reactive oxygen and nitrogen species as major factors involved in neurodegenerative disease development." Free Radic Biol Med 26(9-10): 1346-55.

Gao, H. M. and J. S. Hong (2008). "Why neurodegenerative diseases are progressive: uncontrolled inflammation drives disease progression." Trends Immunol 29(8): 357-65.

Gao, H. M., J. Jiang, et al. (2002). "Microglial activation-mediated delayed and progressive degeneration of rat nigral dopaminergic neurons: relevance to Parkinson's disease." J Neurochem 81(6): 1285-97.

Gao, H. M., B. Liu, et al. (2003). "Critical role for microglial NADPH oxidase in rotenone-induced degeneration of dopaminergic neurons." J Neurosci 23(15): 6181-7.

Gao, J., H. Miao, et al. (2011). "Influence of aging on the dopaminergic neurons in the substantia nigra pars compacta of rats." Curr Aging Sci 4(1): 19-24.

Gao, X., H. Chen, et al. (2011). "Use of ibuprofen and risk of Parkinson disease." Neurology 76(10): 863-9.

Gauss, K. A., L. K. Nelson-Overton, et al. (2007). "Role of NF-kappaB in transcriptional regulation of the phagocyte NADPH oxidase by tumor necrosis factor-alpha." J Leukoc Biol 82(3): 729-41.

Ghosh, A., A. Roy, et al. (2007). "Selective inhibition of NF-kappaB activation prevents dopaminergic neuronal loss in a mouse model of Parkinson's disease." Proc Natl Acad Sci U S A 104(47): 18754-9.

Godbout, J. P. and R. W. Johnson (2009). "Age and Neuroinflammation: A Lifetime of Psychoneuroimmune Consequences." Immunology and Allergy Clinics of North America 29(2): 321-337.

Goldberg, M. P., J. H. Weiss, et al. (1987). "N-methyl-D-aspartate receptors mediate hypoxic neuronal injury in cortical culture." J Pharmacol Exp Ther 243(2): 784-91.

Greenamyre, J. T. and C. F. O'Brien (1991). "N-methyl-D-aspartate antagonists in the treatment of Parkinson's disease." Arch Neurol 48(9): 977-81.

Groemping, Y. and K. Rittinger (2005). "Activation and assembly of the NADPH oxidase: a structural perspective." Biochem J 386(Pt 3): 401-16.

Gutierrez, E. G., W. A. Banks, et al. (1993). "Murine tumor necrosis factor alpha is transported from blood to brain in the mouse." J Neuroimmunol 47(2): 169-76.

Halliwell, B. (2006). "Oxidative stress and neurodegeneration: where are we now?" J Neurochem 97(6): 1634-58.

Henrich-Noack, P., J. H. Prehn, et al. (1996). "TGF-beta 1 protects hippocampal neurons against degeneration caused by transient global ischemia. Dose-response relationship and potential neuroprotective mechanisms." Stroke 27(9): 1609-14; discussion 1615.

Herrera, A. J., M. Tomas-Camardiel, et al. (2005). "Inflammatory process as a determinant factor for the degeneration of substantia nigra dopaminergic neurons." J Neural Transm 112(1): 111-9.

Hirsch, E. C. (2000). "Nigrostriatal system plasticity in Parkinson's disease: effect of dopaminergic denervation and treatment." Ann Neurol 47(4 Suppl 1): S115-20; discussion S120-1.

Hirsch, E. C. and S. Hunot (2009). "Neuroinflammation in Parkinson's disease: a target for neuroprotection?" Lancet Neurol 8(4): 382-97.

Hisanaga, K., M. Asagi, et al. (2001). "Increase in peripheral CD4 bright+ CD8 dull+ T cells in Parkinson disease." Arch Neurol 58(10): 1580-3.

Hu, X., D. Zhang, et al. (2008). "Macrophage antigen complex-1 mediates reactive microgliosis and progressive dopaminergic neurodegeneration in the MPTP model of Parkinson's disease." J Immunol 181(10): 7194-204.

Huusko, J., M. Merentie, et al. (2009). "The effects of VEGF-R1 and VEGF-R2 ligands on angiogenic responses and left ventricular function in mice." Cardiovasc Res.

Huxford, T. and G. Ghosh (2009). "A structural guide to proteins of the NF-kappaB signaling module." Cold Spring Harb Perspect Biol 1(3): a000075.

Imamura, K., N. Hishikawa, et al. (2003). "Distribution of major histocompatability complex 1-positive microglia and cytokine profile of Parkinson's disease brains." Acta Neuropathol 106: 518-526.

Jackson-Lewis, V. and S. Przedborski (2007). "Protocol for the MPTP mouse model of Parkinson's disease." Nat Protoc 2(1): 141-51.

Jackson-Lewis, V. and R. J. Smeyne (2005). "MPTP and SNpc DA neuronal vulnerability: role of dopamine, superoxide and nitric oxide in neurotoxicity. Minireview." Neurotox Res 7(3): 193-202.

Jellinger, K. A. (2001). "The pathology of Parkinson's disease." Adv Neurol 86: 55-72.

Jenner, P. and C. W. Olanow (1996). "Oxidative stress and the pathogenesis of Parkinson's disease." Neurology 47(6 Suppl 3): S161-70.

Jenner, P. and C. W. Olanow (1998). "Understanding cell death in Parkinson's disease." Ann Neurol 44(3 Suppl 1): S72-84.

Jenner, P. and C. W. Olanow (2006). "The pathogenesis of cell death in Parkinson's disease." Neurology 66(10 Suppl 4): S24-36.

Ji, S., G. Kronenberg, et al. (2009). "Acute neuroprotection by pioglitazone after mild brain ischemia without effect on long-term outcome." Exp Neurol 216(2): 321-8.

Jiang, H., Y. C. Wu, et al. (2007). "Parkinson's disease genetic mutations increase cell susceptibility to stress: mutant alpha-synuclein enhances H2O2- and Sin-1-induced cell death." Neurobiol Aging 28(11): 1709-17.

Johnston, L. C., X. Su, et al. (2008). "Human interleukin-10 gene transfer is protective in a rat model of Parkinson's disease." Mol Ther 16(8): 1392-9.

Kang, S. S., J. Y. Lee, et al. (2004). "Neuroprotective effects of flavones on hydrogen peroxide-induced apoptosis in SH-SY5Y neuroblostoma cells." Bioorg Med Chem Lett 14(9): 2261-4.

Keeney, P. M., J. Xie, et al. (2006). "Parkinson's disease brain mitochondrial complex I has oxidatively damaged subunits and is functionally impaired and misassembled." J Neurosci 26(19): 5256-64.

Kim, W. G., R. P. Mohney, et al. (2000). "Regional difference in susceptibility to lipopolysaccharide-induced neurotoxicity in the rat brain: role of microglia." J Neurosci 20(16): 6309-16.

Kin, N. W. and V. M. Sanders (2006). "It takes nerve to tell T and B cells what to do." J Leukoc Biol 79(6): 1093-104.

Kipnis, J. and M. Schwartz (2002). "Dual action of glatiramer acetate (Cop-1) in the treatment of CNS autoimmune and neurodegenerative disorders." Trends Mol Med 8(7): 319-23.

Kirk, S. L. and S. J. Karlik (2003). "VEGF and vascular changes in chronic neuroinflammation." Journal of Autoimmunity 21(4): 353-363.

Klockgether, T. (2004). "Parkinson's disease: clinical aspects." Cell Tissue Res 318(1): 115-20.

Knott, C., G. Stern, et al. (2000). "Inflammatory regulators in Parkinson's disease: iNOS, lipocortin-1, and cyclooxygenases-1 and -2." Mol Cell Neurosci 16(6): 724-39.

Koff, W. C., A. V. Fann, et al. (1986). "Catecholamine-induced suppression of interleukin-1 production." Lymphokine Res 5(4): 239-47.

Koh, J. Y. and D. W. Choi (1987). "Effect of anticonvulsant drugs on glutamate neurotoxicity in cortical cell culture." Neurology 37(2): 319-22.

Kohutnicka, M., E. Lewandowska, et al. (1998). "Microglial and astrocytic involvement in a murine model of Parkinson's disease induced by 1-methyl-4-phenyl-1,2,3,6-tetrahydropyridine (MPTP)." Immunopharmacology 39(3): 167-180.

Kortekaas, R., K. L. Leenders, et al. (2005). "Blood-brain barrier dysfunction in parkinsonian midbrain in vivo." Ann Neurol 57(2): 176-9.

Koto, H., J. C. Mak, et al. (1996). "Mechanisms of impaired beta-adrenoceptor-induced airway relaxation by interleukin-1beta in vivo in the rat." J Clin Invest 98(8): 1780-7.

Krige, D., M. T. Carroll, et al. (1992). "Platelet mitochondrial function in Parkinson's disease. The Royal Kings and Queens Parkinson Disease Research Group." Ann Neurol 32(6): 782-8.

Kurkowska-Jastrzebska, I., T. Litwin, et al. (2004). "Dexamethasone protects against dopaminergic neurons damage in a mouse model of Parkinson's disease." Int Immunopharmacol 4(10-11): 1307-18.

Kurkowska-Jastrzebska, I., A. Wronska, et al. (1999). "The inflammatory reaction following 1-methyl-4-phenyl-1,2,3, 6-tetrahydropyridine intoxication in mouse." Exp Neurol 156(1): 50-61.

Langston, J. W., L. S. Forno, et al. (1999). "Evidence of active nerve cell degeneration in the substantia nigra of humans years after 1-methyl-4-phenyl-1,2,3,6-tetrahydropyridine exposure." Ann Neurol 46(4): 598-605.

Lappas, M., M. Permezel, et al. (2002). "Nuclear factor kappa B regulation of proinflammatory cytokines in human gestational tissues in vitro." Biol Reprod 67(2): 668-73.

Latanich, C. A. and L. H. Toledo-Pereyra (2009). "Searching for NF-kappaB-based treatments of ischemia reperfusion injury." J Invest Surg 22(4): 301-15.

Lawrence, T. (2009). "The nuclear factor NF-kappaB pathway in inflammation." Cold Spring Harb Perspect Biol 1(6): a001651.

Lawrence, T. and C. Fong "The resolution of inflammation: anti-inflammatory roles for NF-kappaB." Int J Biochem Cell Biol 42(4): 519-23.

Lee, M., T. Cho, et al. (2010). "Depletion of GSH in glial cells induces neurotoxicity: relevance to aging and degenerative neurological diseases." The FASEB Journal 24(7): 2533-2545.

Lehnardt, S., L. Massillon, et al. (2003). "Activation of innate immunity in the CNS triggers neurodegeneration through a Toll-like receptor 4-dependent pathway." Proc Natl Acad Sci U S A 100(14): 8514-9.

Lin, M. T. and M. F. Beal (2006). "Mitochondrial dysfunction and oxidative stress in neurodegenerative diseases." Nature 443(7113): 787-95.

Litteljohn, D., E. Mangano, et al. (2011). "Inflammatory mechanisms of neurodegeneration in toxin-based models of Parkinson's disease." Parkinsons Dis 2011: 713517.

Liu, B. and J. S. Hong (2003). "Neuroprotective effect of naloxone in inflammation-mediated dopaminergic neurodegeneration. Dissociation from the involvement of opioid receptors." Methods Mol Med 79: 43-54.

Liu, J., N. Gong, et al. (2009). "Neuromodulatory activities of CD4+CD25+ regulatory T cells in a murine model of HIV-1-associated neurodegeneration." J Immunol 182(6): 3855-65.

Liu, L., E. Buchner, et al. (1996). "Amelioration of rat experimental arthritides by treatment with the alkaloid sinomenine." Int J Immunopharmacol 18(10): 529-43.

Liu, L., K. Resch, et al. (1994). "Inhibition of lymphocyte proliferation by the anti-arthritic drug sinomenine." Int J Immunopharmacol 16(8): 685-91.

Liu, Y., L. Qin, et al. (2003). "Dextromethorphan protects dopaminergic neurons against inflammation-mediated degeneration through inhibition of microglial activation." J Pharmacol Exp Ther 305(1): 212-8.

Loeffler, D. A., D. M. Camp, et al. (2006). "Complement activation in the Parkinson's disease substantia nigra: an immunocytochemical study." J Neuroinflammation 3: 29.

Lotan, M. and M. Schwartz (1994). "Cross-talk between the immune system and the nervous system in response to injury: immplications for regeneration." FASEB J 8(13): 1026-1033.

Lucking, C. B., A. Durr, et al. (2000). "Association between early-onset Parkinson's disease and mutations in the parkin gene." N Engl J Med 342(21): 1560-7.

Marshall, K. A., M. Reist, et al. (1999). "The neuronal toxicity of sulfite plus peroxynitrite is enhanced by glutathione depletion: implications for Parkinson's disease." Free Radic Biol Med 27(5-6): 515-20.

Matarese, G., V. De Rosa, et al. (2008). "Regulatory CD4 T cells: sensing the environment." Trends Immunol 29(1): 12-7.

May, M. J., R. B. Marienfeld, et al. (2002). "Characterization of the Ikappa B-kinase NEMO binding domain." J Biol Chem 277(48): 45992-6000.

McGeachy, M. J., K. S. Bak-Jensen, et al. (2007). "TGF-beta and IL-6 drive the production of IL-17 and IL-10 by T cells and restrain T(H)-17 cell-mediated pathology." Nat Immunol 8(12): 1390-7.

McGeer, P. L., S. Itagaki, et al. (1988). "Reactive microglia are positive for HLA-DR in the substantia nigra of Parkinson's and Alzheimer's disease brains." Neurology 38(8): 1285-91.

McGeer, P. L. and E. G. McGeer (2004). "Inflammation and the degenerative diseases of aging." Ann N Y Acad Sci 1035: 104-16.

McGeer, P. L., C. Schwab, et al. (2003). "Presence of reactive microglia in monkey substantia nigra years after 1-methyl-4-phenyl-1,2,3,6-tetrahydropyridine administration." Ann Neurol 54(5): 599-604.

McGeer, P. L., K. Yasojima, et al. (2001). "Inflammation in Parkinson's disease." Adv Neurol 86: 83-9.

McKeage, K. and S. J. Keam (2009). "Salmeterol/fluticasone propionate: a review of its use in asthma." Drugs 69(13): 1799-828.

Mizuno, Y., N. Hattori, et al. (2001). "Familial Parkinson's disease. Alpha-synuclein and parkin." Adv Neurol 86: 13-21.

Mogi, M., M. Harada, et al. (1994). "Interleukin-1 beta, interleukin-6, epidermal growth factor and transforming growth factor-alpha are elevated in the brain from parkinsonian patients." Neurosci Lett 180(2): 147-50.

Mogi, M., M. Harada, et al. (1996). "Interleukin (IL)-1 beta, IL-2, IL-4, IL-6 and transforming growth factor-alpha levels are elevated in ventricular cerebrospinal fluid in juvenile parkinsonism and Parkinson's disease." Neurosci Lett 211(1): 13-6.

Mogi, M., M. Harada, et al. (1994). "Tumor necrosis factor-alpha (TNF-alpha) increases both in the brain and in the cerebrospinal fluid from parkinsonian patients." Neurosci Lett 165(1-2): 208-10.

Monahan, A. J., M. Warren, et al. (2008). "Neuroinflammation and peripheral immune infiltration in Parkinson's disease: an autoimmune hypothesis." Cell Transplant 17(4): 363-72.

Montastruc, J. L., N. Fabre, et al. (1994). "N-methyl-D-aspartate (NMDA) antagonist and Parkinson's disease: a pilot study with dextromethorphan." Mov Disord 9(2): 242-3.

Moore, P. E., T. Lahiri, et al. (2001). "Selected contribution: synergism between TNF-alpha and IL-1 beta in airway smooth muscle cells: implications for beta-adrenergic responsiveness." J Appl Physiol 91(3): 1467-74.

Mosley, R. L., E. J. Benner, et al. (2006). "Neuroinflammation, Oxidative Stress and the Pathogenesis of Parkinson's Disease." Clin Neurosci Res 6(5): 261-281.

Moss, N. C., W. E. Stansfield, et al. (2007). "IKKbeta inhibition attenuates myocardial injury and dysfunction following acute ischemia-reperfusion injury." Am J Physiol Heart Circ Physiol 293(4): H2248-2253.

Nagatsu, T., M. Mogi, et al. (2000). "Changes in cytokines and neurotrophins in Parkinson's disease." J Neural Transm Suppl(60): 277-90.

Nagatsu, T., M. Mogi, et al. (2000). "Cytokines in Parkinson's disease." J Neural Transm Suppl(58): 143-51.

Nagatsu, T. and M. Sawada (2006). "Cellular and molecular mechanisms of Parkinson's disease: neurotoxins, causative genes, and inflammatory cytokines." Cell Mol Neurobiol 26(4-6): 781-802.

Naik, E. and V. M. Dixit (2011). "Mitochondrial reactive oxygen species drive proinflammatory cytokine production." The Journal of Experimental Medicine 208(3): 417-420.

Natarajan, C. and J. J. Bright (2002). "Curcumin inhibits experimental allergic encephalomyelitis by blocking IL-12 signaling through Janus kinase-STAT pathway in T lymphocytes." J Immunol 168(12): 6506-13.

Negi, G., A. Kumar, et al. (2011). "Melatonin modulates neuroinflammation and oxidative stress in experimental diabetic neuropathy: effects on NF-κB and Nrf2 cascades." Journal of Pineal Research 50(2): 124-131.

Neuwelt, E. A. and W. K. Clark (1978). "The immune system and the nervous system." Neurosurgery 3(3): 419-430.

Nguyen, M. D., T. D'Aigle, et al. (2004). "Exacerbation of motor neuron disease by chronic stimulation of innate immunity in a mouse model of amyotrophic lateral sclerosis." J Neurosci 24(6): 1340-9.

Nguyen, M. D., J. P. Julien, et al. (2002). "Innate immunity: the missing link in neuroprotection and neurodegeneration?" Nat Rev Neurosci 3(3): 216-27.

Nguyen, Q. D., S. Tatlipinar, et al. (2006). "Vascular endothelial growth factor is a critical stimulus for diabetic macular edema." Am J Ophthalmol 142(6): 961-9.

Niehaus, I. and J. H. Lange (2003). "Endotoxin: is it an environmental factor in the cause of Parkinson's disease?" Occup Environ Med 60(5): 378.

Oeckinghaus, A. and S. Ghosh (2009). "The NF-kappaB family of transcription factors and its regulation." Cold Spring Harb Perspect Biol 1(4): a000034.

Orr, C. F., D. B. Rowe, et al. (2002). "An inflammatory review of Parkinson's disease." Prog Neurobiol 68(5): 325-40.

Orr, C. F., D. B. Rowe, et al. (2005). "A possible role for humoral immunity in the pathogenesis of Parkinson's disease." Brain 128(Pt 11): 2665-74.

Owen, A. D., A. H. Schapira, et al. (1996). "Oxidative stress and Parkinson's disease." Ann N Y Acad Sci 786: 217-23.

Pachter, J. S., H. E. de Vries, et al. (2003). "The blood-brain barrier and its role in immune privilege in the central nervous system." J Neuropathol Exp Neurol 62(6): 593-604.

Pan, W. and A. J. Kastin (2002). "TNF[alpha] Transport across the Blood-Brain Barrier Is Abolished in Receptor Knockout Mice." Experimental Neurology 174(2): 193-200.

Panina-Bordignon, P., D. Mazzeo, et al. (1997). "Beta2-agonists prevent Th1 development by selective inhibition of interleukin 12." J Clin Invest 100(6): 1513-9.

Park, K. M. and W. J. Bowers (2010). "Tumor necrosis factor-alpha mediated signaling in neuronal homeostasis and dysfunction." Cell Signal 22(7): 977-83.

Pearce, R. K., A. Owen, et al. (1997). "Alterations in the distribution of glutathione in the substantia nigra in Parkinson's disease." J Neural Transm 104(6-7): 661-77.

Pei, Z., H. Pang, et al. (2007). "MAC1 mediates LPS-induced production of superoxide by microglia: the role of pattern recognition receptors in dopaminergic neurotoxicity." Glia 55(13): 1362-73.

Pereira, S. G. and F. Oakley (2008). "Nuclear factor-kappaB1: regulation and function." Int J Biochem Cell Biol 40(8): 1425-30.

Pisani, V., V. Moschella, et al. (2010). "Dynamic changes of anandamide in the cerebrospinal fluid of Parkinson's disease patients." Movement Disorders 25(7): 920-924.

Polymeropoulos, M. H., C. Lavedan, et al. (1997). "Mutation in the alpha-synuclein gene identified in families with Parkinson's disease." Science 276(5321): 2045-7.

Pope, L. E., M. H. Khalil, et al. (2004). "Pharmacokinetics of dextromethorphan after single or multiple dosing in combination with quinidine in extensive and poor metabolizers." J Clin Pharmacol 44(10): 1132-42.

Prehn, J. H. and J. Krieglstein (1994). "Opposing effects of transforming growth factor-beta 1 on glutamate neurotoxicity." Neuroscience 60(1): 7-10.

Qian, L., M. L. Block, et al. (2006). "Interleukin-10 protects lipopolysaccharide-induced neurotoxicity in primary midbrain cultures by inhibiting the function of NADPH oxidase." J Pharmacol Exp Ther 319(1): 44-52.

Qian, L. and P. M. Flood (2008). "Microglial cells and Parkinson's disease." Immunol Res 41(3): 155-64.

Qian, L., P. M. Flood, et al. (2010). "Neuroinflammation is a key player in Parkinson's disease and a prime target for therapy." J Neural Transm 117(8): 971-9.

Qian, L., X. Gao, et al. (2007). "NADPH oxidase inhibitor DPI is neuroprotective at femtomolar concentrations through inhibition of microglia over-activation." Parkinsonism Relat Disord 13 Suppl 3: S316-20.

Qian, L., K. S. Tan, et al. (2007). "Microglia-mediated neurotoxicity is inhibited by morphine through an opioid receptor-independent reduction of NADPH oxidase activity." J Immunol 179(2): 1198-209.

Qian, L., S. J. Wei, et al. (2008). "Potent anti-inflammatory and neuroprotective effects of TGF-beta1 are mediated through the inhibition of ERK and p47phox-Ser345 phosphorylation and translocation in microglia." J Immunol 181(1): 660-8.

Qian, L., H. M. Wu, et al. (2011). "{beta}2-Adrenergic Receptor Activation Prevents Rodent Dopaminergic Neurotoxicity by Inhibiting Microglia via a Novel Signaling Pathway." J Immunol. 186: 4443-4454.

Qian, L., Z. Xu, et al. (2007). "Sinomenine, a natural dextrorotatory morphinan analog, is anti-inflammatory and neuroprotective through inhibition of microglial NADPH oxidase." J Neuroinflammation 4: 23.

Qin, L., Y. Liu, et al. (2004). "NADPH oxidase mediates lipopolysaccharide-induced neurotoxicity and proinflammatory gene expression in activated microglia." J Biol Chem 279(2): 1415-21.

Qin, L., X. Wu, et al. (2007). "Systemic LPS causes chronic neuroinflammation and progressive neurodegeneration." Glia 55(5): 453-62.

Qureshi, G. A., S. Baig, et al. (1995). "Increased cerebrospinal fluid concentration of nitrite in Parkinson's disease." Neuroreport 6(12): 1642-4.

Ransohoff, R. M. and V. H. Perry (2009). "Microglial physiology: unique stimuli, specialized responses." Annu Rev Immunol 27: 119-45.

Reale, M., N. H. Greig, et al. (2009). "Peripheral chemo-cytokine profiles in Alzheimer's and Parkinson's diseases." Mini Rev Med Chem 9(10): 1229-41.

Reuther-Madrid, J. Y., D. Kashatus, et al. (2002). "The p65/RelA subunit of NF-kappaB suppresses the sustained, antiapoptotic activity of Jun kinase induced by tumor necrosis factor." Mol Cell Biol 22(23): 8175-83.

Reynolds, A. D., R. Banerjee, et al. (2007). "Neuroprotective activities of CD4+CD25+ regulatory T cells in an animal model of Parkinson's disease." J Leukoc Biol 82(5): 1083-94.

Reynolds, A. D., D. K. Stone, et al. (2010). "Regulatory T cells attenuate Th17 cell-mediated nigrostriatal dopaminergic neurodegeneration in a model of Parkinson's disease." J Immunol 184(5): 2261-71.

Reynolds, A. D., D. K. Stone, et al. (2009). "Nitrated {alpha}-synuclein-induced alterations in microglial immunity are regulated by CD4+ T cell subsets." J Immunol 182(7): 4137-49.

Rite, I., A. Machado, et al. (2007). "Blood-brain barrier disruption induces in vivo degeneration of nigral dopaminergic neurons." J Neurochem 101(6): 1567-82.

Roebuck, K. A. (1999). "Regulation of interleukin-8 gene expression." J Interferon Cytokine Res 19(5): 429-38.

Roebuck, K. A., L. R. Carpenter, et al. (1999). "Stimulus-specific regulation of chemokine expression involves differential activation of the redox-responsive transcription factors AP-1 and NF-kappaB." J Leukoc Biol 65(3): 291-8.

Rudolph, D., W. C. Yeh, et al. (2000). "Severe liver degeneration and lack of NF-kappaB activation in NEMO/IKKgamma-deficient mice." Genes Dev 14(7): 854-62.

Ruocco, A., O. Nicole, et al. (1999). "A transforming growth factor-beta antagonist unmasks the neuroprotective role of this endogenous cytokine in excitotoxic and ischemic brain injury." J Cereb Blood Flow Metab 19(12): 1345-53.

Ryu, J. K. and J. G. McLarnon (2008). "VEGF receptor antagonist Cyclo-VEGI reduces inflammatory reactivity and vascular leakiness and is neuroprotective against acute excitotoxic striatal insult." J Neuroinflammation 5: 18.

Sairam, K., K. S. Saravanan, et al. (2003). "Non-steroidal anti-inflammatory drug sodium salicylate, but not diclofenac or celecoxib, protects against 1-methyl-4-phenyl pyridinium-induced dopaminergic neurotoxicity in rats." Brain Res 966(2): 245-52.

Sawada, M., K. Imamura, et al. (2006). "Role of cytokines in inflammatory process in Parkinson's disease." J Neural Transm Suppl(70): 373-81.

Schapira, A. H. (1994). "Mitochondrial function and neurotoxicity." Curr Opin Neurol 7(6): 531-4.

Schapira, A. H. (2006). "Etiology of Parkinson's disease." Neurology 66(10 Suppl 4): S10-23.

Schapira, A. H., J. M. Cooper, et al. (1989). "Mitochondrial complex I deficiency in Parkinson's disease." Lancet 1(8649): 1269.

Schwartz, M. (2004). "Protective autoimmunity and prospects for therapeutic vaccination against self-perpetuating neurodegeneration." Ernst Schering Res Found Workshop(47): 133-54.

Sekut, L., B. R. Champion, et al. (1995). "Anti-inflammatory activity of salmeterol: down-regulation of cytokine production." Clin Exp Immunol 99(3): 461-6.

Sen, R. and D. Baltimore (1986). "Inducibility of kappa immunoglobulin enhancer-binding protein Nf-kappa B by a posttranslational mechanism." Cell 47(6): 921-8.

Sen, R. and D. Baltimore (1986). "Multiple nuclear factors interact with the immunoglobulin enhancer sequences." Cell 46(5): 705-16.

Severn, A., N. T. Rapson, et al. (1992). "Regulation of tumor necrosis factor production by adrenaline and beta-adrenergic agonists." J Immunol 148(11): 3441-5.

Sherer, T. B., R. Betarbet, et al. (2002). "Environment, mitochondria, and Parkinson's disease." Neuroscientist 8(3): 192-7.

Singh, S., K. Singh, et al. (2008). "Nicotine and caffeine-mediated modulation in the expression of toxicant responsive genes and vesicular monoamine transporter-2 in 1-methyl 4-phenyl-1,2,3,6-tetrahydropyridine-induced Parkinson's disease phenotype in mouse." Brain Res 1207: 193-206.

Sizemore, N., A. Agarwal, et al. (2004). "Inhibitor of kappaB kinase is required to activate a subset of interferon gamma-stimulated genes." Proc Natl Acad Sci U S A 101(21): 7994-8.

Sizemore, N., N. Lerner, et al. (2002). "Distinct roles of the Ikappa B kinase alpha and beta subunits in liberating nuclear factor kappa B (NF-kappa B) from Ikappa B and in phosphorylating the p65 subunit of NF-kappa B." J Biol Chem 277(6): 3863-9.

Smeyne, M., Y. Jiao, et al. (2005). "Glia cell number modulates sensitivity to MPTP in mice." Glia 52(2): 144-52.

Smith, A. D. and M. J. Zigmond (2003). "Can the brain be protected through exercise? Lessons from an animal model of parkinsonism." Exp Neurol 184(1): 31-9.

Smith, T. W., U. DeGirolami, et al. (1992). "Neuropathology of immunosuppression." Brain Pathol 2(3): 183-194.

Sofic, E., K. W. Lange, et al. (1992). "Reduced and oxidized glutathione in the substantia nigra of patients with Parkinson's disease." Neurosci Lett 142(2): 128-30.

Spencer, J. P., P. Jenner, et al. (1998). "Conjugates of catecholamines with cysteine and GSH in Parkinson's disease: possible mechanisms of formation involving reactive oxygen species." J Neurochem 71(5): 2112-22.

Stamatovic, S. M., R. F. Keep, et al. (2008). "Brain endothelial cell-cell junctions: how to "open" the blood brain barrier." Curr Neuropharmacol 6(3): 179-92.

Strle, K., J. H. Zhou, et al. (2001). "Interleukin-10 in the brain." Crit Rev Immunol 21(5): 427-49.

Suidan, G. L., J. W. Dickerson, et al. (2010). "CD8 T cell-initiated vascular endothelial growth factor expression promotes central nervous system vascular permeability under neuroinflammatory conditions." J Immunol 184(2): 1031-40.

Sun, M., J. C. Latourelle, et al. (2006). "Influence of heterozygosity for parkin mutation on onset age in familial Parkinson disease: the GenePD study." Arch Neurol 63(6): 826-32.

Szczepanik, M., M. Tutaj, et al. (2005). "Epicutaneously induced TGF-beta-dependent tolerance inhibits experimental autoimmune encephalomyelitis." J Neuroimmunol 164(1-2): 105-14.

Tak, P. P. and G. S. Firestein (2001). "NF-kappaB: a key role in inflammatory diseases." J Clin Invest 107(1): 7-11.

Tanaka, K. F., H. Kashima, et al. (2002). "Existence of functional beta1- and beta2-adrenergic receptors on microglia." J Neurosci Res 70(2): 232-7.

Tanner, C. M. (2003). "Is the cause of Parkinson's disease environmental or hereditary? Evidence from twin studies." Adv Neurol 91: 133-42.

Tansey, M. G., M. K. McCoy, et al. (2007). "Neuroinflammatory mechanisms in Parkinson's disease: potential environmental triggers, pathways, and targets for early therapeutic intervention." Exp Neurol 208(1): 1-25.

Tashkin, D. P. and C. B. Cooper (2004). "The role of long-acting bronchodilators in the management of stable COPD." Chest 125(1): 249-59.

Taylor, D. L., F. Jones, et al. (2005). "Stimulation of microglial metabotropic glutamate receptor mGlu2 triggers tumor necrosis factor alpha-induced neurotoxicity in concert with microglial-derived Fas ligand." J Neurosci 25(11): 2952-64.

Teismann, P. and J. B. Schulz (2004). "Cellular pathology of Parkinson's disease: astrocytes, microglia and inflammation." Cell Tissue Res 318(1): 149-61.

Tetrud, J. W., J. W. Langston, et al. (1989). "Mild parkinsonism in persons exposed to 1-methyl-4-phenyl-1,2,3,6-tetrahydropyridine (MPTP)." Neurology 39(11): 1483-7.

Thomas, M. P., K. Chartrand, et al. (2007). "Ion channel blockade attenuates aggregated alpha synuclein induction of microglial reactive oxygen species: relevance for the pathogenesis of Parkinson's disease." J Neurochem 100(2): 503-19.

Tortella, F. C., J. W. Ferkany, et al. (1988). "Anticonvulsant effects of dextrorphan in rats: possible involvement in dextromethorphan-induced seizure protection." Life Sci 42(24): 2509-14.

Tsoulfas, G. and D. A. Geller (2001). "NF-kappaB in transplantation: friend or foe?" Transpl Infect Dis 3(4): 212-9.

Unsicker, K. and K. Krieglstein (2002). "TGF-betas and their roles in the regulation of neuron survival." Adv Exp Med Biol 513: 353-74.

Van der Heiden, K., S. Cuhlmann, et al. "Role of nuclear factor kappaB in cardiovascular health and disease." Clin Sci (Lond) 118(10): 593-605.

van der Poll, T., J. Jansen, et al. (1994). "Noradrenaline inhibits lipopolysaccharide-induced tumor necrosis factor and interleukin 6 production in human whole blood." Infect Immun 62(5): 2046-50.

Van Snick, J. (1990). "Interleukin-6: an overview." Annu Rev Immunol 8: 253-78.

Vandenbroeck, K., I. Alloza, et al. (2004). "Inhibiting cytokines of the interleukin-12 family: recent advances and novel challenges." J Pharm Pharmacol 56(2): 145-60.

Verhagen Metman, L., P. J. Blanchet, et al. (1998). "A trial of dextromethorphan in parkinsonian patients with motor response complications." Mov Disord 13(3): 414-7.

Verhagen Metman, L., P. Del Dotto, et al. (1998). "Dextromethorphan improves levodopa-induced dyskinesias in Parkinson's disease." Neurology 51(1): 203-6.

Vilar, R., H. Coelho, et al. (2007). "Association of A313 G polymorphism (GSTP1*B) in the glutathione-S-transferase P1 gene with sporadic Parkinson's disease." Eur J Neurol 14(2): 156-61.

Wada, K., H. Arai, et al. (2006). "Expression levels of vascular endothelial growth factor and its receptors in Parkinson's disease." Neuroreport 17(7): 705-9.

Wang, M. S., S. Boddapati, et al. "Curcumin reduces alpha-synuclein induced cytotoxicity in Parkinson's disease cell model." BMC Neurosci 11: 57.

Webster, S. D., M. D. Galvan, et al. (2001). "Antibody-mediated phagocytosis of the amyloid beta-peptide in microglia is differentially modulated by C1q." J Immunol 166(12): 7496-503.

Weng, Y. H., Y. H. Chou, et al. (2007). "PINK1 mutation in Taiwanese early-onset parkinsonism : clinical, genetic, and dopamine transporter studies." J Neurol 254(10): 1347-55.

Werling, L. L., E. C. Lauterbach, et al. (2007). "Dextromethorphan as a potential neuroprotective agent with unique mechanisms of action." Neurologist 13(5): 272-93.

Whitton, P. S. (2007). "Inflammation as a causative factor in the aetiology of Parkinson's disease." Br J Pharmacol 150(8): 963-76.

Wu, D. C., V. Jackson-Lewis, et al. (2002). "Blockade of microglial activation is neuroprotective in the 1-methyl-4-phenyl-1,2,3,6-tetrahydropyridine mouse model of Parkinson disease." J Neurosci 22(5): 1763-71.

Wyss-Coray, T. and L. Mucke (2002). "Inflammation in neurodegenerative disease--a double-edged sword." Neuron 35(3): 419-32.

Xia, Y., M. E. Pauza, et al. (1997). "RelB regulation of chemokine expression modulates local inflammation." Am J Pathol 151(2): 375-87.

Yamada, T., J. K. Chong, et al. (1993). "Concentration of neural thread protein in cerebrospinal fluid from progressive supranuclear palsy and Parkinson's disease." Jpn J Psychiatry Neurol 47(3): 631-5.

Yamada, T., P. L. McGeer, et al. (1992). "Lewy bodies in Parkinson's disease are recognized by antibodies to complement proteins." Acta Neuropathol 84(1): 100-4.

Yang, S., D. Zhang, et al. (2008). "Curcumin protects dopaminergic neuron against LPS induced neurotoxicity in primary rat neuron/glia culture." Neurochem Res 33(10): 2044-53.

Yazdani, U., D. C. German, et al. (2006). "Rat model of Parkinson's disease: chronic central delivery of 1-methyl-4-phenylpyridinium (MPP+)." Exp Neurol 200(1): 172-83.

Zhang, F., L. Qian, et al. (2010). "Inhibition of IkappaB kinase-beta protects dopamine neurons against lipopolysaccharide-induced neurotoxicity." J Pharmacol Exp Ther 333(3): 822-33.

Zhang, S. X., J. J. Wang, et al. (2006). "Pigment epithelium-derived factor (PEDF) is an endogenous antiinflammatory factor." FASEB J 20(2): 323-5.

Zhang, W., S. Dallas, et al. (2007). "Microglial PHOX and Mac-1 are essential to the enhanced dopaminergic neurodegeneration elicited by A30P and A53T mutant alpha-synuclein." Glia 55(11): 1178-88.

Zhang, W., L. Qin, et al. (2005). "3-hydroxymorphinan is neurotrophic to dopaminergic neurons and is also neuroprotective against LPS-induced neurotoxicity." FASEB J 19(3): 395-7.

Zhang, W., E. J. Shin, et al. (2006). "3-Hydroxymorphinan, a metabolite of dextromethorphan, protects nigrostriatal pathway against MPTP-elicited damage both in vivo and in vitro." FASEB J 20(14): 2496-511.

Zhang, W., T. Wang, et al. (2004). "Neuroprotective effect of dextromethorphan in the MPTP Parkinson's disease model: role of NADPH oxidase." FASEB J 18(3): 589-91.

Zhang, Z. G., L. Zhang, et al. (2000). "VEGF enhances angiogenesis and promotes blood-brain barrier leakage in the ischemic brain." J Clin Invest 106(7): 829-38.

Zhou, Y., Y. Wang, et al. (2005). "Microglial activation induced by neurodegeneration: a proteomic analysis." Mol Cell Proteomics 4(10): 1471-9.

Zhu, Y., G. Y. Yang, et al. (2002). "Transforming growth factor-beta 1 increases bad phosphorylation and protects neurons against damage." J Neurosci 22(10): 3898-909.

Zlokovic, B. V. (2008). "The blood-brain barrier in health and chronic neurodegenerative disorders." Neuron 57(2): 178-201.

4

Mathematical Models: Interactions Between Serotonin and Dopamine in Parkinson's Disease

Janet Best[1], Grant Oakley[1], Michael Reed[2] and H. Frederik Nijhout[2]
[1]*Ohio State University*
[2]*Duke University*
USA

1. Introduction

Parkinson's disease (PD) has traditionally been thought of as a dysfunction in the dopamine (DA) signaling system caused primarily by cell death in the substantia nigra pars compacta (SNc). However, strong evidence has been accumulating that the serotonin (5-HT) signaling system is also involved. First, 5-HT influences normal motor function through a dense innervation of the striatum. Second, substantial cell death of serotonergic neurons occurs in PD and in some cases may occur earlier than DA cell death. And, finally, there are indications that interactions between the 5-HT system and the DA system may be responsible for some of the symptoms of PD and some of the side effects of treatment by levodopa. Some of the evidence for these assertions is reviewed below.

The 5-HT system is itself very complex. The serotonergic neurons in the raphe nuclei (RN) send ascending projections to a large number of different brain regions including medial prefrontal cortex (mPFC), motor cortex, hypothalamus, hippocampus, amygdala, and the basal ganglia. And, some of these brain regions, substantia nigra, amygdala, mPFC, and hypothalamus send projections back to the RN (Monti, 2010). Thus it is not surprising that 5-HT is linked to so many behaviors including feeding and body-weight regulation, social hierarchies, aggression and suicidality, obsessive compulsive disorder, alcoholism, anxiety, and affective disorders (Feldman et al., 1997). Since the pharmacology and the electrophysiology of both the serotonergic and the dopaminergic systems are only partially understood, it is a daunting task to understand how these two systems affect one another. This is particularly true in the presence of a degenerative disease that involves massive cell death in both systems.

In this complicated situation, mathematical models can potentially provide insight into mechanisms and interactions. The purpose of the models is not to summarize what is already known. The purpose is to provide a platform for *in silico* biological experimentation. Using models one can try out ideas, validate or refute hypotheses, settle disputes in the literature, and sometimes discover new phenomena. Of course, to be useful the models have to be well-grounded in real physiology and the creation of such models is not easy. However, if one has a model that represents (part of) the underlying physiology well, then *in silico* experiments are quick and inexpensive. The model provides a quantitative way of thinking about the phenomena being investigated and may suggest new hypotheses that can be checked by animal experiments. Thus, modeling, when combined with animal experiments and clinical trials, can shed some light on the complicated pharmacological, electrophysiological, and behavioral issues in PD.

In Section 2, we discuss the evidence for the role of 5-HT in PD and the side effects of levodopa therapy and in Section 3 we discuss possible mechanisms. In Section 4, we describe a mathematical model that we recently created to study homeostatic mechanisms in serotonergic signaling. In Section 5 we use the model, and a previous model of a DA terminal, to discuss the effects of gene polymorphisms, the stability of extracellular DA in the striatum in the face of cell death in the substantia nigra, and the mechanism of action of selective serotonin reuptake inhibitors. Finally, in Section 6 we outline how we plan to use existing models and new models to investigate the interactions between the 5-HT system and the DA system in PD.

2. PD and the serotonergic system

Tremor, rigidity, and bradykinesia, the classical motor symptoms of ideopathic PD, primarily result from loss of dopaminergic neurons in the SNc. However, neural degeneration also occurs in other sites of the brain, ranging from the brain stem to cortex, as the synaptic protein α-synuclein accumulates pathologically to form Lewy bodies (LB) or Lewy neurites. The clinical diagnosis of PD is based upon presence of the motor symptoms indicating dopamine deficiency (Chaudhuri et al., 2006; Jankovic, 2008). Postmortem analysis finds LB not only in remaining substantia nigra cells but in other specific brain regions where cells are lost (Gibb & Lees, 1988). Braak and colleagues (Braak et al., 2003) have proposed a scheme of six stages describing the development of ideopathic PD, characterized by the spatial extent of LB inclusions. Braak stage 1 involves LB inclusions in the region of the brain stem; neurodegeneration of the substantia nigra does not begin until stage 3. Braak's hypothesis concerning the progression of PD predicts that symptoms such as diminished olfactory sensitivity (Lim et al., 2009) or REM behavior disorder (Ahlskog, 2004) should precede the cardinal motor symptoms of the disease, a pattern observed in some but not all cases of PD (Linazasoro, 2007). Indeed, the retrospective nature of Braak's study obscures the actual course of progression (Halliday & McCann, 2010). In a longitudinal study, Halliday & McCann (2010) found that approximately half of ideopathic PD cases follow Braak's scheme. In all cases studied by Halliday and McCann, LB occurred not only in the substantia nigra but also in other brain areas including brain stem. Thus, extra-nigral aspects are always present in PD, and their significance can rival that of the cardinal motor symptoms (Chaudhuri et al., 2006).

Ahlskog (2004) reports that LB have been found in pontomedullary neurons of brains without substantia nigra pathology but that the reverse has not been observed. Among the nondopaminergic systems profoundly affected in PD is the serotonergic system. The extent of damage to the serotonergic system in PD is variable and is less severe than the loss of dopamine: Kish found that, while striatal dopamine concentrations decreased by more than 80%, serotonin markers decreased by less than 70% (Kish et al., 2008). It has not been clearly established to what extent this reduction in serotonin markers is due to raphe cell loss

(Jellinger, 1991), serotonergic terminal loss in the striatum, or molecular regulatory changes (Kish et al., 2008).

In post-mortem analyses of brains from PD patients, Kish et al. (2008) found that serotonin and dopamine have substantially different patterns of loss within the striatum. Serotonin markers show greater loss in the caudate than in putamen, while the dopamine loss is greater in the putamen. Thus the striatal subdivision with the more severe dopamine loss (putamen) was less affected by loss of serotonin markers, possibly reflecting compensatory sprouting of 5-HT terminals (Maeda et al., 2003). Serotonergic responses to dopamine depletion may also be evident in changes in the electrical activity of serotonergic neurons. Zhang et al. (2007) reports that, in an animal model of PD, raphe neurons have altered firing rates and fire bursts more frequently. Under levodopa administration, DA may also be released in bursts from these serotonergic neurons.

One of the clearest and best-studied involvements of 5-HT in PD symptoms is in the motor symptoms, including tremor and especially levodopa induced dyskinesias (LID). Experiments have found that the serotonergic system plays an essential role in both symptoms. Brooks (2007) reports that in order to generate tremors with the characteristic PD frequency of 3-5 Hz in animal models it is necessary to lesion not just nigro-striatal dopaminergic projections but also the midbrain tegmentum, which contains serotonergic cell bodies in the median raphe, rubrospinal, and dentatothalamic tracts. He also notes that loss of midbrain serotonin $5\text{-}HT_{1A}$ binding correlates with tremor severity in PD, unlike loss of striatal dopaminergic function. He speculates that this may explain why some parkinsonian tremors are relatively resistant to dopaminergic medications. 5-HT may not be equally involved in all motor symptoms of PD: it has been observed clinically that rigidity and bradykinesia are more responsive to dopaminergic drugs than is tremor (Fox et al., 2009).

Upon diagnosis of PD, patients can often use levodopa to effectively relieve symptoms for several years. However, more than 50% of patients develop motor complications in response to levodopa administration within 5 years (Olanow et al., 2000); after 10 years, the percentage is approximately 90% (Ahlskog & Muenter, 2001). These complications include a narrowing of the temporal window of efficacy (*i.e.*, the duration of benefit after a given dose of levodopa becomes progressively shorter until it approximates the plasma half-life of levodopa) (Olanow et al., 2006), sudden failures of efficacy known as "on-off fluctuations" (Nicholson & Brotchie, 2002) and, most troublesome, the appearance of involuntary movements (LID) (Carta et al., 2008; Nicholson & Brotchie, 2002).

3. Possible mechanisms of serotonergic involvement in PD motor symptoms

In order to understand the emergence of LID, it is useful to first review how levodopa may achieve therapeutic effect. The idea of administering levodopa is to provide dopamine replacement therapy. Dopamine itself is unable to pass the blood brain barrier, but its immediate precursor, levodopa, is able to reach the brain following peripheral administration when given in combination with a decarboxylase inhibitor to prevent metabolism while in the blood stream (Carta et al., 2008). The motor symptoms of PD typically emerge when a sufficient proportion of dopaminergic cells in SNc have been lost that dopaminergic terminals in the striatum are no longer able to maintain a high enough concentration of extracellular DA. Supplemental levodopa can be taken into the remaining dopaminergic terminals, converted to DA and stored in vesicles for synaptic release.

As the number of remaining dopaminergic cells continues to decrease, the levodopa may increasingly be taken up by other cell types including serotonergic neurons and glial cells. Serotonergic cells may play a special role here, as they also express the enzymes used in dopaminergic cells to convert levodopa to DA (amino acid aromatic decarboxylase, AADC) and to package DA into vesicles (vesicular monoamine transporter 2, MAT). Indeed, experiments have verified that serotonergic cells can store and release DA in vivo and in vitro (Nicholson & Brotchie, 2002). Evidence that serotonergic cells may be playing a role in LID comes from animal models of PD. (Tanaka et al., 1999) showed that, in levodopa treatment of a hemiparkinsonian rat, extracellular DA (eDA) decreased substantially when the serotonergic system was lesioned. Glial cells also contain AADC and so could contribute to the conversion of levodopa to DA; however, experiments by Kannari et al. (2000) in which he used reserpine to block vesicular packaging showed a great reduction of eDA, suggesting that most of the levodopa-derived DA is released by exocytosis of vesicles rather than by glia, at least at physiological levels of levodopa administration. Carta et al. (2007) have provided further evidence implicating serotonergic cells in LID in a rat model by showing that either toxic lesion of the serotonergic system or pharmacological impairment of the system with selective serotonin autoreceptor ($5\text{-}HT_{1A}$ and $5\text{-}HT_{1B}$) agonists resulted in a nearly complete elimination of LID.

The observation that LID becomes increasingly problematic as the disease progresses suggests that LID may result from the fact that DA released from serotonergic cells is not subject to the DA homeostatic mechanisms present in dopaminergic cells. Many approaches to eliminating LID therefore tend to focus instead on manipulating factors that regulate serotonergic cell activity, such as serotonergic autoreceptors that participate in serotonergic homeostatic mechanisms. Simply decreasing serotonergic cell activity by administering serotonin autoreceptor agonists has the drawback of also reducing the amount of dopamine released into the extracellular space, tending to worsen PD symptoms (Iravani et al., 2006). Carta et al. (2008) argue that it is reasonable to use 5-HT autoreceptor agonists especially because the DA intermixed with the 5-HT released by the serotonergic cell effectively lowers the binding of 5-HT to 5-HT autoreceptors and induces the cells to be over-active. A more detailed look at the serotonergic system, using mathematical models, may help suggest more nuanced approaches.

There are many types of serotonin receptors. $5\text{-}HT_{1A}$ receptors are present on the cell body and dendrites of serotonergic neurons in the dorsal and median raphe; they function as autoreceptors and they decrease firing as extracellular 5-HT (e5-HT) goes up. $5\text{-}HT_{1B}$ receptors are present on axon terminals in serotonin projection regions where they function as autoreceptors and decrease the release of serotonin as e5-HT goes up in the terminal region. Applying agonists only to $5\text{-}HT_{1A}$ or only to $5\text{-}HT_{1B}$ autoreceptors in a rat model of PD treated with levodopa can partially reduce LID (Bibbiani et al., 2001; Jackson et al., 2004). Carta et al. (2007) found that providing subthreshold doses of both $5\text{-}HT_{1A}$ and $5\text{-}HT_{1B}$ agonists (that is, doses that would have little or no effect alone) could completely eliminate LID. This is very strong evidence that the absence of the normal control mechanisms by the DA autoreceptors is connected to LID.

Post-synaptic mechanisms may play a role in LID. Given that serotonergic cells may be responsible for releasing much of the levodopa-derived DA in advanced PD and that these cells lack DA homeostatic mechanisms, the intermittent administration of levodopa may result in large swings in the extracellular concentration of DA. The resulting pulsatile stimulation of striatal DA receptors may be the proximate cause of abnormal movements (de la Fuente-Fernandez et al., 2001) and may induce post-synaptic changes. In animal models of PD, alterations have been identified in the D_1 signaling pathway as well as in NMDA and AMPA receptor function and distribution (Bibbiani et al., 2005; Hallett et al., 2005; Robelet et al., 2004), and these changes have been linked to the induction and maintenance of abnormal movements (Gardoni et al., 2006; Hallett et al., 2005; Picconi et al., 2008; Santini et al., 2007). In fact, studies utilizing pumps to provide a fairly continuous dosing with levodopa or DA agonists have found fewer side effects (Nutt et al., 2000).

Changes in gene expression also have been found following treatment with levodopa (Santini et al., 2007), and these may relate to the phenomenon of priming. Some PD patients can be treated with DA receptor agonists without developing dyskinesias. But eventually, as the disease progresses, they generally need to add levodopa in order to achieve relief from symptoms. The phenomenon of priming is that patients started on levodopa and then moved to DA agonists will exhibit dyskinesias even if placed on DA agonists without levodopa (Nicholson & Brotchie, 2002).

4. Mathematical modeling of dopaminergic and serotonergic systems

As a first step in using mathematics to help understand the serotonergic and dopaminergic systems, we have created mathematical models of a serotonin terminal (Best et al., 2010b) and a dopamine terminal (Best et al., 2009). Here we briefly describe the model for a serotonin terminal and in the next section give applications. The substrates in the model are indicated in Figure 1 by the pink boxes and the blue ellipses contain the acronyms of enzymes or transporters. Blood tryptophan is considered a (possibly time-varying) input to the model and there are differential equations for the other nine substrates. Each differential equation is just a quantitative expression of mass balance; i.e. the rate of change of the concentration of a substrate is simply the sum of the rates of the reactions by which it is made minus the sum of the rates of the reactions in which it is used. For example, the concentration of 5-hydroxytryptophan, [5htp], satisfies:

$$\frac{d[5htp]}{dt} = V_{\text{TPH}}(trp, bh4, e5ht) - V_{\text{AADC}}(5htp) \tag{1}$$

where V_{TPH} is the velocity of the TPH reaction and V_{AADC} is the velocity of the AADC reaction. One must specify exactly how these velocities depend on the current values of various substrates. V_{TPH} is given by:

$$V_{\text{TPH}} = \frac{V_{max}(trp)(bh4)}{(K_{trp} + (trp) + \frac{(trp)^2}{K_i})(K_{bh4} + (bh4))} \cdot \left(1.5 - \frac{(e5ht)^2}{((.000768)^2 + (e5ht)^2)}\right). \tag{2}$$

The first term on the right is of Michaelis-Menten form and gives the dependence of the velocity on the concentrations of trp and $bh4$. The enzyme TPH shows substrate inhibition (Best et al., 2010a; Friedman et al., 1974; McKinney et al., 2005), which is the reason for the $(trp)^2$ term in the denominator. The second term on the right expresses how the concentration of extracellular 5-HT influences the rate of synthesis via the autoreceptors. At normal e5-HT concentration (.768 nM) this factor equals one. As e5-HT goes up the factor can go as low as 0.5

and as e5-HT goes down, the factor can go as high as 1.5. We chose K_m and K_i values from the literature and chose the V_{max} so that the normal velocity of the the TPH reaction is in the range given by experiments. The form of the second factor is more speculative. Though it is certain that increasing extracellular concentrations of 5-HT inhibit synthesis via the autoreceptors (Adell et al., 2002), there is relatively little information in the literature about the range of e5-HT concentrations over which the effect takes place and about the strength of the effect in the low nanomolar range. Here, as in other choices of parameters and functional forms, we base our choices as much as possible on the experimental literature. Full details of the model can be found in Best et al. (2010b).

The model can be used to show how the steady state values of concentrations and rates change if parameters, like serotonin transporter (SERT) density, or inputs, like serum tryptophan, change. One can also compute the time courses of the concentrations and rates on long time scales (hours) or very short time scales (msec) as the system responds to the release of 5-HT due to individual action potentials. However, the model has limitations. Various physiological processes known to be important are not included, for example the movement of vesicles or SERTs from the interior of the terminal to and from the synaptic membrane. The detailed biophysics of the autoreceptors is not included; instead the model has terms that represent the effect of e5-HT on TPH and on release from the vesicles. And finally, this is a model for a terminal and thus has limited value in studying network questions about the full serotonergic system.

It is important to keep in mind that there is no such thing as *the* serotonergic terminal. Important parameters vary considerably from one projection region to another. For example, SERT density (which corresponds roughly to the V_{max} of V_{SERT}) varies by about a factor of 5 (Bunin et al., 1998; Daws et al., 2005; Lin et al., 2004). And, functional polymorphisms for the TPH, SERT, and MAO genes are known to exist. Indeed, one of the strengths of the model is that it can be used to study the likely effects of such variations on the functional behavior of serotonergic terminals.

5. Applying the models

In this section we describe several applications of our 5-HT and DA terminal models to show how they can be used. The DA terminal model is similar in structure to the 5-HT model, though the details of the kinetics are different (Best et al., 2009).

5.1 Homeostatic effects of the autoreceptors

It is clear that the 5-HT autoreceptors create homeostasis by providing a kind of end-product inhibition. If firing rate goes up, then e5-HT will go up, which reduces synthesis and release via the autoreceptors. If firing rate goes down, then e5-HT will go down, which increases synthesis and release via the autoreceptors. Thus, the autoreceptors ensure that the average extracellular 5-HT in projections regions due to tonic firing of dorsal raphe neurons does not change very much.

It has been much less remarked in the literature that the autoreceptors provide another kind of homeostasis. The genes for many of the key proteins in the 5-HT system, for example TPH2, SERT, and MAO, have common functional polymorphisms. However, because of the autoreceptors, the polymorphisms have a much smaller effect on e5-HT than one might think. For, example the P449R polymorphism and the R441H polymorphism of TPH2 reduce its

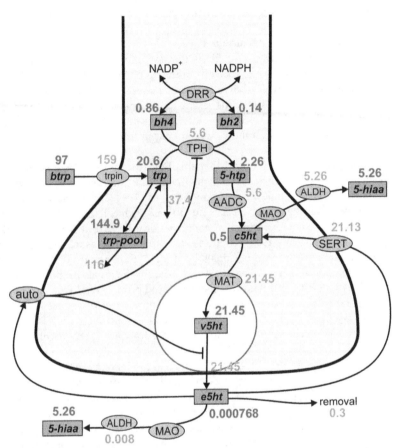

Fig. 1. Steady state concentrations and fluxes in the 5-HT terminal model. The figure shows the reactions in the model. The pink rectangular boxes indicate substrates and blue ellipses contain the acronyms of enzymes or transporters; steady state values in the model are indicated. Concentrations (red) have units of μM and rates (blue) have units of μM/hr. Full names of the substrates are: bh2, dihydrobiopterin; bh4, tetrahydrobiopterin; trp, tryptophan; btrp, serum tryptophan; 5htp, 5-hydroxytryptophan; c5ht, cytosolic 5-HT; v5ht, vesicular 5-HT; e5ht; extracellular 5-HT; 5-hiaa, 5-hydroxyindoleacetic acid; $trp-pool$, the tryptophan pool. Names of enzymes and transporters are: Trpin, neutral amino acid transporter; DRR, dihydrobiopterin reductase; TPH, tryptophan hydroxylase; AADC, aromatic amino acid decarboxylase; MAT, vesicular monoamine transporter; SERT, 5-HT reuptake transporter; auto, 5-HT autoreceptors; MAO, monoamine oxidase; ALDH, aldehyde dehydrogenase. Removal means uptake by capillaries or glial cells or diffusion out of the system.

activity to 65% and 19% of wild type, respectively. But the model predicts that e5-HT will decrease to 90% and 45% of wild type in these two cases; see Figure 4 of (Best et al., 2010b). Similarly, we show in (Best et al., 2009) that the D2 autoreceptors make extracellular DA much less sensitive to the expression level or activity of tyrosine hydroxylase (TH).

5.2 Passive stabilization of DA in the striatum

An interesting and important feature of PD is that symptoms do not appear until a very large percentage (typically 60-90%) of the cells in the SNc have died (Agid, 1991; Zygmond et al., 1990). Animal models have shown that tissue levels of DA in the striatum decline proportionally to cell loss, but eDA remains essentially normal until 85% of the SNc cells have died (Bergstrom & Garris, 2003; Bezard et al., 2001; Dentresangle et al., 2001), and this is widely believed to be the reason that symptoms do not appear until very late in the degeneration of the SNc.

A number of researchers have proposed that this homeostasis of eDA results from active adaptive mechanisms such as increased DA synthesis and the formation of new terminals (Hornykiewicz, 1966; Stanic et al., 2003; Zygmond et al., 1990; 1984). However, Garris and co-workers proposed that the homeostasis is due to passive mechanisms such as release and reuptake and provided some experimental confirmation (Bergstrom & Garris, 2003; Garris et al., 1997; Garris & Wightman, 1994). Their idea is as follows. DA is released in the striatum and is then taken back up into the terminals by the DA transporters (DATs). As the cells in the SNc die the amount of DA released in the striatum decreases proportionally, but the number of DATs available for reuptake has also decreased proportionally. Thus a released DA molecule will spend about the same amount of time in the extracellular space no matter how many SNc cells have died. Garris and co-workers called this "passive stabilization." They did not explain why this homeostasis breaks down when the fraction, f, of SNc cells that are alive becomes small.

We investigated these proposals with our mathematical model of a DA terminal (Reed et al., 2009). We found that the passive stabilization mechanism proposed by Garris works as proposed and we determined why the mechanism breaks down when f is small. Not all released DA molecules are put back into DA terminals by the DATs. Some are taken up by glial cells or blood vessels and some diffuse out of the striatum. As SNc cells die and the DA terminals in the striatum become more sparse, a greater percentage of released DA is lost through these mechanisms. This is why the Garris passive stabilization mechanism breaks down when f is small. We provided quantitative calculations about these effects and showed that passive stabilization itself keeps eDA almost constant when f is between $\frac{1}{2}$ and 1. When more than half of the SNc cells have died, the terminal autoreceptors contribute substantially to the homeostasis of eDA. And, only when f is as low as .15 or .1 are the combined homeostatic effects of passive stabilization and the autoreceptors overwhelmed by the removal of DA from the striatum by the mechanisms discussed above. For details, see (Reed et al., 2009).

5.3 Burst firing in the raphe nuclei and SSRIs

The etiology of depressive illness remains unknown despite a large body of research. A hypothesis that has been central to much work in pharmacology and electrophysiology is that depression is caused by dysfunction in the serotonergic signaling system (Feldman et al.,

1997; Schildkraut, 1965). This hypothesis led to the development of monoamine oxidase inhibitors (MAOIs), tricyclic anti-depressants and the selective serotonin reuptake inhibitors (SSRIs). The idea of the MAOIs is that by preventing the degradation of 5-HT, more will be available for packaging into synaptic vesicles. The idea of the tri-cyclics and the SSRIs is that they block SERTs and inhibit reuptake of 5-HT from the extracellular space, therefore increasing "serotonergic signaling." These drugs have shown some efficacy in the treatment of depression, but the causal chain of events and the reasons why they benefit some patients and not others are unknown.

The simple hypothesis that SSRIs would raise the level of 5-HT in serotonergic synapses by blocking reuptake was thrown into doubt by the discovery that the cell bodies of most 5-HT neurons also release 5-HT and have SERTs. Furthermore, increased e5-HT in the RN decreases the tonic firing rate of those cells via the $5\text{-}HT_{1A}$ autoreceptors (Adell et al., 2002; Gartside et al., 1995). Thus, there are two conflicting effects. Blocking the SERTs in the terminal region would tend to raise e5-HT there, and blocking the SERTs in the raphe nuclei (RN) would tend to decrease e5-HT in the terminal region. The balance between the two effects will depend on the densities of $5\text{-}HT_{1A}$ autoreceptors on different 5-HT populations in the RN and on the densities of SERTs in different projection regions, both quite variable. Thus one would expect that experimental results would depend on dose and on the projection regions being studied, and this was found to be true (Bel & Artigas, 1992; Hervas & Artigas, 1998; Malagie et al., 1995). In some cases, acute doses of SSRIs even decreased e5-HT in projection regions.

The next hypothesis focused on the $5\text{-}HT_{1A}$ autoreceptors on the RN cell bodies. It was shown that giving $5\text{-}HT_{1A}$ antagonists or knocking out the autoreceptors entirely potentiates the SSRI-induced increase of e5-HT in projection regions. Similarly, $5\text{-}HT_{1A}$ knockouts show increased release in projection regions (Chaput et al., 1986; Knobelman et al., 2001). Furthermore, a number of studies showed that chronic treatment with SSRIs desensitizes the $5\text{-}HT_{1A}$ autoreceptors in the RN (Blier et al., 1987; Chaput et al., 1986; Hervas et al., 2001; Invernizzi et al., 1992). And thus, one could explain the improvements of patients on the time scale of 3-6 weeks by the slow desensitization of autoreceptors. However, when e5-HT was measured in projection regions during the entire course of chronic SSRI treatment, it was found that e5-HT concentrations went up initially and then plateaued or declined somewhat over the course of treatment (Anderson et al., 2005; Smith et al., 2000). Thus the autoreceptor desensitization hypothesis seems unlikely to explain the delay of beneficial effects of SSRI treatments.

In (Best et al., 2011) we propose a new hypothesis for the efficacy of SSRIs and provide calculations with the 5-HT terminal model to support our ideas. The 5-HT cells in the RN fire tonically at about 1 Hz and occasionally individual spikes are replaced by short bursts (Feldman et al., 1997; Hajos et al., 1995; Heyn et al., 1982). Our physiological point of view is that tonic firing by the 5-HT neurons in the RN maintains 5-HT tone in target tissues by volume transmission and burst firing conveys specific information to one-on-one synapses that are known to exist (Maley et al., 1990; Parnavelas & Papadopoulos, 1989). Our hypothesis is that chronic treatment of depressed patients with SSRIs returns the response to bursts arriving in terminal regions to normal and we show that this is true in our model. The model behavior depends on the down regulation of SERTs on terminal membranes known to be caused by chronic exposure to SSRIs (Benmansour et al., 2002; Gould et al., 2003; Lau et al., 2008; Mizra et al., 2007). For details, see (Best et al., 2011).

6. Future work

We indicate briefly here some of the ideas that we plan to pursue. We plan to use our current model of a 5-HT terminal described above to investigate the consequences of levodopa uptake by 5-HT terminals. Both 5-HTP and levodopa will compete for AADC that will turn them into 5-HT and DA respectively, and the monoamine transporter will package them together into vesicles. Since there is leakage out of the vesicles driven by concentration gradients, the competition will limit the amounts of 5-HT and DA available for release. Our physiological point of view is that normal 5-HT or DA neurons maintain 5-HT or DA tone in target tissues by volume transmission and convey specific information via burst firing. The autoreceptors on DA neurons inhibit release when the extracellular concentration of DA goes up due to a burst, bringing the concentration back to the normal tonic level rapidly. However, levodopa therapy partially turns 5-HT neurons into DA neurons that do not have DA autoreceptors and one expects that stimulation of the 5-HT system will therefore cause larger than normal swings in extracellular DA in the striatum after levodopa therapy. This effect will be compounded by the fact that cell death in the SNc implies that there will be many fewer DATs in the striatum to take up the released DA. We plan to investigate this situation with our model. Finally, we are currently extending our models to include the competition between tyrosine, tryptophan, leucine, isoleucine, and valine at the blood-brain barrier. When this is completed we can study the tryptophan depletion and tryptophan loading experiments described in (Scholtissen et al., 2006).

We are particularly interested in how levodopa therapy could produce dyskinesis and have some ideas that can be tried out through mathematical modeling. (Carta et al., 2007) provided strong evidence that release of DA from 5-HT neurons causes LID by showing that $5\text{-}HT_{1A}$ agonists that reduce RN firing and/or $5\text{-}HT_{1B}$ agonists that reduce release in the striatum both reduce the incidence of LID in an animal model. We plan to extend our 5-HT terminal model to include the cell body in the RN so that we can study release of DA in the striatum in the presence of either $5\text{-}HT_{1A}$ or $5\text{-}HT_{1B}$ agonists (or both) after cell death in the SNc reduces the number of DATs. This will provide a platform for trying out *in silico* the experiments in (Carta et al., 2007).

There is another intriguing possibility that we plan to investigate by modeling. Recall that the 5-HT neurons in the raphe nuclei release 5-HT from their cell bodies when they fire. The released 5-HT binds to the $5\text{-}HT_{1A}$ autoreceptors on the cell bodies and inhibits RN firing (Adell et al., 2002). This is a kind of lateral inhibition in the RN that limits total firing. However, in the presence of levodopa, the cell bodies will release a combination of 5-HT and DA, and the lower extracellular concentration of 5-HT will provide much less lateral inhibition. Thus is it likely that the 5-HT neurons in the RN fire more frequently after levodopa therapy and there is evidence for altered firing patterns (Zhang et al., 2007). This would have the effect of releasing more DA in the striatum. Notice, however, that raphe neurons project to many brain regions that send inhibitory projections back to the RN (for example the mPFC; see (Celada et al., 2001)). Such negative feedback systems often exhibit oscillations if they are forced hard enough, and such oscillations would mean periodic oscillations in the amount of firing of 5-HT neurons in the RN and thus periodic oscillations in the amount of DA released in the striatum. It is tempting to speculate that such oscillations may contribute to LID and that they could be initiated by intermittent levodopa therapy (Nutt et al., 2000; Olanow et al., 2006; 2000). We plan to investigate this hypothesis by developing mathematical models of the lateral inhibition by diffusion of extracellular 5-HT in the RN and a model of the projections to the mPFC with negative feedback from the mPFC to the RN.

Finally, it is well-known that the brain is capable of rewiring itself after injury to use available neurons for new purposes. Note that, in a certain sense, that is what levodopa therapy is stimulating, the use of 5-HT neurons as DA neurons. And, it is known that lesioning the SNc causes hyperinnervation by 5-HT neurons in the striatum (Maeda et al., 2003). Such retraining and rewiring takes time, of course, and it is possible that it can't happen fast enough to compensate for the degeneration in PD, but the possibility is intriguing. Not enough is known presently for mathematical modeling to be helpful here. However, if and when anatomical and electrophysiological information becomes available about such compensatory processes, mathematical models, developed along the lines that we have indicated, could perhaps suggest treatment strategies that would facilitate the compensatory processes.

7. Acknowledgements

This work was supported by NSF grants DMS-061670 (MR,HFN) and EF-1038593 (HFN,MR), NSF CAREER grant DMS-0956057 (JB), and NSF agreement 0112050 through the Mathematical Biosciences Institute (JB, MR). JB is an Alfred P. Sloan Research Foundation Fellow. The authors thank Shira Rubin for a close reading of the manuscript.

8. References

Adell, A., Celada, P., Abella, M. T. & Artigasa, F. (2002). Origin and functional role of the extracellular serotonin in the midbrain raphe nuclei, *Brain Res Rev* 39: 154–180.

Agid, Y. (1991). Parkinson's disease: pathophysiology, *Lancet* 337: 1321–1324.

Ahlskog, J. E. (2004). Challenging conventional wisdom: The etiologic role of dopamine oxidative stress in Parkinson's disease, *Movement Disorders* 20(3): 271–282.

Ahlskog, J. E. & Muenter, M. D. (2001). Frequency of levodopa-related dyskinesias and motor fluctuations as estimated from the cumulative literature, *Movement Disorders* 16(3): 448–458.

Anderson, G. M., Barr, C. S., Lindell, S., Durham, A. C., Shifrovich, I. & Higley, J. D. (2005). Time course of the effects of the serotonin-selective reuptake inhibitor sertraline on central and peripheral serotonin neurochemistry in the rhesus monkey, *Phycopharma* 178: 339–346.

Bel, N. & Artigas, F. (1992). Fluoxetine preferentially increases extracellular 5-hydroxytryptamine in the raphe nuclei: an in vivo microdialysis study, *Eur. J. Pharmacol.* 229: 101–103.

Benmansour, S., Owens, W. A., Cecchi, M., Morilak, D. & Frazer, A. (2002). Serotonin clearance in vivo is altered to a greater extent by antidepressant-induced downregulation of the serotonin transporter than by acute blockade of the transporter, *J. Neurosci.* 22(15): 6766–6772.

Bergstrom, B. & Garris, P. (2003). 'Passive stabilization' of striatal extracellular dopamine across the lesion spectrum encompassing the presymptomatic phase of Parkinson's disease: a voltametric study in the 6-OHDA-lesioned rat, *J. Neurochem* 87: 1224–36.

Best, J. A., Nijhout, H. F. & Reed, M. C. (2009). Homeostatic mechanisms in dopamine synthesis and release: a mathematical model, *Theor Biol Med Model* 6: 21.

Best, J. A., Nijhout, H. F. & Reed, M. C. (2010a). Models of dopaminergic and serotonergic signaling, *Pharmacopsychiatry* 43(Supp. 1): 561–566.

Best, J. A., Nijhout, H. F. & Reed, M. C. (2010b). Serotonin synthesis, release and reuptake in terminals: a mathematical model, *Theor Biol Med Model* 7: 34–.

Best, J., Reed, M. & Nijhout, H. F. (2011). Bursts and the efficacy of selective serotonin reuptake inhibitors, *Pharmacopsychiatry* 44(Suppl.1):S76-S83.

Bezard, E., Dovero, S., C, C. P., Ravenscroft, P., Chalon, S., Guilloteau, D., Crossman, A. R., Bioulac, B., Brotchie, J. M. & Gross, C. E. (2001). Relationship between the appearance of symptoms and the level nigrostriatal degeneration in a progressive 1-methyl-4-phenyl-1,2,3,6-tetrahydropyridine-lesioned macaque model of Parkinson's disease, *J Neurosci* 21: 6853–6861.

Bibbiani, F., Oh, J. D. & Chase, T. N. (2001). Serotonin 5-HT1a agonist improves motor complications in rodent and primate Parkinsonian models, *Neurology* 57: 1829–1834.

Bibbiani, F., Oh, J. D., Kielaite, A., Collins, M. A., Smith, C. & Chase, T. N. (2005). Combined blockade of AMPA and NMDA glutamate receptors reduces levodopa-induced motor complications in animal models of PD, *Experimental Neurology* 196: 422–429.

Blier, P., de Montigny, C. & Chaput, Y. (1987). Modifications of the serotonin system by antidepressant treatment: implications for the therapeutic response in major depression, *J. Clin. Psychoharmacol*. 7: 24S–35S.

Braak, H., Rüb, U., Gai, W. & Tredici, K. D. (2003). Idiopathic Parkinson's disease: possible routes by which vulnerable neuronal types may be subject to neuroinvasion by an unknown pathogen, *J Neural Transmission* 110: 517–536.

Brooks, D. J. (2007). Imaging non-dopaminergic function in Parkinson's disease, *Molecular Imaging and Biology* 9: 217–222.

Bunin, M., Prioleau, C., Mailman, R. & Wightman, R. (1998). Release and uptake rates of 5-hydroxytryptamine in the dorsal raphe and substantia nigra of the rat brain, *J Neurochem* 70: 1077–1087.

Carta, M., Carlsson, T., Kirik, D. & Björklund, A. (2007). Dopamine released from 5-HT terminals is the cause of l-dopa-induced dyskinesia in Parkinsonian rats, *Brain* 130: 1819–1833.

Carta, M., Carlsson, T., Muñoz, A., Kirik, D. & Björklund, A. (2008). Serotonin–dopamine interaction in the induction and maintenance of l-dopa-induced dyskinesias, *Prog. Brain Res.* 172: 465–478.

Celada, P., Puig, M. V., Casanovas, J. M., Guillazo, G. & Artigas, F. (2001). Control of dorsal raphe serotonergic neurons by the medial prefrontal cortex: Involvement of serotonin-1a, GABAa, and glutamate receptors, *J. Neurosci* 15: 9917–9929.

Chaput, Y., Blier, P. & de Montigny, C. (1986). In vivo electrophysiological evidence for the regulatory role of autoreceptors on serotonergic terminals, *J. Neurosci* 6(10): 2796–2801.

Chaudhuri, K. R., Healy, D. G. & Schapira, A. H. V. (2006). Non-motor symptoms of Parkinson's disease: diagnosis and management, *Lancet/Neurology* 5: 235–245.

Daws, L., Montenez, S., Owens, W., Gould, G., Frazer, A., Toney, G. & Gerhardt, G. (2005). Transport mechanisms governing serotonin clearance in vivo revealed by high speed chronoamperometry, *J Neurosci Meth* 143: 49–62.

de la Fuente-Fernandez, R., Lu, J.-Q., Sossi, V., Jivan, S., Schulzer, M., Holden, J. E., Lee, C. S., Ruth, T. J., Donald, Calne, B. & Stoessl, A. J. (2001). Biochemical variations in the synaptic level of dopamine precede motor fluctuations in Parkinson's disease: PET evidence of increased dopamine turnover, *Annals of Neurology* 49(3): 298–303.

Dentresangle, C., Cavorsin, M. L., Savasta, M. & Leviel, V. (2001). Increased extracellular DA and normal evoked DA release in the rat striatum after a partial lesion of the substantia nigra, *Brain Res* 893(178-185).

Feldman, R., Meyer, J. & Quenzer, L. (1997). *Principles of Neuropharmacology*, Sinauer Associates, Inc, Sunderland, MA.

Fox, S. H., Chuang, R. & Brotchie, J. M. (2009). Serotonin and Parkinson's disease: On movement, mood, and madness, *Movement Disorders* 24: 1255–1266.

Friedman, P. A., Kappelman, A. H. & Kaufman, S. (1974). Partial purification and characterization of tryptophan hydroxylase from rabbit hindbrain, *J Biol Chem* 247: 1465–1473.

Gardoni, F., Picconi, B., Ghiglieri, V., Polli, F., Bagetta, V., Bernardi, G., Cattabeni, F., Luca, M. D. & Calabresi, P. (2006). A critical interaction between NR2B and MAGUK in l-dopa induced dyskinesia, *The Journal of Neuroscience* 26(11): 2914–2922.

Garris, P., Walker, Q. & Wightman, R. (1997). Dopamine release and uptake both decrease in the partially denervated striatum in proportion to the loss of dopamine terminals, *Brain Res* 753: 225–234.

Garris, P. & Wightman, R. (1994). Different kinetics govern dopaminergic neurotransmission in the amygdala, prefrontal cortex, and striatum: an in vivo voltametric study, *J. Neurosci* 14: 442–450.

Gartside, S. E., Umbers, V., Hajos, M. & Sharp, T. (1995). Interaction between a selective 5-HT1a receptor antagonist and an SSRI in vivo: effects on 5-HT cell firing and extracellular 5-HT, *Br. J. Pharmacol.* 115: 1064–1070.

Gibb, W. R. G. & Lees, A. J. (1988). The relevance of the Lewy body to the pathogenesis of idiopathic Parkinson's disease, *J of Neurology, Neurosurgery, and Psychiatry* 51: 745–752.

Gould, G. G., Pardon, M. C., Morilak, D. A. & Frazer, A. (2003). Regulatory effects of reboxetine treatment alone, or following paroxetine treatment, on brain noradrenergic and serotonergic systems., *Neuropsychopharmacology* 28: 1633–1644.

Hajos, M., Gartside, S. E., Villa, A. E. P. & Sharp, T. (1995). Evidence for a repetitive (burst) firing pattern in a sub-population of 5-hydroxytryptamine neurons in the dorsal and median raphe nuclei of the rat, *Neuroscience* 69: 189–197.

Hallett, P. J., Dunah, A. W., Ravenscroft, P., Zhou, S., Bezard, E., Crossman, A. R., Brotchie, J. M. & Standaert, D. G. (2005). Alterations of striatal NMDA receptor subunits associated with the development of dyskinesia in the MPTP-lesioned primate model of Parkinson's disease, *Neuropharmacology* 48: 503–516.

Halliday, G. M. & McCann, H. (2010). The progression of pathology in Parkinson's disease, *Ann. N.Y. Acad. Sci.* 1184: 188–195.

Hervas, I. & Artigas, F. (1998). Effect of fluoxetine on extracellular 5-hydroxytryptamine in rat brain. Role of 5HT autoreceptors., *Eur. J. Pharmacol.* 358: 9–18.

Hervas, I., Velaro, M. T., Romero, L., Mengod, G. & Artigas, F. (2001). Desensitization of 5-HT1a autoreceptors by a low chronic fluoxetine dose. Effect of the concurrent administration of WAY-100635, *Neuropsychopharmacology* 24: 11–20.

Heyn, J., Steinfels, G. F. & Jacobs, B. J. (1982). Activity of serotonin-containing neurons in the nucleus raphe pallidus of freely moving cats, *Brain Res.* 251: 259–276.

Hornykiewicz, O. (1966). Dopamine (3-hydroxytyramine) and brain function, *Pharmacol. Rev.* 18: 925–964.

Invernizzi, R., Bramante, M. & Samanin, R. (1992). Citalopram's ability to increase the extracellular concentrations of serotonin in the dorsal raphe prevents the drug's effect in the frontal cortex, *Brain Res.* 260: 322–324.

Iravani, M. M., Tayarani-Binazir, K., Chu, W. B., Jackson, M. J. & Jenner, P. (2006). In MPTP treated primates, the selective 5-HT1a agonist (R)- (+)-8-hydroxy-DPAT inhibits levodopa-induced dyskinesia but only with increased motor disability, *J Pharmacology and Experimental Therapeutics* 319: 1225–1234.

Jackson, M. J., Al-Barghouthy, G., Pearce, R. K. B., Smith, L., Hagan, J. J. & Jenner, P. (2004). Effect of 5-HT1b/d receptor agonist and antagonist administration on motor function in haloperidol and MPTP-treated common marmosets, *Pharmacology, Biochemistry and Behavior* 79: 391–400.

Jankovic, J. (2008). Parkinson's disease: clinical features and diagnosis, *J Neurol Neurosurg Psychiatry* 79: 368–376.

Jellinger, K. A. (1991). Pathology of Parkinson's disease: Changes other than the nigrostriatal pathway, *Molecular and Chemical Neuropathology* 14: 153–197.

Kannari, K., Tanaka, H., Maeda, T., Tomiyama, M., Suda, T. & Matsunaga, M. (2000). Reserpine pretreatment prevents increases in extracellular striatal dopamine following l-dopa administration in rats with nigrostriatal denervation, *J Neurochem* 74: 263–269.

Kish, S. J., Tong, J., Hornykiewicz, O., Rajput, A., Chang, L.-J., Guttman, M. & Furukawa, Y. (2008). Preferential loss of serotonin markers in caudate versus putamen in Parkinson's disease, *Brain* 131: 120–131.

Knobelman, D. A., Hen, R. & Lucki, I. (2001). Genetic regulation of extracellular serotonin by 5-hydroxtryptamine-1a and 5-hydroxytryptamine-1b autoreceptors in different brain regions of the mouse, *J. Pharmacol. Exper. Therap.* 298: 1083–1091.

Lau, T., Horschitz, S., Berger, S., Bartsch, D. & Schloss, P. (2008). Antidepressant-induced internalization of the serotonin transporter in serotonergic neurons, *FASEB J* 22: 1702–1714.

Lim, S.-Y., Fox, S. H. & Lang, A. E. (2009). Overview of the extranigral aspects of Parkinson disease, *Arch. Neurol.* 66(2): 167–172.

Lin, K.-J., Yen, T.-C., Wey, S.-P., Hwang, J.-J., Ye, X.-X., Tzen, K.-Y., Fu, Y.-K. & Chen, J.-C. (2004). Characterization of the binding sites 123I-ADAM and the relationship to the serotonin transporter in rat and mouse brains using quantitative autoradiography, *J. Nuc. Med.* 45: 673–681.

Linazasoro, G. (2007). Classical Parkinson disease versus Parkinson complex – reflections against staging and in favour of heterogeneity, *European Journal of Neurology* 14: 721–728.

Maeda, T., Kannari, K., H, H. S., Arai, A., Tomiyama, M., Matsunaga, M. & Suda, T. (2003). Rapid induction of serotonergic hyperinnervation in the adult rat striatum with extensive dopaminergic denervation., *Neurosci. Lett.* 343: 17–20.

Malagie, I., Trillat, A. C., Jacquot, C. & Gardier, A. M. (1995). Effects of acute fluoxetine on extracellular serotonin levels in the raphe: an in vivo microdialysis study, *Eur. J. Pharmacol.* 286: 213–217.

Maley, B. E., Engle, M. G., Humphreys, S., Vascik, D. A., Howes, K. A., Newton, B. W. & Elde, R. P. (1990). Monoamine synaptic structure and localization in the central nervous system, *J. Electron Micros. Tech.* 15: 20–33.

McKinney, J., Knappskog, P. M. & Haavik, J. (2005). Different properties of the central and peripheral forms of human tryptophan hydroxylase, *J Neurochem* 92: 311–320.

Mizra, N. R., Nielson, E. O. & Troelsen, K. B. (2007). Serotonin transporter density and anxiolytic-like effects of antidepressants in mice, *Prog. Neuropsycho. Biol. Psych.* 31: 858–866.

Monti, J. M. (2010). The structure of the dorsal raphe nucleus and its relevance to the regulation of sleep and wakefulness, *Sleep Med. Rev.* 14: 307–317.

Nicholson, S. L. & Brotchie, J. M. (2002). 5-hydroxytryptamine (5HTt, serotonin) and Parkinson's disease - opportunities for novel therapeutics to reduce problems of levodopa therapy, *European Journal of Neurology* 9(Suppl. 3): 1–6.

Nutt, J., Obesio, J. A. & Stocchi, F. (2000). Continuous dopamine-receptor stimulation in advanced Parkinson's disease, *TINS* 23: S109–S115.

Olanow, C. W., Obeso, J. A. & Stocchi, F. (2006). Continuous dopamine-receptor treatment of Parkinson's disease: scientific rationale and clinical implications, *Lancet/Neurology* 5: 677–687.

Olanow, C. W., Schapira, A. H. V. & Rascol, O. (2000). Continuous dopamine-receptor stimulation in early Parkinson's disease, *TINS* 23: S117–S126.

Parnavelas, J. G. & Papadopoulos, G. C. (1989). The monoaminergic innervation of the cerebral cortex is not diffuse and non-specific, *TINS* 12: 315–319.

Picconi, B., Paillé, V., Ghiglieri, V., Bagetta, V., Barone, I., Lindgren, H. S., Bernardi, G., Cenci, M. A. & Calabresi, P. (2008). L-dopa dosage is critically involved in dyskinesia via loss of synaptic depotentiation, *Neurobiology of Disease* 29: 327–335.

Reed, M., Best, J. & Nijhout, H. (2009). Passive and active stabilization of dopamine in the striatum, *BioScience Hypotheses* 2: 240–244.

Robelet, S., Melon, C., Guillet, B., Salin, P. & Goff, L. K.-L. (2004). Chronic l-dopa treatment increases extracellular glutamate levels and GLT1 expression in the basal ganglia in a rat model of Parkinson's disease, *European Journal of Neuroscience* 20: 1255–1266.

Santini, E., Valjent, E., Usiello, A., Carta, M., Borgkvist, A., Girault, J.-A., Hervé, D., Greengard, P. & Fisone, G. (2007). Critical involvement of CAMP/DARPP-32 and extracellular signal-regulated protein kinase signaling in l-dopa-induced dyskinesia, *The Journal of Neuroscience* 27(26): 6995–7005.

Schildkraut, J. J. (1965). The catecholamine hypothesis of affective disorders: a review of supporting evidence, *Amer. J. Psych.* 122: 509–522.

Scholtissen, B., Verhey, F. R. J., Steinbusch, H. W. M. & Leentjens, A. F. G. (2006). Serotonergic mechanisms in Parkinson's disease: opposing results from preclinical and clinical data, *J. Neural Trans.* 113: 59–73.

Smith, T., Kuczenski, R., George-Friedman, K., Malley, J. D. & Foote, S. L. (2000). In vivo microdialysis assessment of extracellular serotonin and dopamine levels in awake monkeys during sustained fluoxetine administration, *Synapse* 38: 460–470.

Stanic, D., Parish, C. L., Zhu, W. L., Krstew, E. V., Lawrence, A. J., Drago, J. & Finkelstein, D. I. (2003). Changes in function and ultrastructure of striatal dopaminergic terminals that regenerate following partial lesions of the SNpc, *J Neurochem* 86(329-343).

Tanaka, H., Kannari, K., Maeda, T., Tomiyama, M., Suda, T. & Matsunaga, M. (1999). Role of serotonergic neurons in l-dopa- derived extracellular dopamine in the striatum of 6-OHDA-lesioned rats, *NeuroReport* 10: 631–634.

Zhang, Q.-J., Gao, R., Liu, J., Liu, Y.-P. & Wang, S. (2007). Changes in the firing activity of serotonergic neurons in the dorsal raphe nucleus in a rat model of Parkinson's disease, *Acta Physiologica Sinica* 59(2): 183–189.

Zygmond, M., Abercrombie, E. D., Berger, T. W., Grace, A. A. & Stricker, E. M. (1990). Compensation after lesions of central dopaminergic neurons: some clinical and basic implications, *TINS* 13: 290–296.

Zygmond, M. J., Acheson, A. L., Stachowiak, M. K. & Stricker, E. M. (1984). Neurochemical compensation after nigrostriatal bundle injury in an animal model of preclinical Parkinsonism, *Arch. Neurol.* 41: 856–861.

5

Dopaminergic Control of the Neurotransmitter Release in the Subthalamic Nucleus: Implications for Parkinson's Disease Treatment Strategies

Ben Ampe, Anissa El Arfani, Yvette Michotte and Sophie Sarre
Vrije Universiteit Brussel,
Belgium

1. Introduction

A critical role of the subthalamic nucleus (STN) in the control of movement has been proposed based on the observations that its lesion or high-frequency stimulation, aimed at altering its activity, is effective in alleviating clinical features of Parkinson's disease (Bergman et al,. 1990; Bennazouz et al., 1993; Pollak et al., 1993, Benazzouz et al., 2000). Indeed, overactivity of the subthalamic neurons due to the loss of midbrain dopaminergic neurons is believed to be a key feature in Parkinson's disease. Several studies indicate that the activity of STN neurons can be influenced directly by dopamine and its receptor agonists/antagonists. Indeed, the STN receives a direct dopaminergic input arising in the substantia nigra pars compacta (SNc) and both dopamine D1- and D2-like receptors are present in the STN (Canteras et al., 1990; Hassani et al., 1997; Flores et al., 1999). Understanding the position of the STN within the basal ganglia and the possible direct effects of dopamine and its ligands at the level of this nucleus in normal and parkinsonian states may be important in the development of new therapies for Parkinson's disease. The purpose of this chapter is to give an overview of the current position of the STN in the basal ganglia motorloop and to clarify the role of dopamine at the level of the STN in both normal conditions and in parkinsonian experimental animal models.

2. The subthalamic nucleus and its connections

Despite the small size of this biconvex-shaped structure, the STN has an important role in the modulation of the basal ganglia output and thus movement control (DeLong & Wichmann, 2007; Obeso et al., 2008; Gubbelini et al., 2009). Indeed, together with the striatum, the STN forms the major input to the basal ganglia and is considered an important relay nucleus of the indirect pathway. In this section, the role of the STN within the basal ganglia and its connections are described.

2.1 The subthalamic nucleus as a part of the basal ganglia

The basal ganglia consist of five interconnected nuclei including the caudate nucleus, the putamen [which forms together with the caudate nucleus the striatum], the globus pallidus (pars interna (GPi) and externa (GPe)) the SN (SNc and substantia nigra pars reticulata (SNr)) and the STN (DeLong, 1990; Blandini et al., 2000). Albin and DeLong proposed a schematic view of the basal ganglia organisation which has been used for many years as a reference for understanding their functioning in physiological and pathological conditions (Albin et al., 1989; DeLong, 1990; Gubellini et al., 2009). Currently, this view has been replaced by a more recent representation of the organisation of the basal ganglia based on novel anatomical, neurochemical and physiological data (Levy et al., 1997; Gubellini et al., 2009). In this representation, the striatum and STN are considered as the two major input structures of the basal ganglia. Both nuclei receive input from the cerebral cortex, whereas the GPi and SNr provide output of the basal ganglia to the thalamus and brainstem (DeLong & Wichmann, 2007; Obeso et al., 2008). The striatum is connected with these output structures via a monosynaptic direct pathway and a polysynaptic indirect pathway which includes the GPe and the STN. The striatal direct pathway neurons also receive input from the intralaminar nuclei of the thalamus. The STN is directly connected with the output nuclei.

Besides motor functions, the basal ganglia are involved in cognition and emotion (Alexander et al., 1990; Smith et al., 1998). Indeed, the basal ganglia can be functionally divided into different cortico-subcortical circuits: the motor loop, the associative loop and the limbic loop. Each circuit originates from individual cortical areas, innervates the respective regions of the striatum, GP and SN and, via the thalamus, terminates in their respective cortical areas of origin (Hamani et al., 2004; DeLong & Wichmann, 2007). Like the other structures of the basal ganglia, the STN is subdivided into different major parts: a motor, an associative and a limbic part (Hamani et al., 2004; Benarroch, 2008). The motor part is represented by the large dorsolateral portion of the STN whereas the associative and the limbic part are represented by respectively the ventromedial portion and the medial tip of the STN. Currently, the best characterized cortico-subcortical circuit is the motor circuit.

The motor loop (figure 1) originates from the motor cortex and sends glutamatergic projections to both input nuclei, the striatum and the STN (DeLong & Wichmann, 2007; Obeso et al., 2008). Striatal efferent neurons are γ-aminobutyric acid (GABA)-ergic and are connected, as mentioned before, with the output nuclei, GPi and SNr, by the direct or the indirect pathway. Neurons from the direct pathway, which bear dopamine D1 receptors (excitatory receptors), project directly to the output nuclei. Neurons from the indirect pathway express dopamine D2 receptors (inhibitory receptors) and send GABA-ergic projections to the GPe. The GPe in turn influences the STN by GABA-ergic projections. The STN, which is a glutamatergic structure, provides excitatory input to the output nuclei of the basal ganglia. The balance within the basal ganglia is regulated by the dopaminergic neurons from the SNc. Release of dopamine in the striatum leads to an increase in activity of the direct pathway via the D1 receptors, whereas the activity of the indirect pathway is decreased via the D2 receptors. This dopamine release results in a reduction in the activity of the output nuclei and thus facilitates movement. In Parkinson's disease, nigrostriatal degeneration leads to hyperactivity of the STN and thus to an increase of the output nuclei activity which in turn results in inhibition of ongoing movement.

2.2 Subthalamic nucleus afferents and efferents

As described above, the STN has a pivotal position in the motor circuitry. Indeed, it is part of a complex organisation within the basal ganglia and is connected with a wide range of structures. It is the only glutamatergic nucleus of the basal ganglia (Smith & Parent, 1988; Blandini et al., 2000; Hamani et al., 2004). The STN provides a strong excitatory input to the two output structures, GPi and SNr, but also to the GPe. Via its excitatory input to the SNc, it influences the regulation of the dopamine release (Smith et al., 1990; Parent & Hazrati, 1995; Hamani et al., 2004). Besides the main efferent projections described above, the STN is

Dopaminergic Control of the Neurotransmitter Release in the Subthalamic Nucleus: Implications for
Parkinson's Disease Treatment Strategies

87

connected with the peduncolopontine nucleus and the ventral tegmental area through
which it influences the processing of emotional information (Smith et al., 1990; Parent &
Hazrati, 1995; Haegelen et al., 2009). Furthermore, the STN sends poor glutamatergic
projections to the striatum and the motor cortex (Smith et al., 1990; Blandini et al., 2000).

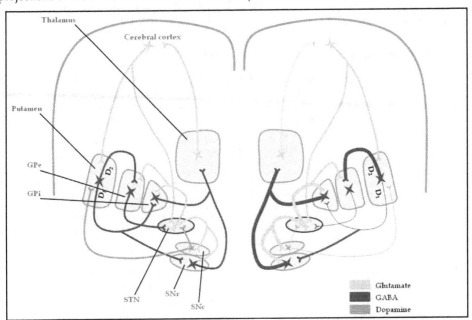

Fig. 1. Left brain hemisphere: motor loop in a normal condition. Right brain hemisphere:
motor loop in Parkinson's disease. The motor loop originates from the motor cortex and
sends glutamatergic projections to both input nuclei, the striatum and the STN. Striatal
neurons from the direct pathway (contain D1 receptors) project directly to the output nuclei
whereas neurons from the indirect pathway (contain D2 receptors) send GABA-ergic
projections to the GPe. The GPe in turn influences the STN by GABA-ergic projections. The
STN provides excitatory input to the output nuclei. Release of dopamine in the striatum
leads to an increase in activity of the direct pathway via the D1 receptors whereas the
activity of the indirect pathway is decreased via the D2 receptors. Dopamine release results
in a reduction in the activity of the output nuclei and, via the thalamus, leads to
glutamatergic projections to the cortex which facilitates movement. In Parkinson's disease,
dopaminergic degeneration of the SNc leads to hyperactivity of the STN and thus an
increase of the output nuclei activity which in turn results in inhibition of ongoing
movement. The thickness of the depicted projections reflects their activity.

Neurons of the STN receive two major projections: a direct excitatory glutamatergic input
from the cerebral cortex and an important inhibitory GABA-ergic innervation from the GPe
(Blandini et al., 2000; Hamani et al., 2004; DeLong & Wichmann, 2007). It also receives
inhibitory projections from the GPi, SNr and striatum. Another source of excitatory input to
the STN is the centromedian-parafascicular nucleus of the thalamus. Furthermore,
glutamatergic and cholinergic projections arise from the pedunculopontine nucleus to the
STN. Besides the main glutamatergic and GABA-ergic afferents to the STN, dopaminergic
neurons from the SNc also innervate the STN (Campbell et al., 1985; Canteras et al., 1990;

Hassani et al., 1996). These neurons modulate the activity of glutamatergic and GABA-ergic afferents arising from respectively the cortex and the pallidum to the STN. In addition, the STN receives serotonergic projections from the dorsal raphe nucleus which may also be involved in the modulation of the STN activity (Blandini et al., 2000; Hamani et al., 2004; DeLong & Wichmann, 2007). In this chapter, the importance of the dopaminergic input from the SNc to the STN will be described.

3. Dopamine receptors in the subthalamic nucleus

Because of their relevance in Parkinson's disease, large research efforts have been made to investigate the presence and localisation of dopamine receptors in the central nervous system, especially since the mid to late eighties (Wamsley et al., 1989). These receptors consist of a large family of D1-like dopamine receptors, divided into D1 and D5 receptors, and D2-like dopamine receptors, divided into D2, D3 and D4 receptors (Niznik, 1987; Niznik et al., 1992; Sibley et al., 1992; Gingrich et al., 1993). In general, D1 receptors are known to be positively coupled to adenylatecyclase via a Gs protein, whereas D2 receptors are either uncoupled or negatively coupled to adenylatecyclase (Onali et al., 1985; Memo et al., 1986). Both the D1-like and the D2-like dopamine receptors are known to be abundantly expressed and widely distributed throughout different basal ganglia nuclei. A series of experimental studies indicate that functional dopamine receptors are expressed and localised in the STN but there is still debate concerning the receptor subtypes.

The occurance of D1 receptors in the STN has been reported in a number of histological studies (Brown et al., 1979; Dubois et al., 1986; Fremeau et al., 1991; Mansour et al., 1992). However, Johnson et al. reported that D1 receptors are not located within the borders of the STN but are situated in the cerebral peduncles (Johnson et al., 1994). By means of autoradiography in rats, Kreiss et al. confirmed the presence of D1 dopamine receptors along the ventral edge of the STN which borders the cerebral peduncle. This was confirmed in a morphological study showing that the dendrites of STN neurons extend across the ventral STN borders into the peduncles (Kita et al., 1983). D1 receptors were not observed in the dorsal regions of the STN (Kreiss et al., 1996). Another autoradiographic study confirmed the presence of D1 receptors in the STN and found that there was a clear dorsoventral gradient in D1 binding sites at the level of the STN (Flores et al., 1999). Dopamine D2 receptors have also been shown to be present at the level of the rat STN by several groups (Boyson et al., 1986; Bouthenet et al., 1987; Johnson et al., 1994). Flores et al. were able to show the presence of all three subtypes of the D2-like receptors, although the amounts of D3 dopamine receptors were very low (Flores et al., 1999). However, no dopamine D1, D2, D3 nor D4 mRNA was detected by several investigators in both rat and human STN (Fremeau et al., 1991; Mansour et al., 1992; Augood et al., 2000). Nevertheless, Bouthenet et al. showed the presence of both D2 and D3 mRNA at the level of the STN with in situ histochemistry (Bouthenet et al., 1991). Moreover, using reverse transcriptase polymerase chain reaction the presence of D1 receptor mRNA was confirmed (Flores et al., 1999), together with the expression of the mRNA encoding for D2 and D3 receptors. By means of in situ hybridisation, high levels of D5 dopamine receptor mRNA were found at the level of the STN (Svenningson & Le Moine, 2002). However, they were unable to detect mRNA levels for all other dopamine receptor subtypes. Baufreton et al. also showed the presence of D5 dopamine receptors on burst competent STN neurons with single-cell reverse transcription-PCR profiling. They also used an antibody raised against a peptide sequence of cloned D5 receptor and detected immunoreactivity in the STN cell bodies (Baufreton et al., 2003).

Dopaminergic Control of the Neurotransmitter Release in the Subthalamic Nucleus: Implications for
Parkinson's Disease Treatment Strategies

89

Thus, using an array of techniques, all dopamine receptor subtypes have been detected in STN. However, the data remain inconsistent and more research is warranted.

4. Role of dopamine at the level of the subthalamic nucleus

Numerous studies in the past have suggested a direct role of dopamine and its receptor ligands at the level of the STN. As described above, the presence of both D1- and D2-like dopamine receptors in the STN has been demonstrated. Several anatomical studies provided evidence for a direct and substantial nigrosubthalamic dopaminergic projection in rats (Campbell et al., 1985; Canteras et al., 1990; Hassani et al., 1996). Moreover, we and others have shown that dopamine is released within the STN in vivo (Cragg et al., 2004; Ampe et al., 2007). However, despite numerous investigations, many discrepancies still exist with regard to the effect of dopamine and its receptor agonists on the activity of STN neurons. In the classical model of the basal ganglia motorloop, dopamine is widely assumed to exert an inhibitory influence on STN neuronal activity (Albin et al., 1995) and dopamine should reduce excitability of STN neurons in parkinsonian brain (DeLong, 1990; Bergman et al., 1994). A variety of in vitro an in vivo experimental studies have addressed this issue.

Several in vitro electrophysiological studies have shown inhibitory effects of dopamine on STN neuronal activity (Campbell et al., 1985; Hassani et al., 1999). However, others have found dopaminergic agonists to excite the activity of STN neurons. Indeed, Zhu et al. (2002a) showed that a dopamine bath application significantly increased the firing rates of STN neurons in a concentration-dependent fashion in both intact and 6-hydroxydopamine (6-OHDA) lesioned rats. They also showed that this excitatory effect of dopamine was largely mimicked by application of the dopamine D2 receptor agonist quinpirole. The dopamine D1 receptor agonist SKF-38393 showed a trend towards an increase in STN firing rate, but this effect was only significant in the 6-OHDA lesioned group. They concluded that dopamine exerts an excitatory influence on STN neuronal activity and that this effect is likely to be established by stimulation of D2 receptors. They also observed that dopamine, in 6-OHDA lesioned rats, in addition to the firing rates, also changes the irregular firing pattern into a more regular pacemaker pattern at the level of the STN (Zhu et al., 2002a). The same group also demonstrated that dopamine increases the firing rates of action potentials and produces inward currents in STN neurons. Together with the fact that these inward currents persisted when excitatory synaptic transmission was blocked, illustrated that dopamine exerted a direct excitatory effect at the level of the STN (Zhu et al., 2002b). In another in vitro electrophysiological study, Tofighy et al. (2003) showed that dopamine caused modest, but reliable, increases in the firing rates of STN neurons and considered this effect likely to be a direct excitatory action on STN neurons. The dopamine D2 receptor agonists quinpirole and bromocriptine caused concentration-dependent increases in the firing rates of STN neurons, whereas the mixed dopamine D1/D2 receptor agonist apomorphine caused only weak and less reproducible responses in STN firing rates. The dopamine D1 receptor agonist, SKF 38393 was without effect on STN firing rates. These results initially suggested an excitatory effect of dopamine on the STN neurons through a direct D2 receptor mediated mechanism. However, due to the fact that the effective concentration of all agonists was high, the authors stated that the effects could well be non-specific. This, together with the inconsistent effects of apomorphine and the inability of dopamine D2 (nor D1) receptor antagonists to reduce the observed excitatory effects led the authors to conclude that these effects probably cannot be assigned to dopamine receptors but to non-catecholaminergic receptors (Tofighy et al., 2003). Baufreton et al., by means of in vitro electrophysiological recordings, showed that activating D1 and D2 dopamine receptors with D1 and D2 agonists promotes pace making at the level of the STN by increasing the firing frequency of neurons that exhibit tonic firing capacity and by changing firing in burst-competent and spontaneously burst-firing neurons. Moreover, they also showed that D5 dopamine receptors may potentiate burst-firing in STN neurons by modulating L-type calcium channels in the absence of dopamine (Baufreton et al., 2003; Baufreton et al., 2005). Finally, Loucif et al. showed that dopamine clearly produces subthalamic membrane depolarisation leading towards an increase in firing rate. This effect seemed to be due to action on D1-like dopamine receptor mediated activation of a cyclic-nucleotide gated non-specific cation conductance. This conductance also contributed to the membrane depolarisation changing STN neuronal bursting towards a regular activity (Loucif et al., 2008). Thus, in vitro studies suggest that dopamine at the level of the STN exerts excitatory effects, possibly via D2 receptors. More recent studies, however, suggest D1-like mediated effects.

Several in vivo studies showed an inhibitory effect of dopamine on the activity of STN neurons. Campbell et al., using horseradish peroxidase and microiontophoresis, suggested that dopamine suppresses STN activity (Campbell et al., 1985). Injection of the mixed D1/D2 agonist apomorphine into the STN of intact rats decreased the mean firing rates of STN neurons significantly. However, an increase of firing rates was observed in 6-OHDA lesioned rats (Hassani et al., 1999). The selective D1 dopamine receptor agonist SKF 82958, when injected into the STN, decreased the activity of STN neurons in both intact and 6-OHDA lesioned rats. Injection of the selective D2 dopamine receptor agonist quinpirole decreased the firing rate of STN neurons, whereas in 6-OHDA lesioned animals it significantly increased firing rates. Hassani and colleagues concluded that dopamine receptor agonists probably have an inhibitory effect on STN neurons of intact rats via a D1 dopamine receptor mediated mechanism, whereas in 6-OHDA lesioned animals dopamine receptor agonists stimulate the STN via D2 dopamine receptors and inhibit activity via D1 dopamine receptors (Hassani et al., 1999). On the other hand, several other in vivo studies suggested a facilitatory effect of dopamine at the level of the STN. Glucose utilization was decreased in the STN following systemic administration of the dopamine D1 receptor antagonist SCH23390 (Trugman et al., 1993) whereas it was increased following systemic administration of the mixed D1/D2 dopamine receptor agonist apomorphine or following amphetamine (Brown et al., 1978; Wechsler et al., 1979; Trugman et al., 1993). Kreiss et al. described predominantly D1 mediated excitatory effects since neuronal firing rates in the STN of intact rats was increased following a systemic administration of apomorphine. Systemic administration of the dopamine D2 receptor agonist quinpirole did not alter STN firing rates, whereas the dopamine D1 receptor agonists SKF 38393 and SKF 82958 clearly increased STN firing rates. Local administration of the dopamine D1 receptor agonist SKF 82958 also increased firing rates (Kreiss et al, 1996). Using microiontophoresis, a clear excitatory effect of dopamine on the majority of STN neurons in both intact and 6-OHDA lesioned rats was observed (Ni et al., 2001). The excitatory effect of dopamine in the 6-OHDA lesioned rats was similar to that in intact rats. Their results were in good agreement with previous studies using the same technique also showing that dopamine induced an increase in firing rate of almost all STN neurons of intact rats (Mintz et al, 1986). Selective dopamine depletion by injection of 6-OHDA in the STN resulted in a clear decrease of the firing rate together with a change in firing pattern, reinforcing the evidence of an excitatory effect of dopamine at the level of the STN (Ni et al. 2001). Finally, we were the first to study the in vivo release of dopamine and glutamate in the STN using in vivo microdialysis (Ampe et al., 2007). We were able to establish that perfusion of the STN with NMDA enhanced dopamine and glutamate release in a concentration dependent manner. We

Dopaminergic Control of the Neurotransmitter Release in the Subthalamic Nucleus: Implications for
Parkinson's Disease Treatment Strategies

91

showed that this release was dependent on both D1 and D2 receptors since the NMDA-mediated effects were blocked by local perfusion of both the dopamine D1 receptor antagonist SCH 23390 and the dopamine D2 receptor antagonist raclopride, confirming the presence of this type of receptors in the STN. The importance of the dopaminergic innervation to the STN in these effects was demonstrated by the fact that depletion of dopamine by 6-OHDA lesioning of the SNc resulted in an absence of the effects of NMDA in the STN (Ampe et al., 2007). More recently, we showed that perfusion of the STN with dopamine or its D1 receptor agonist SKF38393 results in excitation of the STN since extracellular glutamate is increased. Again, 6-OHDA lesioning abolished these effects (Ampe et al., submitted elsewhere). Taken together, the majority of the available in vivo data clearly suggest an excitatory effect of dopamine on STN neurons that is mediated via dopamine D1 receptors.

	Intact		6-OHDA	
	STN inhibition	**STN activation**	**STN inhibition**	**STN activation**
In Vitro	**DA** *Campbell et al., 1985* *Hassani et al., 1999*	**DA** *Zhu et al., 2002a* *Zhu et al., 2002b* **D2 - quinpirole** *Zhu et al., 2002a* *Tofighy et al., 2003* **D1/D5-** **SKF82958;SKF** **81297** *Baufreton et al., 2003*		**DA** *Zhu et al., 2002b* **D2 - quinpirole** *Zhu et al., 2002a* *Baufreton et al.,* *2005* **D1/D5-** **SKF38393 ;** **SKF82958;** **SKF 81297** *Baufreton et al.,* *2005* *Loucif et al, 2008*
In Vivo	**DA** *Campbell et al., 1985* **amphetamine** *Welchsler et al.,1979* **D1/D2 -** **apomorphine** *Brown et al., 1978* *Hassani et al., 1999* **D1/D5 – SKF82958** *Hassani et al., 1999* **D2 - quinpirole** *Hassani et al., 1999*	**DA** *Mintz et al., 1986* *Ni et al., 2001* **D1/D2 -** **apomorphine** *Trugmann et al.,1993* *Kreiss et al., 1996* **D1/D5-SKF38393 ;** **SKF82958** *Ni et al., 2001* *Kreiss et al., 1996*	**D1/D5 – SKF82958** *Hassani et al., 1999*	**DA** *Ni et al., 2001* **D2 - quinpirole** *Hassani et al., 1999* *Ni et al., 2001* **D1/D5-SKF38393** *Ni et al., 2001*

Table 1. Overview of different publications regarding the effects of dopamine and its agonists on subthalamic activity in both intact and 6-OHDA lesioned rats.

5. Implications for Parkinson's disease treatment strategies

The existence of a direct nigrosubthalamic dopaminergic pathway is nowadays a well established fact. Moreover, dopamine receptors of both D1 and D2 like families have been shown to be present at the level of the STN. Otheiatal level, it is now clear that dopamine exerts direct effects at the level of other basal ganglia nuclei of which the STN plays a pivotal role in Parkinson's disease. Since altered neuronal output from the STN plays a central role in the pathophysiology of Parkinson's disease and overactivity of subthalamic neurons due to the loss of dopaminergic neurons contributes to increased excitation of the main output nuclei, effects of dopaminergic drugs (still the main drug treatment for Parkinson's disease) on subthalamic neuronal activity is highly important. It has been shown in different studies that dopamine and its agonists can alter subthalamic activity in both intact and parkinsonian animals. However, discrepancies still exist regarding the effects of dopaminergic stimulation. In the pathological state, most in vitro and in vivo studies agree on an excitatory effect of dopamine at the subthalamic level. Surprisingly, this opposes the current hypothesis that dopamine receptor stimulation alleviates symptoms of Parkinson's disease by reducing STN output (DeLong, 1990). The receptor subtypes by which dopamine exerts these excitatory effects differ between studies and different effects are seen depending on the receptor subtype. Moreover, not only effects on firing rates but also effects on subthalamic firing patterns were seen after dopamine application, further strengthening the hypothesis that dopamine clearly alters neuronal output at the subthalamic level. Dopamine replacement therapy remains the standard therapy for Parkinson's disease. Most of the dopamine agonists used to treat the symptoms of Parkinson's disease are non-specific for one or the other receptor subtype. We also know that after the so-called "honeymoon period" the effective response to dopamine wears off, and that undesirable side effects, like dyskinesia, occur. Further investigation towards an even better understanding of the effects of dopamine at the subthalamic level, and the receptor subtypes involved in these effects, can lead towards the development of better targeted drugs for the treatment of Parkinson's disease. Therefore, future studies investigating the effects of selective ligands of different dopamine receptor subtypes in experimental Parkinson's disease models, combining investigation towards electrophysiological effects and effects on neurotransmitter release of these ligands at the level of the STN, are necessary for developing more specific and selective drugs to treat different stages of Parkinson's disease.

6. References

Albin, R.L.; Young, A.B. & Penney, J.B. (1989). The functional anatomy of basal ganglia disorders. *Trends in neurosciences*, Vol.12, No.10, (October 1989), pp. 366-75, ISSN 0166-2236

Albin, R.L.; Young, A.B. & Penney, J. B. (1995). The functional anatomy of disorders of the basal ganglia. *Trends in neurosciences*, Vol.18, No.2, (February 1995), pp. 63-4, ISSN 0166-2236

Alexander, G.E.; Crutcher, M.D. & DeLong, M.R. (1990). Basal ganglia-thalamocortical circuits: parallel substrates for motor, oculomotor, "prefrontal" and "limbic" functions. *Progress in brain research*, Vol.85, (1990), pp. 119-46, ISSN 0079-6123

Ampe, B.; Massie, A.; D'Haens, J.; Ebinger, G.; Michotte, Y. & Sarre, S. (2007). NMDA-mediated release of glutamate and GABA in the subthalamic nucleus is mediated by dopamine: an in vivo microdialysis study in rats. *Journal of neurochemistry*, Vol.103, No.3, (November 2007), pp. 1063-74, ISSN 0022-3042

Augood, S.J.; Hollingsworth, Z.R.; Standaert, D.G.; Emson, P.C. & Penney, J.B. Jr. (2000). Localization of dopaminergic markers in the human subthalamic nucleus. *The Journal of comparative neurology*, Vol.421, No.2, (May 2000), pp. 247-55., ISSN 0021-9967

Dopaminergic Control of the Neurotransmitter Release in the Subthalamic Nucleus: Implications for
Parkinson's Disease Treatment Strategies

93

Baufreton, J.; Garret, M.; Rivera, A.; de la Calle, A.; Gonon, F.; Dufy, B.; Bioulac, B. &
Taupignon, A.L. (2003). A D5 (not D1) dopamine receptors potentiate burst-firing
in neurones of the subthalamic nucleus by modulating an L-type calcium
conductance. *Journal of Neuroscience*, Vol.23, No.3, (February 2003), pp. 816–825,
ISSN 0270-6474

Baufreton, J.; Zhu, Z.T.; Garret, M.; Bioulac, B.; Johnson, S.W. & Taupignon, A.L. (2005).
Dopamine receptors set the pattern of activity generated in subthalamic neurons.
The FASEB Journal, Vol.19, No.13, (November 2005), pp. 1771-7, ISSN 0892-6638

Benarroch, E.E. (2008). Subthalamic nucleus and its connections: Anatomic substrate for the
network effects of deep brain stimulation. *Neurology*, Vol.70, No.21, (May 2008), pp.
1991-5, ISSN 0028-3878

Benazzouz, A.; Gross, C.; Féger, J.; Boraud, T. & Bioulac, B. (1993). Reversal of rigidity and
improvement in motor performance by subthalamic high-frequency stimulation in
MPTP-treated monkeys. *The European journal of neuroscience*, Vol.5, No.4, (April
1993), pp. 382-9, ISSN 0953-816X

Benazzouz, A.; Piallat, B.; Ni, Z.G.; Koudsie, A.; Pollak, P. & Benabid, A.L. (2000)
Implication of the subthalamic nucleus in the pathophysiology and pathogenesis of
Parkinson's disease. *Cell Transplant 9*, 215-221, 0963-6897.

Bergman, H.; Wichmann, T. & DeLong, M.R. (1990). Reversal of experimental parkinsonism
by lesions of the subthalamic nucleus. *Science*, Vol.249, No.4975, (September 1990),
pp. 1436-8, ISSN 0036-8075

Bergman, H.; Wichmann, T.; Karmon, B. & DeLong, M.R. (1994). The primate subthalamic
nucleus. II. Neuronal activity in the MPTP model of parkinsonism. *Journal of
neurophysiology*, Vol.72, No.2, (August 1994), pp. 507–20, ISSN 0022-3077

Bouthenet, M.L.; Matres, M.P.; Sales, N. & Schwartz, J.C. (1987). A detailed mapping of
dopamine D2 receptors in rat central nervous system by autoradiography with
(125I)iodosulpiride. *Neuroscience*, Vol.20, No. 1, (January 1987), pp. 117-55, ISSN
0306-4522

Bouthenet, M.L.; Souil, E.; Matres, M.P.; Sokoloff, P.; Giros, B. & Schwartz, J.C. (1991).
Localisation of dopamine D3 receptor mRNA in the rat brain using in situ
histochemistry: comparison with dopamine D2 receptor mRNA. *Brain research*, Vol.
564, No.2, (November 1991), pp. 203-19, ISSN:0006-8993

Boyson, S.J.; McGonigle, P. & Molinoff, P.B. (1986). Quantitative autoradiographic
localization of the D1 and D2 subtypes of dopamine receptors in rat brain. *The
Journal of neuroscience*, Vol. 6, No.11, (November 1986), pp. 3177-88, ISSN 0270-6474

Blandini, F.; Nappi, G.; Tassorelli, C. & Martignoni, E. (2000). Functional changes of the
basal ganglia circuitry in Parkinson's disease. *Progress in neurobiology*, Vol.62, No.1,
(September 2000), pp. 63-88, ISSN 0555-4047

Brown, L.L. & Wolfson, L.I. (1978). Apomorphine increases glucose utilization in the
substantia nigra, subthalamic nucleus, and corpus striatum of rat. *Brain research*,
Vol.140, No.1, (January 1978), pp. 188-93, ISSN 0006-8993

Brown, L.L.; Maakman, M.H.; Wolfson, L.I.; Dvorkin, B.; Warner C. & Katzman, R. (1979). A
direct role of dopamine in the rat subthalamic nucleus and an adjacent
intrapeduncular area. *Science*, Vol.206, No.4425, (December 1979), pp. 1416-8, ISSN
0036-8075

Campbell, G.A.; Eckardt, M.J. & Weight, F.F. (1985). Dopaminergic mechanisms in the
subthalamic nucleus of rat: analysis using horseradish peroxidase and

microiontophoresis. *Brain Research,* Vol.333, No.2, (May 1985), pp. 261-70, ISSN 0006-8993

Canteras, N.S.; Shammah-Lagnado, S.J.; Silva, B.A. & Ricardo, J.A. (1990). Afferent connections of the subthalamic nucleus: a combined retrograde and anterograde horseradish peroxidase study in the rat. *Brain Research,* Vol.513, No.1, (April 1990), pp. 43-59, ISSN 0006-8993

Cragg, S.J.; Baufreton, J.; Xue, Y.;Bolam, J.P. & Bevan, M.D. (2004). Synaptic release of dopamine in the subthalamic nucleus. *European Journal of Neuroscience,* Vol.20, No.7, (October 2004), pp. 1788-802, ISSN 0953-816X

DeLong, M.R. (1990). Primate models of movement disorders of basal ganglia origin. *Trends in Neuroscience,* Vol.13, No.7, (July 1990), pp. 281-5, ISSN 0166-2236

DeLong, M.R. & Wichmann, T. (2007). Circuits and circuit disorders of the basal ganglia. *Archives of neurology,* Vol.64, No.1, (January 2007), pp. 20-4, ISSN 0003-9942

Dubois, A.; Savasta, M.; Curet, O. & Scatton, B. (1986). Autoradiographic distribution of the D1 agonist (3H)SKF38393 in the rat brain and spinal cord. Comparison with the distribution of D2 receptors. *Neuroscience,* Vol.19, No.1, (September 1986), pp. 125-37, ISSN 0306-4522

Flores, G.; Liang, J.J.; Sierra, A.; Martinez-Fong, D.; Quiron, R.; Aceves, J. & Srivastava, L.K. (1999). Expression of dopamine receptors in the subthalamic nucleus of the rat: characterisation using reverse transcriptase-polymerase chain reaction and autoradiography. *Neuroscience,* Vol.91, No.2, (1999), pp. 549-56, ISSN 0306-4522

Fremeau, R.T.; Duncan, G.E.; Fornaretto, M.G; Dearry, A.; Gingrich, J.A.; Breese, G.R. & Caron, M.G. (1991). Localization of D1 dopamine receptor mRNA in brain supports a role in cognitive, affective and neuroendocrine aspects of dopaminergic neurotransmission. *Proceedings of the National Academy of Sciences of the United States of America,* Vol.88, No.9, (May 1991), pp. 3772-6, ISSN 0027-8424

Gingrich, J.A. and Caron, M.G. (1993). Recent advances in the molecular biology of dopamine receptors. *Annual review of neuroscience,* Vol.16, (1993), pp. 299-321, ISSN 0147-006X

Gubellini, P.; Salin, P.; Kerkerian-Le Goff, L. & Baunez, C. (2009). Deep brain stimulation in neurological diseases and experimental models: from molecule to complex behavior. *Progress in neurobiology,* Vol.89, No.1, (September 2009), pp. 79-123, ISSN 0555-4047

Haegelen, C.; Rouaud, T.; Darnault, P. & Morandi, X. (2009). The subthalamic nucleus is a key-structure of limbic basal ganglia functions. *Medical hypotheses,* Vol.72, No.4, (April 2009), pp. 421-6, ISSN 0306-9877

Hamani, C.; Saint-Cyr, JA.; Fraser, J.; Kaplitt, M. & Lozano, AM. (2004). The subthalamic nucleus in the context of movement disorders. *Brain,* Vol.127, No. 1, (January 2004), pp. 4-20, ISSN 0006-8950

Hassani, O.K.; Mouroux, M. & Féger, J. (1996). Increased subthalamic neuronal activity after nigral dopaminergic lesion independent of disinhibition via the globus pallidus. *Neuroscience,* Vol.72, No.1, (May 1996), pp. 105-15, ISSN 0306-4522

Hassani, O.K.; Francois, C.; Yelnik, J.; Féger J. (1997) Evidence for a dopaminergic innervation of the subthalamic nucleus in the rat. *Brain Res.* 749, 88-94, ISSN 0006-8993.

Hassani, O.K. & Féger, J. (1999). Effects of intra-subthalamic injection of dopamine receptor agonists on subthalamic neurones in normal and 6-hydroxydopamine lesioned rats:

Dopaminergic Control of the Neurotransmitter Release in the Subthalamic Nucleus: Implications for
Parkinson's Disease Treatment Strategies

95

an electrophysiological and C-Fos study. *Neuroscience,* Vol.92, No.2, (1999), pp. 533-43, ISSN 0306-4522

Johnson, A.E; Coirini, H.; Kallstrom, L. & Wiesel, F.A. (1994). Characterization of dopamine receptor binding sites in the subthalamic nucleus. *Neuroreport,* Vol.5, No.14, (September 1994), pp. 1836-8, ISSN 0959-4965

Kita, H.; Chang, H.T. & Kitai, S.T. (1983). The morphology of intracellulary labeled rat subthalamic neurons; a light microscopic analysis. *The Journal of comparative neurology,* Vol.215, No.3, (April 1983), pp. 245-57, ISSN 0021-9967

Kreiss, D.S.; Anderson, L.A. & Walters, J.R. (1996). Apomorphine and dopamine D(1) receptor agonists increase the firing rates of subthalamic nucleus neurons. *Neuroscience,* Vol.72, No.3, (June 1996), pp. 863-76, ISSN 0306-4522

Levy, R.; Hazrati, L.N.; Herrero, M.T.; Vila, M.; Hassani, O.K.; Mouroux, M.; Ruberg, M.; Asensi, H.; Agid, Y.; Féger, J.; Obeso, J.A.; Parent, A. & Hirsch, E.C. (1997). Re-evaluation of the functional anatomy of the basal ganglia in normal and Parkinsonian states. *Neuroscience,* Vol.76, No.2, (January 1997), pp. 335-43, ISSN 0306-4522

Loucif, A.J.; Woodhall, G.L.; Sehirli, U.S.; Stanford, I.M. (2008). Depolarisation and suppression of burst activity in the mouse subthalamic nucleus by dopamine D1/D5 receptor activation of a cyclic-nucleotide gated non-specific cation conductance. *Neuropharmacology,* Vol. 55, No.1 (July 2008), pp. 94-105, ISSN 0028-3908

Mansour, A.; Meador-Woodruff, J.H.; Zhou, Q.; Civello, O.; Akil, H. & Watson, S.J. (1992). A comparison of D1 receptor binding and mRNA in rat brain using receptor autoradiography and in situ hybridization techniques. *Neuroscience,* Vol.46, No.4, (1992), pp. 959-71, ISSN 0306-4522

Memo, M.; Missale, C.; Carruba, M.O. & Spano, P.F. (1986). D2 dopamine receptors associated with inhibition of dopamine release from rat neostriatum are independent of cyclic AMP. *Neuroscience letters,* Vol.71, No.2, (November 1986), pp. 192-6, ISSN 0304-3940

Mintz, I.; Hammond, C. & Féger, J. (1986). Excitatory effect of iontophoretically applied dopamine on identified neurones of the rat subthalamic nucleus. *Brain Research,* Vol.375, No.1, (June 1986), pp. 172-5, ISSN 0006-8993

Ni, Z.G.; Gao, D.M.; Bouali-Benazzouz, R.; Benabid, A.L. & Benazzouz, A. (2001). Effect of microionotophoretic application of dopamine on subthalamic nucleus neuronal activity in normal rats and in rats with unilateral lesion of the nigrostriatal pathway. *European Journal of Neuroscience,* Vol.14, No.2, (July 2001), pp. 373-81, ISSN 0953-816X

Niznik, H.B. (1987). Dopamine receptors: molecular structure and function. *Molecular and cellular endocrinology,* Vol.54, No.1, (November 1987), pp. 1-22, ISSN 0303-7207

Niznik, H.B. & Van Tol, H.H. (1992). Dopamine receptor genes: new tools for molecular psychiatry. *Journal of psychiatry & neuroscience : JPN,* Vol.17, No.4, (October 1992), pp. 158-80, ISSN 1180-4882

Obeso, J.A.; Rodríguez-Oroz, M.C.; Benitez-Temino, B.; Blesa, F.J.; Guridi, J.; Marin, C. & Rodriguez, M. (2008). Functional organization of the basal ganglia: therapeutic implications for Parkinson's disease. *Movement disorders : official journal of the Movement Disorder Society,* Vol.23, No.3, (2008), pp. 548-59, ISSN 0885-3185

Onali, P.; Olianas, M.C. and Gessa, G.L. (1985). Characterization of dopamine receptors mediating inhibition of adenylatecyclase in rat striatum. *Molecular pharmacology*, Vol.28, No.2, (August 1985), pp. 138-45, ISSN 0026-895X

Parent, A. & Hazrati, L.N. (1995). Functional anatomy of the basal ganglia. II. The place of subthalamic nucleus and external pallidum in basal ganglia circuitry. *Brain research reviews*, Vol.20, No.1, (January 1995), pp. 128-54, ISSN 0165-0173

Pollak, P.; Benabid, A.L.; Gervason, C.L.; Hoffmann, D.; Seigneuret, E. & Perret, J. (1993). Long-term effects of chronic stimulation of the ventral intermediate thalamic nucleus in different types of tremor. *Advances in neurology*, Vol.60, (1993), pp. 408-13, ISSN 0091-3952

Sibley, D.R. & Monsma, F.J. Jr. (1992). Molecular biology of dopamine receptors. *Trends in pharmacological sciences*, Vol.13, No.2, (February 1992), pp. 61-9, ISSN 0165-6147

Smith, Y. & Parent, A. (1988). Neurons of the subthalamic nucleus in primates display glutamate but not GABA immunoreactivity. *Brain research*, Vol.453, No.1-2, (June 1988), pp. 353-6, ISSN 0006-8993

Smith, Y.; Hazrati, L.N. & Parent, A. (1990). Efferent projections of the subthalamic nucleus in the squirrel monkey as studied by the PHA-L anterograde tracing method. *The Journal of comparative neurology*, Vol.294, No.2, (April 1990), pp. 306-23, ISSN 0021-9967

Smith, Y.; Bevan, M.D.; Shink, E. & Bolam, J.P. (1998). Microcircuitry of the direct and indirect pathways of the basal ganglia. *Neuroscience*, Vol.86, No.2, (September 1998), pp. 353-87, ISSN 0306-4522

Svenningsson, P. & Le Moine, C. (2002). Dopamine D1/5 receptor stimulation induces c-fos expression in the subthalamic nucleus: possible involvement of local D5 receptors. *The European journal of neuroscience*, Vol.15, No.1, (January 2002), pp. 133-42, ISSN 0953-816X

Tofighy, A.; Abbott, A.; Centonze, D.; Cooper, A.J.; Noor, E.; Pearce, S.M.; Puntis, M.; Stanford, I.M.; Wigmore, M.A. & Lacey, M.G. (2003). Excitation by dopamine of rat subthalamic nucleus neurones in vitro – a direct action with unconventional pharmacology. *Neuroscience*, Vol.116, No.1, (2003), pp. 157-66, ISSN 0306-4522

Trugman, J.M. and James, C.L. (1993). D1 dopamine agonist and antagonist effects on regional cerebral glucose utilization in rats with intact dopaminergic innervation. *Brain research*, Vol.607, No.1-2, (April 1993), pp. 270-4, ISSN 0006-8993

Wamsley, J.K.; Gehrelt, D.R.; Filloux, F.M. & Dawson, T.M. (1989). Comparison of the distribution of D1 and D2 dopamine receptors in the rat brain. *Journal of chemical neuroanatomy*, Vol.2, No.3, (May-June 1989), pp. 119-37, ISSN 0891-0618

Wechsler, L.R.; Savaki, H.E. & Sokoloff, L. (1979). Effects of D-and L-amphetamine on local cerebral glucose utilization in the conscious rat. *Journal of neurochemistry*, Vol.32, No.1, (January 1979), pp. 15-22, ISSN 0022-3042

Zhu, Z.; Bartol, M.; Shen, K. & Johnson, S.W. (2002a). Excitatory effects of dopamine on subthalamic nucleus neurones: in vitro study of rats pretreated with 6-hydroxydopamine and levodopa. *Brain Research*, Vol.945, No.1, (July 2002), pp. 31-40, ISSN 0006-8993

Zhu, Z.T.; Shen, K.Z. & Johnson, S.W. (2002b). Pharmacological identification of inward current evoked by dopamine in rat subthalamic neurones in vitro. *Neuropharmacology*, Vol.42, No.6, (May 2002), pp. 772-81, ISSN 0028-3908

6

Role of Lysosomal Enzymes in Parkinson's Disease: Lesson from Gaucher's Disease

Tommaso Beccari et al.*
*Dipartimento di SEEA, Università di Perugia,
Italy*

1. Introduction

The lysosome, initially discovered by Christian de Duve in 1955, is an intracellular organelle responsible of the ordered degradation of proteins, glycoproteins, proteoglycans, lipids, and other macromolecules originated from autophagy, endocytosis and phagocytosis. It is characterize by a limiting external membrane containing intraluminal vesicles. These organelles are estimated to contain 50-60 soluble acidic hydrolases (Journet et al., 2002), 55 membrane-associated proteins and 215 integral membrane proteins (Bagshaw et al., 2005). The macromolecules are scomposed by acid hydrolases in small molecules that are transported back in the cytosol by specific transporter proteins and then catabolized or re-used by anabolic processes. Lysosomal hydrolases are synthetized as N-glycosylated precursors in the endoplasmatic reticulum and are transported to the lysosomes via a vectorial transport dependent on mannose 6-phosphate. Lysosomes are involved in many cellular processes like cholesterol homeostasis, autophagy, membrane repair, pathogen defense, cell signaling, apoptosys and bone/tissue remodelling; it is a fundamental organelle for cell life and not only the wastebasket of the cell. Microscopic identification of lysosomes is hard due to heterogeneity of organelles morphology dependent on their function as digestive organelles. The size and quantity of lysosomes varies in different cell types and can increase when the lysosomes accumulate non-digested material. Functional deficit of hydrolases, membrane-associated or integral membrane proteins causes lysosomal storage disorders (LSDs), a group of inherited metabolic pathologies characterized by intralysosomal deposition of undegraded macromolecules and by multisystemic phenotype (Saftig, 2006). The absence or reduced activity of a specific lysosomal hydrolase or other lysosomal proteins cause an abnormal function of the entire endosomal/lysosomal system (Bellettato & Scarpa, 2010).

More than 50 lysosomal storage disorders (LSD) are known with a total incidence of 1:7,000-1:9,000 (Fletcher, 2006). Two thirds of them involve the central nervous system (Meikle et al.,

*Chiara Balducci[1], Silvia Paciotti[1], Emanuele Persichetti[1], Davide Chiasserini[2], Anna Castrioto[2], Nicola Tambasco[2], Aroldo Rossi[2], Paolo Calabresi[2], Veronica Pagliardini[3], Bruno Bembi[4] and Lucilla Parnetti[2]
[1]Dipartimento di SEEA, Università di Perugia, Italy
[2]Clinica Neurologica, Ospedale S. Maria della Misericordia, Università di Perugia, Italy
[3]Dipartimento di Pediatria, Università di Torino, Italy
[4]Centro Regionale per le malattie Rare, Ospedale Universitario 'Santa Maria della Misericordia', Italy*

1999). The LSD can be classified in sphingolipidoses, mucopolysaccharidoses, mucolipidoses, lipid storage disease, glycogen storage disease type II and lysosomal transport defects. Different LSD displayed different symptoms severity and different age onset and it depend on the organs affected and the residual enzyme activity. Generally, mutation leaving very low residual enzyme activity cause the most severe onset form of the pathologies; contrary higher residual enzyme activity delays disease onset (Kolter & Sandhoff, 1999). The disease course and severity are different in late-onset forms and can be variable even among affected siblings in the same family (Zhao & Grabowski, 2002). LSDs are often multisystemic disorders and many of these displayed a severe, progressive and untreatable neurological impairment. Almost all LSDs are related to devastating, progressive and untreatable effects on central nervous system (CNS). Neuronal loss occurs in the advanced stages of the diseases and is due to apoptosis or necrosis. The neurological symptoms are mental retardation, progressive neurodegeneration, dementia. Most LSDs show CNS involvment althought the undegraded material concentration is lower in the brain than in other organs. It seems that neurons are more vulnerable than other cellular type probably for a limited cell regeneration potential or for the absence of compensatory pathways (Bellettato & Scarpa, 2010). The Neuronal Ceroid Lipofuscinoses (NCLs) are lysosomal storage diseases affecting the CNS, with progressive loss of vision, decreasing cognitive and motor skills, epileptic seizures and premature death, with dementia without visual loss prominent in the rarer adult forms (Kohan et al., 2011). GM1 type 3 Gangliosidosis is an autosomal recessive lysosomal storage disorder caused by β-galactosidase deficiency, patients were recently found to be affected by generalized dystonia associated to akinetic-rigid parkinsonism (Roze et al., 2005). The San Filippo Syndrome type B is a LSDs due to mutation in the gene encoding α-N-acetylglucosaminidase with an accumulation of heparan sulfate. Affected children shown mental retardation, dementia, behavior problems. The analysis of mutant mice showed cytoplasmic inclusion of P-tau aggregates, characteristic of tauopathies, a group of age-related dementia that include Alzheimer disease (Ohmi et al., 2009).

In some adult neurodegenerative disorders like Alzheimer's disease, Parkinson's disease and Huntington' s disease the clical features are similar to those found in LSDs: accumulation of undegraded material, abnormal inflammatory response in the brain and changes in neurons morphology and functionality (Bellettato et al., 2010). In Parkinson's disease was found an involvement of cathepsin D, a lysosomal enzyme, in α-synuclein degradation and formation of carboxy-terminally truncated α-synuclein. Recent works suggest that impaired cathepsin D activity would result in incresed a-synuclein levels that cause its aggregation (Sevlever et al., 2008). In Huntington's disease N-terminal mutant huntingtin fragments form inclusions that lead to cell death. Some protease, like cathepsin D, B and L, help to degrade mutant huntingtin but increase N-terminal fragment formation and inclusions deposition inducing neuronal disruption (Kim et al., 2006).

2. Gaucher's disease: An overview

Gaucher's disease (GD) is an inherited autosomal recessive metabolic disorder, resulting from a deficiency of the lysosomal enzyme β-glucocerebrosidase (also called acid β-glucosidase, GCase) (EC 3.2.1.45).

GD was first described as a systemic disease by Philippe Gaucher in 1882, but only in 1965 this disorder was related to the deficiency of β-glucocerebrosidase (Patrick, 1965; Brady et al.

1965). This enzyme is involved in the catabolic pathway of glycosphingolipids and is responsible for the cleavage of the β-glucosidic bond on the glucosylceramide (or glucocerebroside) (Fig. 1).

The human β-glucosidase is encoded by a gene (GBA) located on chromosome 1 (1q21) (Barneveld et al., 1983) which comprises 11 exons and 10 introns, spanning 7.6 kb of sequence. A non processed pseudogene (GBAP), which shares 96% exonic sequence homology, is located 16 kb downstream of the functional β-glucocerebrosidase gene (Horowitz et al., 1989).

The lack of GCase activity leads to accumulation of glycolipid substrates, primarily glucocerebroside and its nonacylated analog, glucosylsphingosine, in all organs, particularly in spleen, liver, lungs and bone marrow (Cox & Shofield, 1997; Beutler & Grabowski, 2001). The material stored is the product of the arrested breakdown of gangliosides, glycosphingolipids and globosides, which derived from the cellular turnover of membranes.

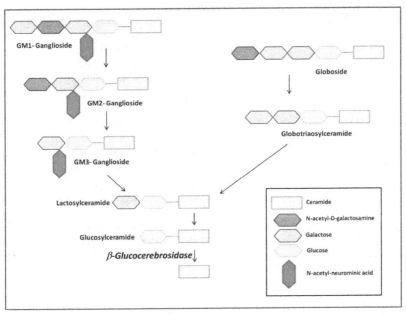

Fig. 1. Involvement β-glucocerebrosidase in the catabolic pathway of glycosphingolipids

Although in the patients the GCase is inactive in all cells, glucocerebroside accumulation occurs principally within the lysosomes of macrophages which adopt a characteristic "Gaucher's cell" morphology. Disease manifestations are related to the migration and accumulation of the Gaucher's cells, which displace healthy cells in the tissues. Furthermore the abnormal material stored in the cells of the reticuloendothelial system induces the release of inflammatory factors, including chemokines and cytokines, which leads to the cascade of pathological changes (Beutler & Grabowski, 2001; Cox, 2001; Aerts & Hollak, 1997; Moran et al., 2000; Jmoudiak & Futerman, 2005; Nilsson & Svennerhol, 1982; Pelled et al., 2005; Futerman & van Meer, 2004) (Table 1).

Gaucher's disease may occur at any age in any human population (Beutler & Grabowski, 2001; Zimran et al., 1992; Cox & Shofield, 1997; Erikson, 1986). Although the birth frequency of Gaucher's disease is one case per 60,000 live births in the general population (Meikle et al., 1999), it is the most frequent genetic disease in the Ashkenazi Jewish people where epidemiological data, based on estimated gene frequencies, show a prevalence of one case per 850 live births (Beutler et al., 1993).

GD has a highly variable phenotype, and even though a recent trend is to consider GD as a continuum of disease states (Goker-Alpan et al., 2003), three basic clinical forms are conventionally distinguished on the basis of the neurological involvement: the non neuronopathic form (type 1), the acutely neuronopathic form (type 2) and the subacute neurophatic form (type 3).

Products	Functions
Lysozyme	Antibacterial
Angiotensin-converting enzyme	Vasopressor
Lysosomal acid hydrolases	Digestion
Interleukin-1b, TNFa	Diverse host defence: fever, weight loss
Interleukin 6	Acute phase response, B-cell stimulation, bone resorption, trophic for mieloma cells
Interleukin 8	Granulocyte chemoattractant
Interleukin 10	Inhibits pro-inflammatory cytokines

Table 1. Macrophage secretory products icreased in Gaucher's disease

Type 1 GD (OMIM 230800) is the most frequent form of Gaucher's disease and account 94% of all registered cases according to Gaucher Registry. It is a chronic multisystem storage disorder which, by definition, does not involve the central nervous system. Nevertheless recent studies have shown a possible correlation between type 1 GD and some neurological manifestations (Sindransky, 2004; Cherin, 2006; Biegstraaten et al., 2008). In a number of cases these symptoms can be the consequence of secondary complications of the primary disease (e.g. compression of bone marrow or root nerve as a result of vertebral crush fractures caused by osteonecrosis), whereas in other ones they can be the product of specific GBA gene mutations, particularly in patients presenting parkinsonian syndromes (Aharon-Peretz et al., 2004; Bembi et al., 2003; Clark et al., 2005; Gan-Or et al., 2008; Machaczka et al., 1999; McKeran et al., 1985; Tayeby et al. 2003; Ziegler et al. 2007).

The type 1 GD course is slowly progressive. Generally the symptoms develop in adulthood even though various clinical manifestation may emerge in childhood. The clinical spectrum is vast and includes the complete absence of symptoms as well as the severe organ involvement with disability and occasionally fatal outcome. The patients show hepatosplenomegaly, with thrombocytopenia, anemia and leucopenia. Although in most patients these complications are not life-threatening and may go unrecognized for many years (some subjects remain asymptomatic up to the age of 70 or 80 years) (Berrebi et al., 1984), in other ones this metabolic defect can cause bruising, bleeding and high risk of infection as consequence of pancytopenia and respiratory insufficiency due to diffuse infiltration of Gaucher's cells into the alveolar spaces, perivascular, peribronchial, and into the septal regions (Schneider et al., 1977; Lee, 1982). Asthenia and fatigability are constant and seem independent of anemia, but rather to reflect an alteration of basal metabolism and cytokine secretion (Allen et al., 1997). Moreover degenerative changes in skeleton are the leading cause of bone pain and disability in patients with type 1 disease. The infiltration of Gaucher's cells in the bone marrow causes osteonecrosis, particularly during growth and leads to impaired function of large joints, including hip, knee, and shoulder. Other bone symptoms include local swelling (Gaucheromas) and osteolysis as well as generalized demineralization and osteoporosis with consequent risk of fractures. Furthermore patients may show abnormal diffuse yellow-brawn skin pigmentation and delays of growth, menarche and dentition. In rare cases there can be also renal involvement, pulmonary hypertension (Theise & Ursell, 1990), and cardiac abnormalities.

Type 2 (OMIM 230900) is the most severe form of Gaucher's disease which accounts for fewer than 1% cases. It manifests in early childhood; neurological deterioration progresses quickly and death generally occurs within the age of two years, in a context of psychomotor decline (Brady et al., 1993). The majority of cases of type 2 GD emerges around age of 3 months. The presenting sign is usually hepatosplenomegaly. By 6 months, neurologic complications develop. The first diagnostic simptoms are frequently supranuclear horizontal oculomotor paralysis or bilateral fixed strabismus accompanied by trismus, retroflection of the head, progressive spasticity, hyperreflexia, positive Babinski signs and other phatologic reflexes. Other symptoms can be dysphagia and difficulty in handling secretions developed, often followed by aspiration pneumonia. Death occurs by either apnea or aspiration pneumonia.

Gaucher's disease type 3 (OMIM 231000) is particularly frequent in Norbottnian Swedes (Erikson, 1986). It leads to subacute neurological symptoms that are less severe than those of type 2 disease. It is characterized by the presence of a later onset and a slow progressive neurological syndrome. The clinical manifestations vary. Systemic symptoms precede neurologic abnormalities and usually are similar to those seen in type 1 GD. Neurologic deterioration includes cerebellar ataxia, spastic paraperesis, psychomotor seizures, horizontal supranuclear ophthalmoplegia, myoclonic epilepsy and dementia.

Over 300 mutations of the β-glucosidase gene have been described (Beutler & Gelbart, 1996; Geabowski & Horowitz, 1997, Hruska et al., 2008). The most common are c.1226A>G (N370S), c.1448T>C (L444P), IVS2+1G>A and 84insG. The frequency and distribution of mutations vary with the population studied; in the Ashkenazi population N370S is found in 78% of patients whereas in non-Jewish populations the most frequent mutation is L444P (36%), followed by N370S (29%) (Beutler, 2006).

Although molecular analysis of the glucocerebrosidase gene in patients with Gaucher's disease has permitted broad correlations between genotype and phenotype, this does not consent a confident prediction of clinical phenotype (Cox & Sholfield, 1997; Germain, 2004). Many studies have shown the enormous clinical variation between patients who have the same genotype including monozygotic twins (Sidransky, 2004; Lachmann et al., 2004). Nevertheless the presence of N370S on one or both alleles is associated with type 1 GD and it seems to protect against neurological symptoms, except for Parkinson-like syndromes (Charrow et al., 2000; Cherin et al., 2006). On the contrary the presence of the L444P/L444P mutation is associated with the development of neurological manifestations, above all in Gaucher's disease type 3 (75% of cases) (Charrow et al., 2000). Other mutations, including 84insG, IVS2+1G>A, c.754T>A (F213I) and c.1297G>T (V394L), are generally responsible for the emergence of a neurological form, when associated with mutation L444P either alone or integrated in a complex allele.

3. Gaucher's and Parkinson's disease: Theories of a link

Parkinson's disease (PD) is the one of the common movement disorders and the second most common human neurodegenerative disease. The major diagnostic neuropathological features of the pathologiy are loss of dopaminergic neurons and the appearance of Lewy bodies (LB), which are intraneuronal inclusions composed by α-synuclein and abnormal ubiquitinated proteins aggregates.

The first associations of the glucocerebrosidase enzyme with parkinsonism were discovered through careful clinical observation of people affecting by GD, who in several cases developed Parkinson's disease. Although in recent years GBA mutations were found to be a major risk factor for the development of Parkinson's disease (Sidransky et al., 2009), it is not clear how these are related. However many findings suggest that GBA protein and α-synuclein are implicated in a common cellular pathway and different hypothesis have been created to explain the linkage between them.

Recent studies have shown as some mutations in the GBA gene can lead to the misfolded protein formation (Sawkar et al., 2005), contributing to parkinsonism by leading to lysosomal insufficiency, as a result of impairing autophagic pathways necessary to prevent the synucleopathies, or by crushing the ubiquitin-proteasome system.

During the life span of a protein, cellular systems continuously check on the quality of the protein and take care of its repair or removal from the cell if there is any abnormality. The advancement during the past decades in understanding the quality control system of cellular proteins has allowed the identification of unequivocal links between malfunctioning of these systems and some severe human pathologies, including major neurodegenerative disease as Parkinson's (PD) and Alzheimer's (AD).

Many newly synthesized proteins are incorrectly translated or wrongly folded as a result of errors in their sequence due to either genetic mutations or alterations during the synthesis process (Wheatley & Inglis, 1980; Vabulas & Hartl, 2005; Shubert et al., 2000; Yewdell, 2005). The role of protein catabolism in protecting cells from defective, misfolded proteins is essential to avoid the risk of long term accumulation of proteins which frequently develop abnormal intermolecular interaction, forming insoluble aggregates toxic for the cells (Squier, 2001; Kourie & Henry, 2001). So it is evident the involvement of the quality control system in maintaining cell homeostasis as well as the association between the alteration of the protein turnover and many disease states (Kundu & Thompson, 2008). The autophagy-lysosome and the ubiquitin-proteasome pathways are the two main routes of the quality control system in eukaryotic.

Autophagy-lysosomal degradation pathway is a complex system tightly regulated by series of signaling events that promote the efficient delivery of macronutrients and organelles to lysosomes for degradation by acidic hydrolases (Levine & Klionsky, 2004). It is implicated in the catabolism and recycling of long-lived proteins and organelles and it is thought to be involved in many physiological processes, including the response to starvation, cell growth control, antiaging mechanisms and innate immunity. Some years ago the authophagy-lysosome pathway was considered as a non selective form of catabolism, while now the view is changed and it is thought as a specialized system that distinguishes the substrates and chooses the route by which they reach the lysosomes. Three types of autophagy have been described: macroautophagy, microautophagy and chaperon mediated autophagy (CMA) (Cuervo, 2004). They share a common endpoint, the lysosome, but differ in substrates targeted, their regulation and the conditions in which each of them is preferentially activated.

Macroautophagy process is activated to generate essential macromolecules and energy in condition of nutritional scarcity (Mizushima, 2005) or as a mechanism to remove the altered intracellular components (Levine & Klionsky, 2004). It can be induced also by hypoxia, neurotrophic factor deprivation, excitotoxins and accumulation of protein aggregates through PI3K and ERK-mediated pathways (Zhu t al., 2007; Boland & Nixon, 2006). Macroautophagy is described as the sequestration of complete regions of the cytosol, including not only soluble proteins, but also complete organelles, into a double membrane vescicle known as autophagosome, which is considered an immature form of autophagic vacuole (AV) (Seglen et al., 1996; Mortimore et al., 1996). The limiting double membrane is thought to arise from the endoplasmatic reticulum, although the Golgi complex has also been indicated as a source (Levine & Klionsky, 2004; Mijaljica et al., 2006). Because these vesicles lack any enzyme, the trapped contents are not degradated until the autophagosome founds with a lysosome, forming a single membrane autophagolysosome.

Macroautophagy is regulated by the action of a family of molecules, known as autophagy-related proteins (Atg), which participates in each of the different steps of this process (Klionsky et al., 2003). A series of conjugation events (protein-to-lipid and protein-to-protein) and several members of intracellular kinase families are involved (Klionsky, 2005; Ohsumi, 2001).

One hypotheses has been proposed to explain the role of dysregulated autophagy in PD pathogenesis, in patients affected to Gaucher's disease. This theory ("offensive metabolite theory") is based on the ceramide activity in the process of autophagic pathway modulation (Scarlatti et al., 2004). Ceramide is a sphingolipid mediator with an essential role in different situations correlated with authophagic system, such as cell growth, cell death, proliferation and stress response (Klionsky & Emr, 2000). Studies have shown as ceramide interferes with the inhibitory class I PI3K signaling pathway and induces the expression of a autophagy-related gene beclin 1, stimuling the autophagyc process.

It's possible that the lack of β-glucocerebrosidase activity and the accumulation of glucocerebroside may interfere with the ceramide modulation system, destroing cellular pathways necessary for autophagic-lysosomal degradation and leading to the LB formation.

The other types of described autophagy are microautophagy and CMA. The first one consists of direct engulfment of small volumes of cytosol (constituted by soluble proteins but also by complete organelles) by lysosomes (Ahlberg et al., 1982) through invaginations or tabulations that "pinch off" from the membrane into the lysosomal lumen where they are rapidly degraded (Marzella et al., 1981). Microautophagy participates in the continuous turnover of long-lived proteins inside many types of cells (Mortimore et al., 1988); in addition a number of studies have shown as a particular form of microautophagy can lead to preferential degradation of peroxisomes (micropexophagy) (Farre and Subramani, 2004; Mukaiyama et al., 2002; Veenhuis et al., 2000).

Chaperon-mediated autophagy is characterized by selectivity; about 30% of cytosolic proteins are degraded by this pathway. Through CMA particular cytosolic proteins are recognized by a chaperone in the cytosol, which delivers the proteins directly to the surface of the lysosome (Dice, 1990; Majeski & Dice, 2004, Massey et al., 2006). A distinctive feature of this pathway is that all substrate proteins contain in their amino acid sequence a motif, biochemically related to the pentapeptide KFERQ, required for targeting to the lysosomal compartment (Dice, 1990). A heat shock protein, hsc73 (Chiang et al., 1989) , recognizes the substrates containing the motif, and brings them to the lysosome membrane, where it binds to the receptor protein, lamp2 (lysosome-associated membrane protein type 2a) (Cuervo & Dice, 1996). The substrate interacts direcly with lamp2, and once unfolded, it is transported in the lysosome lumen (Salvador et al., 2000) where it is degraded.

Substrates for CMA consist of a very heterogeneous pool of cytosolic proteins, different for structure and function, but having all the same KFERQ motif. CMA acts in the degradation of many different substrates (i.e. several glycolitic enzymes, glutathione transferase, ribonuclease A) and damaged proteins: its selective role allows removal of the altered proteins without affecting neighbouring healty ones (Kiffin et al., 2004; Cuervo et al., 1999). Many studies have shown as this autophagic pathway is activated when stress condition occurs in the cells, such as prolonged nutrient deprivation or exposure to toxic compounds (Cuervo & Dice, 1998).

Independently of the autophagic pathway, all substrates are brought to the lysosome lumen where several different lysosomal hydrolases rapidly degrade them. These enzymes are synthesized in the endoplasmatic reticulum, sorted to the trans-Golgi network by mannose-6-phosphate receptors, transported through the endosome to arrive to their lysosomal destination, where they are activated upon the exposure to the acid environment (Jadot et al., 1997). The proteolytic capacity of lysosomes comprises a mixture of endo- and exo-peptidases, called cathepsins, which act in concert to degrade proteins to a mixture of amino acids and dipeptides. Expression, activation and inhibition of these cathepsins are differentially regulated, and individual cathepsins often have non-redundant functions in normal and disease states (Kroemer & Jaattela, 2005). In addition to peptidases activity, intralysosomal conditions and other lysosomal components (i.e. glycosidase, lipases, phospholipases, solphatases, nucleases and phosphatases) are designed to favor the complete degradation of the internalized products.

One route of degradation of the α-synuclein is via CMA pathway (Cuervo et al., 2004). Studies have revealed as impaired lysosomal function seems to be involved in familial forms of PD, as consequence of reduced α-synuclein degradation. So one theory is that disturbances in the lysosome (i.e. the alteration in the GCase function) contribute to reduce α-synuclein degradation and consequently promote its aggregation. This may be possible since ceramide can activate cathepsin D (aspartate protease), which in turn is responsible for the proteolytic activation of other lysosomal proteins (Heinrich et al., 1999). So the reduced activity of one protease can spark off the decremented action of other acid hydrolases causing an α-synuclein accumulation and contributing in LB formation.

The other α-synuclein degradation pathway is the ubiquitin-proteasome system (UPS). It serves as the primary route for the degradation of thousands of short-lived proteins and provides the specificity and temporal control needed for tuning the stady-state levels of many regulatory proteins (Ciechanover et al., 2000). UPS-mediated catabolism is also essential to preserve amino acid pools in acute starvation and contributes significantly to the degradation of defective proteins (Ciechanover & Brudin, 2003; Whealtley & Inglis, 1980; Vabulas & Hartl, 2005). UPS contributes also to diverse cellular processes, such as protein quality control, cell-cycle progression, signal transduction, and development (Kerscher et al., 2006).

Substrates of the ubiquitin/proteasome system (UPS) get post-translationally modified by covalent attachment of multiple ubiquitin molecules at internal lysine residues. This polyubiquitylation of substrate proteins involves three enzymes: ubiquitin-activating enzymes (E1), ubiquitin-conjugating enzymes (E2), and ubiquitin protein ligases (E3). E1 hydrolyses ATP and forms a thioester-linked conjugate between itself and ubiquitin; E2 receives ubiquitin from E1 and forms a similar thioester intermediate with ubiquitin; and E3 binds both E2 and the substrate, and transfers the ubiquitin to the substrate. A chain made of four to six ubiquitin moieties targets the conjugated substrate for degradation by the 26S proteasome (Richly et al., 2005; Zhang et al., 2009).

The UPS can only degrade proteins when they are in a soluble state or as a part of reversible protein complexes that can be disassembled into single protein units (Finkbeiner et al., 2006; Kopito, 2000). So any type of irreversible oligomeric structures, preaggregates, and protein aggregates cannot be handled by UPS, instead they can be degraded by the autophagic-lysosomal pathway.

A different theory ("misfolded protein theory") to explain the linkage between Gaucher's and Parkinson's disease, is that mutant misfolded glucocerebrosidase might overwhelm the UPS, causing a delay in the degradation of accumulated proteins, including α-synuclein (Dawson, 2006). Ron et al. have shown that misfolded GCase endures endoplasmatic reticulum associated degradation (ERAD) (Ron and Horowitz, 2005). In this process, mutant proteins are identified as misfolded by the ER quality control system and retrotraslocated from ER to cytosol, ubiquitinated and eliminated by the ubiquitin-proteasome system. The same authors proposed that mutated GBA protein (but not WT GBA) undergoes parkin (E3-ligase)-mediated ubiquitination, creating an imbalance in protein degradation resulting in secondary toxicity. It is likely that, since GCase is not a natural substrate of parkin, the enduringly ER retention and proteasomal degradation of mutant β-glucosidase, mediated by parkin, affect its activity toward its natural substrates. Accumulation during the years of these proteins can lead to the death of cells in substantia nigra and eventually, to the development of PD.

The theories described above, cannot explain completely the correlation between the diseases. In the "offensive metabolite theory" the reducing of the released ceramide inhibits the autophagic-lysosomal functions. This can explain the development of LB and parkinsonism in Gaucher patients, but not in GBA mutations carriers.

Moreover in Gaucher patients where mutations in GBA result in no protein product (i.e. c.84dupG and IVS2+1G>A) the risk to develop PD is high. So the "misfolded protein theory" also cannot clear fully the question, even if it is probably that very truncated forms of the mutant protein still might induce endoplasmic reticulum stress and guide to crashing of UPS.

4. Genetic studies and neuropathological data

The first indication of a relationship between parkinsonism and GD was due to sporadic case reports in the literarture (Neudorfer et al., 1996; Machaczka et al., 1999; Tayebi et al., 2001). In these papers it was highlighted how in some GD patients the enzyme deficiency itself could predisposed to the susceptibility to parkinsonisms.

These observations of occurrence of Parkinson's disease in some patients with non-neuropathic type 1 Gaucher disease and in their first degree relatives has led to the identification of GBA1 heterozigous mutations as a genetic risk factor for idiopathic Parkinson's disease.

In these subjects the mean age at onset of parkinsonian symptoms is lower than in patients without GD1, becoming evident at an average age of 48 years compared with 71 years in the general population (Elbaz et al., 2003).

These early observations led to several studies which revealed that patients with idiopathic PD had a higher probability of harboring GBA1 mutations compared to the general population.

The first large study was conducted by Lwin et al. (2004), using sequence analyses on brain samples from 57 subjects of different nationality, GBA alterations were detected in 12 sample (21%).

Subsequently Aharon-Peretz et al. (2004), explored the association between six GBA mutations (N370S, L444P, c.84dupG, IVS+1A>G, R496H, V394L) and PD in Ashkenazi Jews population. From the screening of 99 patients and 1,543 healty people they identified these mutations in 31.3% of patients with PD versus 6.2% of healty controls.

Many studies have been conducted in the years, some of these have been screened PD patients for common GBA mutations (Clarck et al., 2005; Sato et al., 2005; Tan et al., 2007; Wu et al., 2007; De Marco et al., 2008; Spitz et al., 2008; Mata et al., 2008; Gan-Or et al., 2008), others have been sequenced the entire GBA gene (Eblan et al., 2006; Ziegler et al., 2007; Clark et al., 2007; Bras & Singleton, 2009; Kalinderi et al., 2009; Neumann et al., 2009).

All of these studies evidenced a higher frequency of GBA mutations among PD patients than in matched controls, but the frequency of GBA mutations varies in relation with the study's design (popolation, number and type of mutations screened or whole GBA scanning).

Toft et al. (2006) searched the association between two mutations (N370S and L444P) and PD in Norwegian population. From the analyses of 311 patients and 474 controls they found these mutations in 2.3% of subjects with PD versus 1.7% of controls.

The frequency of GBA mutations ranges between 10.7% and 31.3% in PD patients from Ashkenazi Jewish and between 2.3% and 9.4% in patients from other populations.

Most of these studies were conducted on sporadic PD patients, recently Nichols et al. (2009) and Mitsui et al. (2009) specifically investigated familial PD. They demonstrated an association between GBA variants and familial PD cases as well as sporadic disease.

Most of these studies have independently reached similar results demonstrating that GBA mutations are found in patients with PD at a higher frequency than expected.

A large meta-analysis was conducted by Sidransky et al. (2009) pooling genotypic data from 16 different centers across the world. A total of 5,691 genotyped patients with Parkinson disease and 4,898 controls were evaluated; full sequencing was performed on 1859 patient and 1674 control samples. Overall, the odds ratio for carryng a GBA mutation in subjects with PD was 5.43 (95% CI 3.89-7.57), selecting mutations in GBA gene as a common risk factor for PD.

Investigators extended their studies to analyses whether GBA mutations are related with other Lewy bodies disorders. Goker-Alpan et al. (2006), analyzing the coding region of GBA gene in 75 brain's sample of autopsy cases with pathologically confirmed Lewy body disorders, found GBA mutations in 23% of LBD patients, 4% of PD patients and none within Multiple System Atrophy patients (MSA).

Afterward Mata et al. (2008), Farrer et al. (2009) and Clark et al. (2009) showed a correlation between GBA mutations and LBD, while was found no significant difference in GBA mutations incidence between MSA patients and controls (Segarane et al., 2009).

Considering the spectrum of PD clinical manifestations in GD1 patients, a wide range of symptoms have been described, varying from the more aggressive, early-onset disease, with poor response to L-dopa therapy, to the more typical PD disease (presenting with asymmetric onset of resting tremor, bradykinesia, rigidity, gait and balance disturbance, weakness, pain, cognitive decline, and depression), responsive to L-dopa (Neudorfer et al., 1996; Tayebi et al, 2003; Bembi et al., 2003; Tayebi et al, 2001; Halperin et al. 2006; Gan-Or et al., 2008; Bultron et al., 2010; Chérin et al., 2010;). The emerging evidence of the association between GBA mutations and a variety of synucleinopathyes may account for the wide phenotype variability (Hruska at al., 2006; Velayati et al, 2010). Even if different studies described early-onset (< 50 years) as an element that characterizes this association, this observation might be influenced by the small number of patients involved in each study.

Trying to find an answer to this issue, Gan-Or et al. (2008) performed a study analysing a large cohort of 420 unrelated Jewish Ashkenazi PD patients, which evidenced a strong correlation between GD1 and early-onset of PD symptoms (average age at onset of 51.2 years, versus 60.7 years of the noncarriers PD population), while GBA carriers showed an average age of 57.2 years at PD onset.

They also analysed the different effects of mutation severity, observing a higher risk for PD in patients carrying severe GBA mutations as well as a decreased age of symptoms onset. Finally, when they analysed clinical PD manifestations among GBA carriers and non-carriers, they observed a reduced presence of rigidity (16.90% vs 28.57%) and an increase of weakness (16.90% vs 7.14%) in GBA carriers.

Another recent large observational study of 444 consecutive GD1 patients (Bultron et al., 2010), aiming to analyse the risk of PD occurrence, showed 11 patients (2.47%) who developed the disease at a mean age of 55.0 ± 8.8 years (range 40-65 years). Analysing GD overall severe score index (SSI) and bone disease score (Hermann score) in the overall population, they found both of them significantly higher in PD patients (SSI: 10.8±0.8 vs 6.9±3.7, p=0.02; Herman score: 4.6±0.5 vs 2.5±1.5, p=0.002).

Moreover, these authors estimated age and gender-adjusted risk to develop PD in three different groups of GD1 patients, finding that the range of risk was increased 11.0 to 31.3 fold in male patients and 5.7 to 13.8 fold in female patients, with an overall relative risk to develop PD in GD1 patients of 21.4 (95% CI, 10.7-38.3).

As regard the clinical response to ERT in GD1 patients with PD, all published experiences demonstrated its effectiveness on hematological and systemic involvement, while they were ineffective in correcting PD symptoms (Neudorfer et al., 1996; Tayebi et al, 2003; Bembi et al., 2003; Tayebi et al, 2001; Itokawa et al., 2006; Bultron et al., 2010). The new era of substrate reducing and chaperone therapies with small molecules that are able to cross the blood-brain barrier may open new perspectives in the treatment of central nervous system involvement in GD, including PD symptoms. A recent report of Hughes et al. (2007) that showed an improvement in the clinical conditions of a PD patient during SRT with Miglustat, introduces a new possible therapeutic approach.

5. Expression of GBA and other lysosomal enzyme in animal models of Parkinson's disease

The majority of sporadic PD cases result from interaction between genes and environment but the age remains the greatest risk factor. The first evidence of a genetic involvement in PD manifestations was the identification of three missense mutations on the α-synuclein gene, SNCA. These mutations (A30P, E46K, A53T) segregate with the disease in unrelated families and caused PD with high penetrance (Polymeropoulos et al., 1997; Kruger et al., 1998; Zarranz et al., 2004). Afterward duplication and triplication of the SNCA gene has been shown to cause PD, suggesting that high level expression of α-synuclein may also be pathogenic (Singleton et al., 2003; Ibanez et al., 2004). The degree of overexpression was found to correlate with the degree of severity of the pathology. The effects of point mutation and duplication-triplication of SNCA gene have been investigated using transgenic technology and viral infection and different mouse models were created. All PD animal models are based on the concept that parkinsonian signs are linked to dopaminergic nigral cell loss and even if they show many of the symptoms of the disease they don't display all the complexity of the neurological pathology. A lot of mouse line expressing wild-type or mutant α-synuclein (Masliah et al., 2000; Lee et al., 2002; Richfield et al., 2002) was found to lead to the develp of granular deposits, but none of these results in the involvment of dopaminergic nerve cellsof the substantia nigra. Previous data demonstrated that truncated α-synuclein (1-120) was aboundantly presents in Lewy bodies extracts (Tofaris et al., 2003). There are two different animal models of Parkinson's disease: the first one is a mouse model that express a truncated human α-synuclein (1-120) under the rat tyrosine hydroxylase promoter on a mouse α-synuclein null background (Tofaris et al., 2006). In this mouse model (TG Syn 120) were found pathological inclusions in substantia nigra and olfactory bulb, a reduction in dopamine levels in the striatum and in spontaneous locomotion and a better response to amphetamine. C-terminally truncated α-synuclein aggregates more quickly than full-lenght protein and has been found in Lewy bodies in human patients. The second one is a rat model (6OH-DA) with the lesion of the ascending nigrostriatal dopamine pathway due to 6-hydroxydopamine injection in the unilateral substantia nigra (Rozas et al., 1997; Picconi et al., 2003). These rats displayed some feautures of parkinsonian pathology. This rat model has been initially used to understand the behavioral functions of the basal ganglia, and to evaluate the brain's ability to compensate for specific neurochemical depletions. Now this model is use has strument to understand the mechanisms of PD pathology and as an experimental basis to develop new antiparkinsonian drugs and treatment strategies, or surgical approaches (Rozas et al., 1997). To deepen the involvement of lysosomal enzyme in Parkinson's disease, a comparative analysis of the activity of β-glucocerebrosidase (EC 3.2.1.45), α-mannosidase (EC 3.2.1.24), β-mannosidase (EC 3.2.1.25), β-hexosaminidase (EC 3.2.1.52) and β-galactosidase (EC 3.2.1.23) have been performed in different brain sections of the two animal's model.

In particular lysosomal enzymatic activities were determined in cerebellum, cortex and brain-stem. The obtained results show a different expression in these sections of central nervous system of TG Syn 120 mouse model compared to control mice, with a decreased activity of all the enzymes in brain-stem, and an increased activity in the cerebellum. In the cortex all the enzymatic activities remain invariated.

		Beta-hexosaminidase	Alpha-mannosidase	Beta-mannosidase	Beta-galactosidase	Beta-glucosidase
brain-stem	Wistar	20.37±4.33	0.45±0.17	0.32±0.08	3.70±1.22	0.15±0.1
	6OH-DA	17.61±5.75	0.31±0.1	0.23±0.1	2.82±0.91	0.15±0.08
cerebellum	Wistar	16.43±3.42	0.51±0.23	0.36±0.13	3.88±0.83	0.1±0.04
	6OH-DA	11.27*±2.5	0.25*±0.05	0.22*±0.05	2.64*±0.81	0.08±0.02
cortico-striatal	Wistar	18.81±3.64	0.3±0.05	0.39±0.29	1.30±0.83	0.1±0.04
	6OH-DA	12.85*±0.92	0.167*±0.03	0.11*±0.03	0.48±0.38	0.05*±0.022

Table 2. Lysosomal enzyme specific activities (μmol min^{-1}/mg total protein x 1000) in, cerebellum, cortico-striatal and brain-stem of control and 6OH-DA rats. Mean ± SD are given. *$p<0.05$ versus control.

A more pronounced differences in lysosomal enzyme expressions were observed in 6OH-DA rats (table 2). A clear reduction of enzyme activities were found in brain-stem, cerebellum and cortico-striatal. The chemical model show a profound involvement of the brain's areas and this is, probably, a consequence of the 6-hydroxydopamine treatment, infact the neurotoxins destroied selectively and rapidly catecholaminergic neurons whereas the PD pathogenensis in human and in the mouse model follows a progressive course over decades. The results obtained in this rat model might explain the reduction on alpha-mannosidase, beta-glucosidase, and beta-mannosidse activities observed in the CSF od PD patients (Balducci et al., 2007).

6. CSF lysosomal enzyme activities as possible marker of synucleinopathies

Recently it became evident that accumulation of unwanted and misfolded protein play a central role in the PD pathogenesis. An involvement of the lysosomal system has been postulated. Lysosomal activity decreased over the lifespan and a lysosomal malfunction has been linked with cronic neurodegenerative disorders (Terman, 2006; Pan et al., 2008). This assumption has been confirmed by the selective inhibition of lysosomal enzyme in different cellular models that leads to protein aggregation, synaptic loss and neuronal death (Felbor et al., 2002; Bendiske & Bahr, 2003). Furthermore, in experimental system, has been noted that α-synuclein aggregation leads to inhibition of lysosomal functions, triggering a vicious cycle (Bennett et al., 2005; Cuervo et al., 2004). On the basis of these evidences was performed a comparative analysis of the activity of β–glucocerebrosidase (EC 3.2.1.45), α-mannosidase (EC 3.2.1.24), β-mannosidase (EC 3.2.1.25), β-hexosaminidase (EC 3.2.1.52) and β-galactosidase (EC 3.2.1.23) in cerebrospinal fluid (CSF) of Parkinson's disease (PD) subjects and age matched controls first (Balducci et al., 2007), and then in Dementia with Lewy bodies (DLB), Alzheimer's disease (AD) and Frontotemporal Dementia (FTD) patients as well as in age matched controls (Parnetti et al., 2009). The framekork is different in the different neurodegenerative diseases, in PD patients a reduced activity of β-glucocerebrosidase, β-mannosidase and α-mannosidase was found, whereas β-galactosidase and β-hexosaminidase remain unchanged. In DLB patients, all the enzymes tested showed a decrease activity with β–glucocerebrosidase with the lower value. In FTD patients, only α-mannosidase activity was lower than controls, while the other enzymes showed unchanged acticities. α-mannosidase and β-hexosaminidase are the only two enzyme that showed reduced activity in AD patients.

The data suggest a significant involvement of the ensosomal-lysosomal system in the neurodegenerative diseases examined. Moreover, the different pattern of lysosomal activity can reflect the diverse implication of the lysosomal apparatous in the distinct neurodegenerative pathologies. It has also been hypotized that ameliorate the activity of the lysosomal system can be a possible therapeutic strategy for these disorders characterized by misfolding and aggregation of wild-type or mutant protein in the cytoplas of neuronal cells (Lee et al., 2004).

7. Conclusion

Clinical and genetic studies suggest that mutations in the glucocerebrosidase gene are an important risk factor for the development of parkinsonism and related didorders. While Gaucher disease is an autosomal inherited disorder, patients with parkinson's disease can be Gaucher heterozygotes or homozygotes. The involvment of the lysosomal system in parkinson's disease has also been further demonstated by the different expression of lysosomal enzymes, such as β-glucosidase, α-mannosidase, β-mannosidase, and β-galactosidase in CSF and in the brain of animal models. The elucidation of the molecular basis of this association may contribute to understand the development of parkinsonism. Anyway it is still unclear which is the common cellular pathway that links Gaucher and Parkinson diseases.

8. References

Aerts, J.M. & Hollak, C.E. (1997). Plasma and metabolic abnormalities in Gaucher's disease. *Bailliere's Clinical Haematology*, Vol.10, No.4, (Dec), pp. 691-709, ISSN 0950-3536

Aharon-Peretz, J., Rosenbaum, H. & Gershoni-Baruch, R. (2004). Mutations in the glucocerebrosidase gene and Parkinson's disease in Ashkenazi Jews. *The New England Journal of Medcine*, Vol.351, No.19 (Nov), pp. 1972-7, ISSN 0028-4793

Ahlberg, J., Marzella, L. & Glaumann, H. (1982). Uptake and degradation of proteins by isolated rat liver lysosomes. Suggestion of a microautophagic pathway of proteolysis. *Laboratory Investigation*, Vol.47, No.6, (Dec), pp. 523-32, ISSN 0023-6837

Allen, M.J., Myer, B.J., Khokher, A.M., Rushton, N. & Cox, T.M. (1997). Pro-inflammatory cytokines and the pathogenesis of Gaucher's disease: increased release of interleukin-6 and interleukin-10. *QJM: monthly journal of the Association of Physicians*, Vol.90, No.1, (Jan), pp. 19-25, ISSN 1460-2725

Altered dynamics of the lysosomal receptor for chaperone-mediated autophagy with age. *Journal of Cell Science*, Vol.120, No.5, (Mar), pp. 782-91, ISSN 0021-9533

Bagshaw, R.D., Mahuran, D.J. & Callahan, J.W. (2005). Lysosomal membrane proteomics and biogenesis of lysosomes. *Molecular Neurobiology*, Vol. 32, No. 1, (Aug), pp. 27-41, ISSN:0893-7648

Balducci, C., Pierguidi, L., Persichetti, E., Parnetti, L., Sbaragli, M., Tassi, C., Orlacchio, A., Calabresi, P., Beccari, T. & Rossi, A. (2007). Lysosomal hydrolases in cerebrospinal fluid from subjects with Parkinson's disease. *Movement Disorder*, Vol.22, No.10, (Jul), pp. 1481-84, ISSN 0885-3185

Barneveld, R.A., Keijzer, W., Tegelaers, F.P., Ginns, E.I., Geurts van Kessel, A., Brady, R.O., Barranger, J.A., Tager, J.M., Galjaard, H., Westerveld, A. & Reuser, A.J. (1983). Assignment of the gene coding for human beta-glucocerebrosidase to the region q21-q31 of chromosome 1 using monoclonal antibodies. *Human Genetics*, Vol.64, No.3, pp. 227-31, ISSN 0340-6717

Bellettato, C.M. & Scarpa, M. (2010). Pathophysiology of neuropathic lysosomal storage disorders. *Journal of Inherited and Metabolic Disorders*, Vol.33, No.4, (Aug), pp. 347-62, ISSN 0141-8955

Bembi, B., Zambito Marsala, S., Sidransky, E., Ciana, G., Carrozzi, M., Zorzon, M., Martini, C., Gioulis, M., Pittis, M.G. & Capus, L. (2003). Gaucher's disease with Parkinson's disease: clinical and pathological aspects. *Neurology*, Vol.61, No.1, (Jul), pp. 99-101, ISSN 0028-3878

Bendiske, J. & Bahr, B.A. (2003). Lysosomal activation is a compensatory response against protein accumulation and associated synaptopathogenesis--an approach for slowing Alzheimer disease? *Journal of Neuropathology and Experimental Neurology,* Vol.62, No.5, (May), pp. 451-463, ISSN 0022-3069

Bennett, E.J., Bence, N.F., Jayakumar, R. & Kopito, R.R. (2005). Global impairment of the ubiquitin-proteasome system by nuclear or cytoplasmic protein aggregates precedes inclusion body formation. *Molecular Cell,* Vol.17, No.3, (Feb), pp. 351-365, ISSN 1097-2765

Berrebi, A., Wishnitzer, R. & Von-der-Walde, U. (1984). Gaucher's disease: unexpected diagnosis in three patients over seventy years old. *Nouvelle Revue Francaise d'Hematologie,* Vol.26, No.3, pp. 201-3, ISSN 0029-4810

Beutler, E., Nguyen, N.J., Henneberger, M.W., Smolec, J.M., McPherson, R.A., West, C. & Gelbart, T. (1993). Gaucher disease: gene frequencies in the Ashkenazi Jewish population. *The American Journal of Human Genetics,* Vol.52, No.1, (Jan), pp. 85-8, ISSN 0002-9297

Beutler, E. & Gelbart, T. (1996). Glucocerebrosidase (Gaucher disease). *Human Mutation,* Vol.8, No.3, pp. 207-13, ISSN 1059-7794.

Beutler, E. & Grabowski, G.A. (2001). Gaucher disease. *The Metabolic and Molecular Basis of Inherited Disease Vol. III, 8th* ed. Scriver CR., Beaudet AL., Sly WS., Valle D., editors, 3635–68, NY, McGraw-Hill, New York

Beutler, E. (2006). Gaucher disease: multiple lessons from a single gene disorder. *Acta Paediatrica Supplement,* Vol.95, No.451, (Apr), pp. 103-9, ISSN 0803-5326

Biegstraaten, M., van Schaik, I.N., Aerts, J.M. & Hollak, C.E. (2008). 'Non-neuronopathic' Gaucher disease reconsidered. Prevalence of neurological manifestations in a Dutch cohort of type I Gaucher disease patients and a systematic review of the literature. *Journal of Inherited Metabolic Disease,* Vol.31, No.3, (Jun), pp. 337-49, ISSN 0141-8955

Boland, B. & Nixon, R.A. (2006). Neuronal macroautophagy: from development to degeneration. *Molecular Aspects of Medicine,* Vol.27, No.5-6, (Oct-Dec), pp. 503-19, ISSN 0098-2997.

Brady, R.O., Kanfer, J.N. & Shapiro, D. (1965). Metabolism of glucocerebrosides. II. Evidence of an Enzymatic deficiency in Gaucher's disease. *Biochemical and Biophysical Research Communication,* Vol.18, pp. 221-5, ISSN 0006-291X

Brady, R.O., Barton, N.W. & Grabowski, G.A. (1993). The role of neurogenetics in Gaucher disease. *Archives of Neurology,* Vol.50, No.11, (Nov), pp. 1212-24, ISSN 003-9942

Bras, J.M. & Singleton, A. (2009). Genetic susceptibility in Parkinson's disease. *Biochimica et biophysica acta,* Vol. 1792, No. 7, (Jul), pp. 597-603, ISSN 0006-3002

Bultron, G., Kacena,K., Pearson, D., Boxer, M., Yang, R., Sathe, S., Pastores, G. & Mistry, P.K. (2010). The risk of Parkinson's disease in type 1 Gaucher disease. *Journal of Inherited Metabolic Disease,* Vol. 33, No. 2 (Apr), pp. 167-73, ISSN 0141-8955

Charrow, J., Andersson, H.C., Kaplan, P., Kolodny, E.H., Mistry, P., Pastores, G., Rosenbloom, B.E., Scott, C.R., Wappner, R.S., Weinreb, N.J. & Zimran, A. (2000). The Gaucher registry: demographics and disease characteristics of 1698 patients with Gaucher disease. *Archives of Internal Medicine,* Vol.160, No.18, (Oct), pp. 2835-43, ISSN 0003-9926

Chérin, P., Sedel, F., Mignot, C., Schupbach, M., Gourfinkel-An, I., Verny, M. & Baumann, N. (2006). Neurological manifestations of type 1 Gaucher's disease: Is a revision of disease classification needed?. *Revue Neurologique*, Vol.162, No.11, (Nov), pp. 1076-83, ISSN 0035-3787

Chérin, P., Rose, C., de Roux-Serratrice, C., Tardy, D., Dobbelaere, D., Grosbois, B., Hachulla, E., Jaussaud, R., Javier, R.M., Noël, E., Clerson, P. & Hartmann, A. (2010). The neurological manifestations of Gaucher disease type 1: the French Observatoire on Gaucher disease (FROG). *Journal of Inherited Metabolic Disease*, Vol. 33, No. 4, (Aug), pp. 331-8, , ISSN 0141-8955

Chiang, H.L., Terlecky, S.R., Plant, C.P. & Dice, J.F. (1989). A role for a 70-kilodalton heat shock protein in lysosomal degradation of intracellular proteins. *Science*. Vol.246, No.4928, (Nov), pp. 382-5, ISSN 0036-8075

Ciechanover, A., Orian, A. & Schwartz, A.L. (2000). Ubiquitin-mediated proteolysis: biological regulation via destruction. *Bioessays*, Vol.22, No.5, (May), pp. 442-51, ISSN 0265-9247

Ciechanover, A. & Brundin, P. (2003). The ubiquitin proteasome system in neurodegenerative diseases: sometimes the chicken, sometimes the egg. *Neuron*, Vol.40, No.2, (Oct), pp. 427-46, ISSN 0896-6273

Clark, L.N., Nicolai, A., Afridi, S., Harris, J., Mejia-Santana, H., Strug, L., Cote, L.J., Louis, E.D., Andrews, H., Waters, C., Ford, B., Frucht, S., Fahn, S., Mayeux, R., Ottman, R. & Marder, K. (2005). Pilot association study of the beta-glucocerebrosidase N370S allele and Parkinson's disease in subjects of Jewish ethnicity. *Movement Disorders*, Vol.20, No.1, (Jan), pp. 100-3, ISSN 0885-3185

Clark, L.N., Ross, B.M., Wang, Y., Mejia-Santana, H., Harris, J., Louis, E.D., Cote, L.J., Andrews, H., Fahn, S., Waters, C., Ford, B., Frucht S., Ottman, R. & Marder, K. (2007). Mutations in the glucocerebrosidase gene are associated with early-onset Parkinson disease. *Neurology*, Vol.18, No.12, (Sep), pp. 1270-1277, ISSN:0028-3878

Clark, L.N., Kartsaklis, L.A., Wolf Gilbert, R., Dorado, B., Ross, B.M., Kisselev, S., Verbitsky, M., Mejia-Santana, H., Cote, L.J., Andrews, H., Vonsattel, J.P., Fahn, S., Mayeux, R., Honig, L.S. & Marder, K. (2009). Association of glucocerebrosidase mutations with dementia with lewy bodies. *Archives of Neurology*, Vol.66, No.5, (May), pp.578-583, ISSN 0003-9942

Cox, T.M. & Schofield, J.P. (1997). Gaucher's disease: clinical features and natural history. *Bailliere's Clinical Haematology*, Vol.10, No.4, (Dec), pp. 657-89, ISSN 0950-3536

Cox, T.M. (2001). Gaucher disease: understanding the molecular pathogenesis of sphingolipidoses. *Journal of Inherited Metabolic Disease*, Vol.24, Suppl.2, pp. 106-21, discussion 87-8, ISSN 0141-8955

Cuervo, A.M. & Dice, J.F.(1996). A receptor for the selective uptake and degradation of proteins by lysosomes. *Science*, Vol.273, No.5274, (Jul), pp. 501-3, ISSN 0036-8075

Cuervo, A.M. & Dice, J.F. (1998). Lysosomes, a meeting point of proteins, chaperones, and proteases. *Journal of Molecular Medicine*, Vol.76, No.1, (Jan), pp. 6-12, ISSN 0377-046X

Cuervo, A.M., Hildebrand, H., Bomhard, E.M. & Dice, J.F. (1999). Direct lysosomal uptake of alpha 2-microglobulin contributes to chemically induced nephropathy. *Kidney International*, Vol.55, No.2, (Feb), pp. 529-45, ISSN 0085-2538

Cuervo, A.M. (2004). Autophagy: many paths to the same end. *Molecular and Cellular Biochemistry*, Vol.263, No.1-2, (Aug), pp. 55-72, ISSN 0300-8177

Cuervo, A.M., Stefanis, L., Fredenburg, R., Lansbury, P.T. & Sulzer, D. (2004). Impaired degradation of mutant alpha-synuclein by chaperone-mediated autophagy. *Science,* Vol.305, No.5688, (Aug), pp. 1292-5, ISSN 0036-8075.

Dawson, T.M. (2006). Parkin and defective ubiquitination in Parkinson's disease. *Journal of Neural Transmission Supplement,* No.70, pp. 209-13, ISSN 0303-6995

De Duve, C., Pressman, B.C., Gianetto, R., Wattiaux, R. & Appelmans, F. (1955). Tissue fractionation studies. 6. Intracellular distribution patterns of enzymes in rat-liver tissue. *The Biochemical Journal,* Vol.60, No.4, (Aug), pp. 604-617, ISSN 0264-6021

De Marco, E.V., Annesi, G., Tarantino, P., Rocca, F.E., Provenzano, G., Civitelli, D., Cirò Candiano, I.C., Annesi, F., Carrideo, S., Condino, F., Nicoletti, G., Messina, D., Novellino, F., Morelli, M. & Quattrone, A. (2008). Glucocerebrosidase gene mutations are associated with Parkinson's disease in southern Italy. *Movement disorders* , Vol.23, No.3, (Feb), pp. 46046-3, ISSN 0885-3185

Dice, J.F. (1990). Peptide sequences that target cytosolic proteins for lysosomal proteolysis. *Trends in Biochemical Science,* Vol.15, No.8, (Aug), pp. 305-9, ISSN 0968-0004

Eblan, M.J., Nguyen, J., Ziegler, S.G., Lwin, A., Hanson, M., Gallardo, M., Weiser, R., De Lucca, M., Singleton, A. & Sidransky, E. (2006). Glucocerebrosidase mutations are also found in subjects with early-onset parkinsonism from Venezuela. *Movement Disorder,* Vol.21, No.2, (Feb), pp. 282-3, ISSN 0885-3185

Elbaz, A., Bower, J.H., Peterson, B.J., Maraganore, D.M., McDonnell, S.K., Ahlskog, J.E., Schaid, D.J. & Rocca, W.A. (2003). Survival study of Parkinson disease in Olmsted County, Minnesota. *Archives of Neurology,* Vol.60, No.1, (Jan), pp. 91-6, ISSN 0003-9942

Erikson, A. (1986). Gaucher disease-Norrbottnian type (III). Neuropaediatric and neurobiological aspects of clinical patterns and treatment. *Acta Paediatric Scandinavica Supplement,* Vol.326, pp. 1-42, ISSN 0300-8843

Farré, J.C. & Subramani, S. (2004). Peroxisome turnover by micropexophagy: an autophagy-related process. *Trends in Cell Biology,* Vol.14, No.9, (Sep), pp. 515-23, ISSN 0962-8924

Farrer,M.J., Williams, L.N., Algom, A.A., Kachergus, J., Hulihan, M.M., Ross, O.A., Rajput, A., Papapetropoulos, S., Mash, D.C. & Dickson, D.W. (2009). Glucosidase-beta variations and Lewy body disorders. *Parkinsonism & related disorders,* Vol.15, No.6, (Jul), pp. 414-6, ISSN 1353-8020

Felbor, U., Kessler, B., Mothes, W., Goebel, H.H., Ploegh, H.L., Bronson, R.T. & Olsen, B.R. (2002). Neuronal loss and brain atrophy in mice lacking cathepsins B and L. *Proceedings of the National Academy of Sciences (USA),* Vol.99, No.12, (Jun), pp. 7883-8, ISSN 0027-8424

Finkbeiner, S., Cuervo, A.M., Morimoto, R.I. & Muchowski, P.J. (2006). Disease-modifying pathways in neurodegeneration. *J Neuroscience,* Vol.26, No.41, (Oct), pp. 10349-57, ISSN 0270-6474

Fletcher, J.M. (2006). Screening for lysosomal storage disorders--a clinical perspective.*Journal of inherited metabolic disease,* Vol.29, No.2-3 (Apr-Jun), pp. 405-8, ISSN 0141-8955

Futerman, A.H. & van Meer, G. (2004). The cell biology of lysosomal storage disorders. *Nature Reviews: Molecular and Cell Biology,* Vol.5, No.7, (Jul), pp. 554-65, ISSN 1471-0072

Gan-Or, Z., Giladi, N., Rozovski, U., Shifrin, C., Rosner, S., Gurevich, T., Bar-Shira, A. & Orr-Urtreger, A. (2008). Genotype-phenotype correlations between GBA mutations and Parkinson disease risk and onset. *Neurology*, Vol.70, No.24, (Jun), pp. 2277-83, ISSN 0028-3878

Gaucher disease and parkinsonism: a phenotypic and genotypic characterization. *Molecular Genetics and Metabolism*, Vol.73, No.4, (Aug), pp. 313-21, ISSN 1096-7192

Germain, D.P. (2004). Gaucher's disease: a paradigm for interventional genetics. *Clinical Genetics*, Vol.65, No.2, (Feb), pp. 77-86, ISSN 0009-9163

Goker-Alpan O., Schiffmann R., Park J.K., Stubblefield B.K., Tayebi N. & Sidransky E. (2003). Phenotypic continuum in neuronopathic Gaucher disease: an intermediate phenotype between type 2 and type 3. *Journal of Pediatrics*, Vol.143, No.2, (Aug), pp. 273-6, ISSN 0022-3476

Goker-Alpan, O., Giasson, B.I., Eblan, M.J., Nguyen, J., Hurtig, H.I., Lee, V.M., Trojanowski, J.Q. & Sidransky, E. (2006). Glucocerebrosidase mutations are an important risk factor for Lewy body disorders. *Neurology*, Vol.67, No.5, (Sep), pp. 908-10, ISSN 0028-3878

Goker-Alpan, O., Lopez, G., Vithayathil, J., Davis, J., Hallett, M. & Sidransky, E. (2008). The spectrum of parkinsonian manifestations associated with glucocerebrosidase mutations. *Archives of Neurology*, Vol. 65, No. 10, (Oct), pp: 1353-7, ISSN 0003-9942

Grabowski, G.A. & Horowitz, M. (1997). Gaucher's disease: molecular, genetic and enzymological aspects. *Bailliere's Clinical Haematology*, Vol.10, No.4, (Dec), pp. 635-56, 0950-3536

Halperin, A., Elstein, D. & Zimran, A. (2006). Increased incidence of Parkinson disease among relatives of patients with Gaucher disease. *Blood Cells, Molecules & Diseases*, Vol. 36, No. 3, (May-Jun), pp. 426-8, ISSN: 1079-9796

Heinrich, M., Wickel, M., Schneider-Brachert, W., Sandberg, C., Gahr, J., Schwandne,r R., Weber, T., Saftig, P., Peters, C., Brunner, J., Krönke, M. & Schütze, S.(1999). Cathepsin D targeted by acid sphingomyelinase-derived ceramide. *EMBO Journal*, Vol.18, No.19, (Oct), pp. 5252-63, ISSN 0261-4189

Horowitz, M., Wilder, S., Horowitz, Z., Reiner, O., Gelbart, T. & Beutler, E. (1989). The human glucocerebrosidase gene and pseudogene: structure and evolution. *Genomics.*, Vol.4, No.1, (Jan), pp. 87-96, ISSN 0888-7543

Hruska, K.S., Goker-Alpan, O. & Sidransky, E. (2006). Gaucher disease and the synucleinopathies. *Journal of biomedicine & biotechnology*, Vol. 3, 78549, ISSN:1110-7243

Hruska, K.S., LaMarca, M.E., Scott, C.R. & Sidransky, E. (2008). Gaucher disease: mutation and polymorphism spectrum in the glucocerebrosidase gene (GBA). *Human Mutation*, Vol.29, No.5, (May), pp. 567-83, ISSN 1059-7794

Hughes, D.A., Ginsberg, L., Bake,r R., Goodwin, S., Milligan, A., Richfield, L. & Mehta, A.B. (2007). Effective treatment of an elderly patient with Gaucher's disease and Parkinsonism: a case report of 24 months' oral substrate reduction therapy with miglustat. *Parkinsonism & related disorders*, Vol. 13, No.6, (Aug), pp. 365-8. ISSN: 1353-8020

Ibáñez, P., Bonnet, A.M., Débarges, B., Lohmann, E., Tison, F., Pollak, P., Agid, Y., Dürr, A. & Brice, A. (2004). Causal relation between alpha-synuclein gene duplication and familial Parkinson's disease. *Lancet,* Vol.364, No.9440, (Sep), pp. 1169-71, ISSN 0140-6736

Itokawa, K., Tamura, N., Kawai, N., Shimazu, K. & Ishii, K. (2006). Parkinsonism in type I Gaucher's disease. *Internal Medicine,* Vol. 45, No.20, pp. 1165-7, ISSN: 0918-2918

Jadot, M., Dubois, F., Wattiaux-De Coninck, S. & Wattiaux, R. (1997). Supramolecular assemblies from lysosomal matrix proteins and complex lipids. *European Journal of Biochemistry,* Vol.249, No.3, (Nov), pp. 862-9, ISSN 0014-2956.

Jmoudiak, M. & Futerman, A.H. (2005). Gaucher disease: pathological mechanisms and modern management. *British Journal of Haematology,* Vol.129, No.2, (Apr), pp. 178-88, ISSN 0007-1048

Journet, A., Chapel, A., Kieffer, S., Roux, F. & Garin, J. (2002). Proteomic analysis of human lysosomes: application to monocytic and breast cancer cells. *Proteomics,* Vol. 2, Np. 8, (Aug), pp. 1026-40, ISSN:1615-9853

Kalinderi, K., Bostantjopoulou, S., Paisan-Ruiz, C., Katsarou, Z., Hardy, J. & Fidani, L. (2009). Complete screening for glucocerebrosidase mutations in Parkinson disease patients from Greece. *Neurosci Letters,* Vol.452, No.2, (Mar), pp. 87-9, ISSN 0304-3940

Kerscher, O., Felberbaum, R. & Hochstrasser, M. (2006). Modification of proteins by ubiquitin and ubiquitin-like proteins. *Annual Review of Cell and Developmental Biology,* Vol.22, pp. 159-80, ISSN 1081-0706.

Kiffin, R., Christian, C., Knecht, E. & Cuervo, A.M. (2004). Activation of chaperone-mediated autophagy during oxidative stress. *Molecular Biology of the Cell,* Vol.15, No.11, (Nov), pp. 4829-40, ISSN 1059-1524

Kim, Y.J., Sapp, E., Cuiffo, B.G., Sobin, L., Yoder, J., Kegel, K.B., Qin, Z.H., Detloff, P., Aronin, N. & Di Figlia, M. (2006). Lysosomal proteases are involved in generation of N-terminal huntingtin fragments. *Neurobiology of Disease,* Vol.22, No.2, (May), pp. 346-56, ISSN 0969-9961

Klionsky, D.J. & Emr,S.D. (2000). Autophagy as a regulated pathway of cellular degradation. *Science,* Vol.290, No.5497, (Dec), pp. 1717-21, ISSN 0036-8075

Klionsky, D.J., Cregg, J.M., Dunn, W.A. Jr, Emr, S.D., Sakai,Y., Sandoval, I.V., Sibirny, A., Subramani, S., Thumm, M., Veenhuis, M. & Ohsumi, Y. (2003). A unified nomenclature for yeast autophagy-related genes. *Developmental Cell,* Vol.5, No.4, (Oct), pp. 539-45, ISSN 1534-5807

Klionsky, D.J. (2005). Autophagy. *Current Biology,* Vol.15, No.8, (Apr), pp. 282-3, ISSN 0960-9822.

Kohan, R., Cismondi, I.A., Oller-Ramirez, A.M., Guelbert, N., Anzolini, T.V., Alonso, G., Mole, S.E., de Kremer, D.R & de Halac, N.I. (2011). Therapeutic Approaches to the Challenge of Neuronal Ceroid Lipofuscinoses. *Current Pharmaceutical Biotechnology,* (Jan) [Epub ahead of print] ISSN 1389-2010

Kolter, T. & Sandhoff, K. (2006). Sphingolipid metabolism diseases. *Biochimica et Biophysica Acta,* Vol.1758, No.12, (Dec), pp. 2057-79, ISSN 0006-3002

Kopito, R.R. (2000). Aggresomes, inclusion bodies and protein aggregation. *Trends Cell Biology,* Vol.10, No.12, (Dec), pp. 524-30, ISSN 0962-8924

Kourie, J.I. & Henry, C.L. (2001). Protein aggregation and deposition: implications for ion channel formation and membrane damage. *Croat Medical Journal.*, Vol.42, No.4, (Aug), pp. 359-74, ISSN 0353-9504

Kroemer, G. & Jäättelä, M. (2005). Lysosomes and autophagy in cell death control. *Nature Reviews. Cancer*, Vol.5, No.11, (Nov), pp. 886-97, ISSN 1474-175X

Krüger, R., Kuhn, W., Müller, T., Woitalla, D., Graeber, M., Kösel, S., Przuntek, H., Epplen,J.T., Schöls, L. & Riess, O. (1998). Ala30Pro mutation in the gene encoding alpha-synuclein in Parkinson's disease. *Nature genetics*, Vol.18, No.2, (Feb), pp. 106-8, ISSN 1061-4036

Kundu, M. & Thompson, C.B. (2008). Autophagy: basic principles and relevance to disease. *Annual Review of Pathology*, Vol.3, pp. 427-55, ISSN 1553-4006

Lachmann, R.H., Grant, I.R., Halsall, D. & Cox, T.M. (2004). Twin pairs showing discordance of phenotype in adult Gaucher's disease. *QJM: monthly journal of the Association of Physicians*, Vol.97, No.4, (Apr), pp. 199-204, ISSN 1460-2725

Lee, H.J., Shin, S.Y., Choi, C., Lee, Y.H. & Lee, S.J.(2002). Formation and removal of alpha-synuclein aggregates in cells exposed to mitochondrial inhibitors. *The Journal of biological chemistry*, Vol.277, No.7, (Feb), pp. 5411-7, ISSN 0021-9258

Lee, H.J., Khoshaghideh, F., Patel, S. & Lee, S.J. (2004). Clearance of alpha-synuclein oligomeric intermediates via the lysosomal degradation pathway. *The Journal of neuroscience*, Vol.24, No.8, (Feb), pp. 1888-96, ISSN 0270-6474

Lee, R.E. (1982). The pathology of Gaucher disease. *Progress in Clinical and Biological Research*, Vol.95, pp. 177-217, ISSN 0361-7742

Levine, B. & Klionsky, D.J. (2004). Development by self-digestion: molecular mechanisms and biological functions of autophagy. *Developmental Cell*, Vol.6, No.4, (Apr), pp. 463-77, ISSN 1534-5807

Lwin, A., Orvisky, E., Goker-Alpan, O., LaMarca, M.E. & Sidransky, E. (2004). Glucocerebrosidase mutations in subjects with parkinsonism. *Molecular genetics and metabolism*, Vol.81, No.1, (Jan), pp. 70-3, ISSN 1096-7192

Machaczka, M., Rucinska, M., Skotnicki, A.B. & Jurczak, W. (1999). Parkinson's syndrome preceding clinical manifestation of Gaucher's disease. *American Journal of Hematology*, Vol.61, No.3, (Jul), pp. 216-7, ISSN 0361-8609

Majeski, A.E. & Dice, J.F. (2004). Mechanisms of chaperone-mediated autophagy. *The International Journal of Biochemistry & Cell Biology*, Vol.36, No.12, (Dec), pp. 2435-44, ISSN 1357-2725

Marzella, L., Ahlberg, J. & Glaumann, H. (1981). Autophagy, heterophagy, microautophagy and crinophagy as the means for intracellular degradation. *Virchows Arch. B, Cell Pathology Including Molecular Pathology*, Vol.36, No.2-3, pp. 219-34, ISSN 0340-6075

Masliah, E., Rockenstein, E., Veinbergs, I., Mallory, M., Hashimoto, M., Takeda, A., Sagara, Y., Sisk, A. & Mucke, L. (2000). Dopaminergic loss and inclusion body formation in alpha-synuclein mice: implications for neurodegenerative disorders. *Science*, Vol.287, No.5456, (Feb), pp. 1265-9, ISSN 0036-8075

Massey, A.C., Zhang, C. & Cuervo, A.M. (2006). Chaperone-mediated autophagy in aging and disease. *Current Topics in Developmental Biology*, Vol.73, pp. 205-35, ISSN 0070-2153

Mata, I.F., Samii, A., Schneer, S.H., Roberts, J.W., Griffith, A., Leis, B.C., Schellenberg, G.D., Sidransky, E., Bird, T.D., Leverenz, J.B., Tsuang, D. & Zabetian, C.P. (2008). Glucocerebrosidase gene mutations: a risk factor for Lewy body disorders. *Archives of neurology*, Vol.65, No.3, (Mar), pp. 379-82, ISSN 0003-9942

McKeran, R.O., Bradbury, P., Taylor, D. & Stern, G. (1985). Neurological involvement in type 1 (adult) Gaucher's disease. *Journal of Neurology, Neurosurgery, and Psychiatry*, Vol.48, No.2, (Feb), pp. 172-5, ISSN 0022-3050

Meikle, P.J., Hopwood, J.J., Clague, A.E. & Carey, W.F. (1999). Prevalence of lysosomal storage disorders. *Journal of American Medical* Association, Vol.281, No.3, (Jan), pp. 249-54, ISSN 0098-7484

Mijaljica, D., Prescott, M. & Devenish, R.J. (2006). Endoplasmic reticulum and Golgi complex: Contributions to, and turnover by, autophagy. *Traffic*, Vol.7, No.12, (Dec), pp. 1590-5, ISSN 1398-9219

Mitsui, J., Mizuta, I., Toyoda, A., Ashida, R., Takahashi, Y., Goto, J., Fukuda, Y., Date, H., Iwata, A., Yamamoto, M., Hattori, N., Murata, M., Toda, T. & Tsuji, S. (2009). Mutations for Gaucher disease confer high susceptibility to Parkinson disease. *Archives of neurology*, Vol.66, No.5, (May), pp. 571-6, ISSN 0003-9942

Mizushima, N. (2005). A(beta) generation in autophagic vacuoles. *The Journal Cell Biology*, Vol.171, No.1, (Oct), pp. 15-7, ISSN 0021-9525

Moran, M.T., Schofield, J.P., Hayman, A.R., Shi, G.P., Young, E. & Cox, T.M. (2000). Pathologic gene expression in Gaucher disease: up-regulation of cysteine proteinases including osteoclastic cathepsin K. *Blood*, Vol.96, No.5, (Sep), pp. 1969-78, ISSN 0006-4971

Mortimore, G.E., Lardeux, B.R. & Adams, C.E. (1988). Regulation of microautophagy and basal protein turnover in rat liver. Effects of short-term starvation. *The Journal of Biological Chemistry*, Vol.263, No.5, (Feb), pp. 2506-12, ISSN 0021-9258

Mortimore, G.E., Miotto, G., Venerando, R. & Kadowaki, M. (1996). Autophagy. *Sub-cellular Biochemistry*, Vol.27, pp. 93-135, ISSN 0306-0225

Mukaiyama, H., Oku, M., Baba, M., Samizo, T., Hammond, A.T., Glick, B.S., Kato, N. & Sakai, Y. (2002). Paz2 and 13 other PAZ gene products regulate vacuolar engulfment of peroxisomes during micropexophagy. *Genes to Cells: devoted to molecular & cellular mechanisms*, Vol.7, No.1, (Jan), pp. 75-90, ISSN 1356-9597

Neudorfer, O., Giladi, N., Elstein, D., Abrahamov, A., Turezkite, T., Aghai, E., Reches, A., Bembi, B. & Zimran, A. (1996). Occurrence of Parkinson's syndrome in type I Gaucher disease. *QJM : monthly journal of the Association of Physicians*, Vol.8, No. 9 (Sep), pp. 691-4, ISSN: 1460-2725

Neumann, J., Bras, J., Deas, E., O'Sullivan, S.S., Parkkinen, L., Lachmann, R.H., Li, A., Holton, J., Guerreiro, R., Paudel, R., Segarane, B., Singleton, A., Lees, A., Hardy, J., Houlden, H., Revesz, T. & Wood, N.W. (2009). Glucocerebrosidase mutations in clinical and pathologically proven Parkinson's disease. *Brain : a journal of neurology*, Vol.132, No.7, (Jul), pp. 1783-94, ISSN 0006-8950

Nichols, W.C., Pankratz, N., Marek, D.K., Pauciulo, M.W., Elsaesser, V.E., Halter, C.A., Rudolph, A., Wojcieszek, J., Pfeiffer, R.F., Foroud, T. & Parkinson Study Group-PROGENI Investigators. (2009). Mutations in GBA are associated with familial

Parkinson disease susceptibility and age at onset. *Neurology*, Vol.72, No.4, (Jan), pp.310-6, ISSN 0028-3878

Nilsson, O. & Svennerholm, L. (1982). Accumulation of glucosylceramide and glucosylsphingosine (psychosine) in cerebrum and cerebellum in infantile and juvenile Gaucher disease. *Journal of Neurochemistry*, Vol.39, No.3, (Sep), pp. 709–718, ISSN 0022-3042

Occurrence of Parkinson's syndrome in type I Gaucher disease. *QJM : monthly journal of the Association of Physicians*, Vol.89, No.9, (Sep), pp. 691-4, ISSN 1460-2725

Ohmi, K., Kudo, L.C., Ryazantsev, S., Zhao, H.Z., Karsten, S.L. & Neufeld, E.F.(2009). Sanfilippo syndrome type B, a lysosomal storage disease, is also a tauopathy. *Proceedings of the National Academy of Sciences of the United States of America*, Vol.106, No.20, (May), pp. 8332-7, ISSN 0027-8424

Ohsumi, Y. (2001). Molecular dissection of autophagy: two ubiquitin-like systems. *Nature Reviews. Molecular Cell Biology*, Vol.2, No.3, (Mar), pp. 211-6, ISSN 1471-0072

Pan, T., Kondo, S., Le, W. & Jankovic, J. (2008). The role of autophagy-lysosome pathway in neurodegeneration associated with Parkinson's disease. *Brain : a journal of neurology*, Vol.131, No.8, (Aug), pp. 1969-78, ISSN 0006-8950

Parnetti, L., Balducci, C., Pierguidi, L., De Carlo, C., Peducci, M., D'Amore, C., Padiglioni, C., Mastrocola, S., Persichetti, E., Paciotti, S., Bellomo, G., Tambasco, N., Rossi, A., Beccari, T. & Calabresi, P. (2009). Cerebrospinal fluid beta-glucocerebrosidase activity is reduced in Dementia with Lewy Bodies. *Neurobiology of Disease*, Review Vol.34, No.3, (Jun), pp. 484-6, ISSN 0969-9961

Patrick, A.D. (1965). Deficiencies of –SH-dependent enzymes in cystinosis. *Clinical Science*, Vol.28, (Jun), pp. 427-43, ISSN 0009-9287

Pelled, D., Trajkovic-Bodennec, S., Lloyd-Evans, E., Sidransky, E., Schiffmann, R. & Futerman, A.H. (2005). Enhanced calcium release in the acute neuronopathic form of Gaucher disease. *Neurobiology of Disease*, Vol.18, No.1,(Feb), pp. 83-8, ISSN 0969-9961

Picconi, B., Centonze, D., Håkansson, K., Bernardi, G., Greengard, P., Fisone, G., Cenci, M.A. & Calabresi, P. (2003) Loss of bidirectional striatal synaptic plasticity in L-DOPA-induced dyskinesia. *Nature neuroscience*, Vol.6, No.5, (May), pp. 501-6, ISSN 1097-6256

Polymeropoulos, M.H., Lavedan, C., Leroy, E., Ide, S.E., Dehejia, A., Dutra, A., Pike, B., Root, H., Rubenstein, J., Boyer, R., Stenroos, E.S., Chandrasekharappa, S., Athanassiadou, A., Papapetropoulos, T., Johnson, W.G., Lazzarini, A.M., Duvoisin, R.C., Di Iorio, G., Golbe, L.I. & Nussbaum, R.L. (1997). Mutation in the alpha-synuclein gene identified in families with Parkinson's disease. *Science*, Vol.276, No.5321, (Jun), pp. 2045-7, ISSN 0193-4511

Richfield, E.K., Thiruchelvam, M.J., Cory-Slechta, D.A., Wuertzer, C., Gainetdinov, R.R., Caron, M.G., Di Monte, D.A. & Federoff, H.J. (2002). Behavioral and neurochemical effects of wild-type and mutated human alpha-synuclein in transgenic mice. *Experimental neurology*, Vol.175, No.1, (May), pp. 35-48, ISSN 0014-4886

Richly, H., Rape, M., Braun, S., Rumpf, S., Hoege, C. & Jentsch, S. (2005). A series of ubiquitin binding factors connects CDC48/p97 to substrate multiubiquitylation and proteasomal targeting. *Cell*, Vol.120, No.1, (Jan), pp. 73-84, ISSN 0092-8674

Ron, I. & Horowitz, M. (2005). ER retention and degradation as the molecular basis underlying Gaucher disease heterogeneity. *Human Molecular Genetics*, Vol.14, No.16, (Aug), pp. 2387-98, ISSN 0964-6906

Ron, I., Rapaport, D. & Horowitz, M. (2010). Interaction between parkin and mutant glucocerebrosidase variants: a possible link between Parkinson disease and Gaucher disease. *Human Molecular Genetics*, Vol.19, No.19, (Oct), pp. 3771-81, ISSN 0964-6906

Rozas, G., Guerra, M.J. & Labandeira-García, J.L. (1997). An automated rotarod method for quantitative drug-free evaluation of overall motor deficits in rat models of parkinsonism. *Brain research. Brain research protocols*, Vol.2, No.1, (Dec), pp. 75-84, ISSN 1385-299X

Roze, E., Paschke, E., Lopez, N., Eck, T., Yoshida, K., Maurel-Ollivier, A., Doummar, D., Caillaud, C., Galanaud, D., Billette de Villemeur, T., Vidailhet, M. & Roubergue, A. (2005). Dystonia and parkinsonism in GM1 type 3 gangliosidosis. *Movement Disorders*, Vol.20, No.10, (Oct), pp. 1366-9, ISSN 0885-3185

Saftig, P. (2006). Physiology of the lysosome, In: *Fabry Disease: Perspectives from 5 Years of FOS*, Mehta A., Beck M., Sunder-Plassmann G., Oxford: Oxford PharmaGenesis; Chapter 3 ISBN-10: 1-903539-03-X, Oxford

Salvador, N., Aguado, C., Horst, M. & Knecht, E. (2000). Import of a cytosolic protein into lysosomes by chaperone-mediated autophagy depends on its folding state. *The Journal of Biological Chemistry*, Vol.275, No.35, (Sep), pp. 27447-56, ISSN 0021-9258

Sato, C., Morgan, A., Lang, A.E., Salehi-Rad, S., Kawarai, T., Meng, Y., Ray, P.N., Farrer, L.A., St George-Hyslop, P. & Rogaeva, E. (2005). Analysis of the glucocerebrosidase gene in Parkinson's disease. *Movement Disorders*, Vol.20, No.3, (Mar), pp. 367-70, ISSN 0885-3185

Sawkar, A.R., Adamski-Werner, S.L., Cheng, W.C., Wong, C.H., Beutler, E., Zimmer, K.P. & Kelly, J.W. (2005). Gaucher disease-associated glucocerebrosidases show mutation-dependent chemical chaperoning profiles. *Chemistry and Biology*, Vol.12, No.11, (Nov), pp. 1235-44, ISSN 1074-5521

Scarlatti, F., Bauvy, C., Ventruti, A., Sala, G., Cluzeaud, F., Vandewalle, A., Ghidoni, R. & Codogno, P. (2004). Ceramide-mediated macroautophagy involves inhibition of protein kinase B and up-regulation of beclin 1. *The Journal of Biological Chemistry*, Vol.279, No.18, (Apr), pp. 18384-91, ISSN 0021-9258

Schneider, E.L., Epstein, C.J., Kaback, M.J. & Brandes, D. (1977). Severe pulmonary involvement in adult Gaucher's disease. Report of three cases and review of the literature. *American Journal of Medicine*, Vol.63, No.3, (Sep), pp. 475-80, ISSN 0002-9343

Schubert, U., Antón, L.C., Gibbs, J., Norbury, C.C., Yewdell, J.W. & Bennink, J.R. (2000). Rapid degradation of a large fraction of newly synthesized proteins by proteasomes. *Nature*, Vol.404, No.6779, (Apr), pp. 770-4, ISSN 0028-0836

Segarane, B., Li, A., Paudel, R., Scholz, S., Neumann, J., Lees, A., Revesz, T., Hardy, J., Mathias, C.J., Wood, N.W., Holton, J. & Houlden, H. (2009). Glucocerebrosidase mutations in 108 neuropathologically confirmed cases of multiple system atrophy. *Neurology*, Vol.72, No.13, (Mar), pp. 1185-6, ISSN 0028-3878

Seglen, P.O., Berg, T.O., Blankson, H., Fengsrud, M., Holen, I. & Strømhaug, P.E. (1996). Structural aspects of autophagy. *Advances in Experimental Medicine and Biology*, Vol.389, pp. 103-11, ISSN 0025-2598

Sevlever, D., Jiang, P. & Yen, S.H. (2008). Cathepsin D is the main lysosomal enzyme involved in the degradation of alpha-synuclein and generation of its carboxy-terminally truncated species. *Biochemistry*, Vol.47, No.36, (Sep), pp. 9678-87, ISSN 0006-2960

Sidransky, E. (2004). Gaucher disease: complexity in a "simple" disorder. *Molecular Genetics and Metabolism*, Vol.83, No.1-2, (Sep-Oct), pp. 6-15, ISSN 1096-7192

Sidransky, E., Nalls, M.A., Aasly, J.O., Aharon-Peretz, J., Annesi G., Barbosa, E.R., Bar-Shira, A., Berg, D., Bras, J., Brice, A., Chen, C.M., Clark, L.N., Condroyer, C., De Marco, E.V., Dürr, A., Eblan, M.J., Fahn, S., Farrer, M.J., Fung, H.C., Gan-Or, Z., Gasser, T., Gershoni-Baruch, R., Giladi, N., Griffith, A., Gurevich, T., Januario, C., Kropp, P., Lang, A.E., Lee-Chen, G.J., Lesage, S., Marder, K., Mata, I.F., Mirelman, A., Mitsui, J., Mizuta, I., Nicoletti, G., Oliveira, C., Ottman, R., Orr-Urtreger, A., Pereira, L.V., Quattrone, A., Rogaeva, E., Rolfs, A., Rosenbaum, H., Rozenberg, R., Samii, A., Samaddar, T., Schulte, C., Sharma, M., Singleton, A., Spitz, M., Tan, E.K., Tayebi, N., Toda, T., Troiano, A.R., Tsuji, S., Wittstock, M., Wolfsberg, T.G., Wu, Y.R., Zabetian, C.P., Zhao, Y. & Ziegler, S.G. (2009). Multicenter analysis of glucocerebrosidase mutations in Parkinson's disease. *The New England Journal of Medicine*, Vol.361, No.17, (Oct), pp. 1651-61, ISSN 0028-4793

Singleton, A.B., Farrer, M., Johnson, J., Singleton, A., Hague, S., Kachergus, J., Hulihan, M., Peuralinna, T., Dutra, A., Nussbaum, R., Lincoln, S., Crawley, A., Hanson, M., Maraganore, D., Adler, C., Cookson, M.R., Muenter, M., Baptista, M., Miller, D., Blancato, J., Hardy, J. & Gwinn-Hardy, K. (2003). alpha-Synuclein locus triplication causes Parkinson's disease. *Science*, Vol.302, No.5646, (Oct), pp. 841, ISSN 0193-4511

Spitz, M., Rozenberg, R., Pereira, L.da V. & Reis Barbosa, E. (2008). Association between Parkinson's disease and glucocerebrosidase mutations in Brazil. *Parkinsonism & related disorders*, Vol.14, No.1, (Aug), pp. 58-62, ISSN 1353-8020

Squier, T.C. (2001). Oxidative stress and protein aggregation during biological aging. *Experimental Gerontolology*, Vol.36, No.9, (Sep), pp. 1539-50, ISSN 0531-5565

Tan, E.K., Tong, J., Fook-Chong, S., Yih, Y., Wong, M.C., Pavanni, R. & Zhao, Y. (2007). Glucocerebrosidase mutations and risk of Parkinson disease in Chinese patients. *Archives of Neurology*, Vol.64, No.7, (Jul), pp. 1056-8, ISSN 0003-9942

Tayebi, N., Callahan, M., Madike, V., Stubblefield, B.K., Orvisky, E., Krasnewich, D., Fillano, J.J. & Sidransky, E. (2001) Gaucher disease and parkinsonism: a phenotypic and genotypic characterization. *Molecular Genetics and Metabolism*, Vol. 73, No 4 (Aug), pp. 313-21, ISSN 1096-7192

Tayebi, N., Walker,J., Stubblefield, B., Orvisky, E., LaMarca, M.E., Wong, K., Rosenbaum, H., Schiffmann, R., Bembi, B. & Sidransky, E. (2003). Gaucher disease with parkinsonian manifestations: does glucocerebrosidase deficiency contribute to a vulnerability to parkinsonism? *Molecular Genetics and Metabolism*, Vol.79, No.2, (Jun), pp. 104-9, ISSN 1096-7192

Terman, A. (2006). Catabolic insufficiency and aging. *Annals of the New York Academy of Sciences*, Vol.1067, (May), pp. 27-36, ISSN 0077-8923

Theise, N.D. & Ursell, P.C. (1990). Pulmonary hypertension and Gaucher's disease: logical association or mere coincidence? *The American Journal of Pediatric Hematology/Oncology*, Vol.12, No.1, (Spring), pp. 74-6, ISSN 0192-8562

Tofaris, G.K., Razzaq, A., Ghetti, B., Lilley, K.S. & Spillantini, M.G. (2003). Ubiquitination of alpha-synuclein in Lewy bodies is a pathological event not associated with impairment of proteasome function. *The Journal of Biological Chemistry*, Vol.278, No.45, (Nov), pp. 44405-11, ISSN 0021-9258

Tofaris, G.K., Garcia, Reitböck, P., Humby, T., Lambourne, S.L., O'Connell, M., Ghetti, B., Gossage, H., Emson, P.C., Wilkinson, L.S., Goedert, M. & Spillantini, M.G.(2006). Pathological changes in dopaminergic nerve cells of the substantia nigra and olfactory bulb in mice transgenic for truncated human alpha-synuclein(1-120): implications for Lewy body disorders. *The Journal of Neuroscience : the Official Journal of the Society for Neuroscience*, Vol.26, No.15, (Apr), pp. 3942-50, ISSN 0270-6474

Toft, M., Pielsticker, L., Ross, O.A., Aasly, J.O. & Farrer, M.J. (2006). Glucocerebrosidase gene mutations and Parkinson disease in the Norwegian population. *Neurology*, Vol.66, No.3, (Feb), pp. 415-7, ISSN 0028-3878

Vabulas, R.M. & Hartl, F.U. (2005). Protein synthesis upon acute nutrient restriction relies on proteasome function. *Science*, Vol. 310, No. 5756, (Dec), pp. 1960-3, ISSN 0193-4511

Veenhuis, M., Salomons, F.A. & Van Der Klei, I.J. (2000). Peroxisome biogenesis and degradation in yeast: a structure/function analysis. *Microscophy Research and Technique*, Vol.51, No.6, (Dec), pp. 584-600, ISSN 1059-910X.

Velayati, A., Yu, W.H. & Sidransky, E. (2010). The role of glucocerebrosidase mutations in Parkinson disease and Lewy body disorders. *Current Neurology and Neuroscience Reports*, Vol. 10, No. 3 (May), pp. 190-8, ISSN: 1528-4042

Wheatley, D.N., & Inglis, M.S. (1980). An intracellular perfusion system linking pools and protein synthesis. *Journal of Theoretical Biology*, Vol. 83, No. 3, (Apr), pp. 437-45, ISSN 0022-5193

Wu, Y.R., Chen, C.M., Chao, C.Y., Ro, L.S., Lyu, R.K., Chang, K.H. & Lee-Chen, G.J. (2007). Glucocerebrosidase gene mutation is a risk factor for early onset of Parkinson disease among Taiwanese. *Journal of Neurology, Neurosurgery, and Psychiatry*, Vol.78, No.9, (Sep), pp. 977-9, ISSN 0022-3050

Yewdell, J.W. (2005). Serendipity strikes twice: the discovery and rediscovery of defective ribosomal products (DRiPS). *Cellulae and Molecular Biology (Noisy-le-grand)* , Vol.51, No.7, (Dec), pp. 635-41, ISSN 0145-5680

Zarranz, J.J., Alegre, J., Gómez-Esteban, J.C., Lezcano, E., Ros, R., Ampuero, I., Vidal, L., Hoenicka, J., Rodriguez, O., Atarés, B., Llorens, V., Gomez Tortosa, E., del Ser, T., Muñoz, D.G. & de Yebenes, J.G. (2004). The new mutation, E46K, of alpha-synuclein causes Parkinson and Lewy body dementia. *Annals of Neurology*, Vol.55, No.2, (Feb), pp. 164-73, ISSN 0364-5134

Zhang, D., Chen, T., Ziv, I., Rosenzweig, R., Matiuhin, Y., Bronner, V., Glickman, M.H. & Fushman, D. (2009). Together, Rpn10 and Dsk2 can serve as a polyubiquitin chain-length sensor. *Molecular Cell*, Vol.36, No.6, (Dec), pp. 1018-33, ISSN 1097-2765

Zhao, H. & Grabowski, G.A. (2002). Gaucher disease: Perspectives on a prototype lysosomal disease. *Cellular and molecular life sciences*, Vol. 59, No. 4, (Apr), pp. 694-707, ISSN:1420-682X

Zhu, J.H., Horbinski, C., Guo, F., Watkins, S., Uchiyama, Y. & Chu, C.T. (2007). Regulation of autophagy by extracellular signal-regulated protein kinases during 1-methyl-4-phenylpyridinium-induced cell death. *The American Journal of Pathology*, Vol.170, No.1, (Jan), pp. 75-86, ISSN 0002-9440

Ziegler, S.G., Eblan, M.J., Gutti, U., Hruska, K.S., Stubblefield, B.K., Goker-Alpan, O., LaMarca, M.E. & Sidransky, E. (2007). Glucocerebrosidase mutations in Chinese subjects from Taiwan with sporadic Parkinson disease. *Molecular Genetics and Metabolism*, Vol.91, No.2, (Jun), pp. 195-200, ISSN 1096-7192

Zimran, A., Gelbart, T., Garver, P., Thurston, D., Saven, A. & Beutler, E. (1992). Gaucher disease. Clinical, laboratory, radiologic, and genetic features of 53 patients. *Medicine (Baltimore)*, Vol.71, No.6, (Nov.), pp. 337-53, ISSN 0025-7974

7

Possible Contribution of the Basal Ganglia Brainstem System to the Pathogenesis of Parkinson's Disease

Kaoru Takakusaki[1], Kazuhiro Obara[1] and Toshikatsu Okumura[2]
[1]Research Center for Brain Function and Medical Engineering,
[2]Department of General Medicine,
Asahikawa Medical University, School of Medicine,
Japan

1. Introduction

Insight into the organization of the motor and non-motor symptoms in Parkinson's disease (PD) is critical for understanding the role of basal ganglia in the control of behavioral expression. Motor symptoms are generally characterized by hypokinesia-bradykinesia, resting tremor, muscular rigidity and posture-gait disabilities (Morris et al., 1994; Murrey et al., 1978). Sleep disturbances are major non-motor symptoms, which include insomnia, narcolepsy-like sleep attack and rapid eye movement (REM) sleep behavioral disorder (RBD) (Ferini-Strambi & Zucconi, 2000; Iranzo et al., 2006; Postuma et al., 2010; Schenck, 1996), in addition to disturbances of emotional expression and impairments of cognitive and executive functions (Aarsland et al., 2010).

It has been well established that the cortico-basal ganglia loops (C-BG loop) contribute to the volitional and intentional control of movements (Delong & Wichmann, 2007). Basal ganglia outflow directly toward to the midbrain of the brainstem (basal ganglia-brainstem system; BG-BS system) has been recently recognized with respect to the regulation of muscle tone and posture-gait synergy (Takakusaki et al., 2003a, 2004c). It has been suggested that the BG-BS may also contribute to the modulation of vigilance states (Takakusaki et al., 2004c, 2005). Fundamental structures involved in the control of posture and locomotion and those in the muscle tone regulation during awake-sleep states exist in the brainstem and spinal cord (Chase & Morales 1990; Takakusaki et al., 1993, 1994, 2004a, 2006). The importance of the midbrain area including the pedunculopontine tegmental nucleus (PPN) has been particularly recognized in relation to these functions (Palphill & Lozano 2000; Datta, 2002; Rye 1997). The PPN and a vicinity of this nucleus (PPN area) receive excitatory projections from the cortical motor areas (Matsumura et al., 2000) and the limbic system via the hypothalamus. The PPN is also a major target of GABAergic projections from the basal ganglia output nuclei (Moriizumi et al., 1988; Rye et al., 1987; Span & Grofova, 1991; Lavoie & Parent 1994).

The purpose of this review is to facilitate understanding the pathophysiological mechanism of motor and non-motor functions in PD. For this, we first refer general framework in the central nervous system for movement control in relation to volitional, emotional and automatic aspects. In the second section we demonstrated recent findings obtained in animal experimentation how BG-BS system controlled postural muscle tone and locomotion. Then we propose hypothetical models that can provide rational explanations of motor disturbances in PD. In the third, final, section, we consider the role of the BG-BS systems in non-motor functions with special reference to the regulation of arousal state and awake-sleep states.

2. General framework of movement control

2.1 Fundamental mechanisms of gait control

Activation of different areas in the forebrain evokes different types of goal directed behaviors. On the basis of findings of our studies (Takakusaki et al., 2004b, 2006) as well as those of previous works (Grillner 1981, Mori 1987, Rossignol 1996), current perception of the neuronal pathways involved in locomotor control is illustrated in Fig.1A.

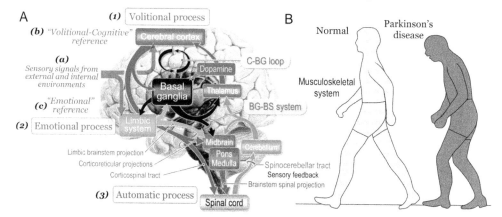

Fig. 1. Fundamental signal flows involved in gait control

A. Schematic illustrations of basic signal flows involved in gait control. (a) - (c) Sensory signals (a) act on the cerebral cortex and the limbic system generate "volitional and cognitive reference" (b) and "emotional reference" (c), respectively. (1) Volitional process requires cortical information processing. (2) Projection from the limbic system to the brainstem is responsible for emotional processes. (3) The brainstem (midbrain, pons and medulla) and spinal cord are involved in automatic processes. The basal ganglia and the cerebellum control volitional and automatic processes via cortico-basal ganglia (C-BG) loop and basal ganglia-brainstem (BG-BS) system, respectively. B. Posture of normal (left) and parkinsonian (right) states.

Motor behaviors require the recruitment of the activities of the entire nervous system (Fig.1A) and musculoskeletal systems (Fig.1B). Sensory signals, derived from both external stimuli and internal visceral information (Fig.1Aa), have the following dual functions (Takakusaki, 2008). One is to generate cognitive information processing that is utilized for working memory to guide future behavior (Fig.1Ab). Another may affect the emotional and arousal states (Fig.1Ac). Accordingly, animals initiate movements depending on either a *"volitional or cognitive reference"* or an *"emotional reference"* (Takakusaki 2008). Goal-directed behaviors therefore may require following the three processes; *"volitional process"* (Fig.1A(1)), *"emotional process"* (Fig.1A(2)) and *"automatic processes"* (Fig.1A(3)). The volitional process is derived from intentionally-elicited motor commands arising from the cerebral cortex based on volitional and cognitive references. This process requires cortical information processing and is executed by the corticoreticular and corticospinal projections. The emotional process is elicited by emotional reference via projections from the limbic-hypothalamus to the brainstem. This contributes to the emotional motor behaviors including fight or flight reactions. Regardless of whether the locomotion is volitional or emotional, it is accompanied by the automatic processes that are evoked by sequential activation of basic motor programs in the brainstem and spinal cord. The cerebellum regulates volitional and automatic processes by acting on the cerebral cortex and the brainstem, respectively. Sensory feedback via spinocerebellar tract plays an important role in this operation. The basal ganglia control these processes via loops with the cerebral cortex, brainstem and the limbic system. Because output of the basal ganglia is altered in basal ganglia disorders, all these movement processes can be disturbed.

2.2 Mechanisms of integrating posture and locomotion by subcortical structures

In animal experiments, decerebrate cat preparation has been used to examine subcortical mechanisms of controlling posture and locomotion. When the decerebration was made at the precollicular-postmammillary level (x in Fig.2A), a cat maintained reflex standing posture due to decerebrate rigidity (mesencephalic cat). Repetitive microelectrical stimulation (50 Hz, 30 μA) applied to the cuneiform nucleus (CNF; a blue point in Fig.2B) bilaterally increased the level of extensor (soleus) muscle tone, and then elicited stepping movements which were developed to locomotion by moving a treadmill (an arrowhead in Fig.2Ba). However the same type of stimuli applied to the ventral part of the PPN (red point in Fig.2B) induced muscular atonia, which lasted even after termination of the stimulation (Fig. 2Bc). Stimulation between these two sites (a green point in Fig.2C) evoked stepping movements followed by muscular atonia (Fig.2Bb). Stimulation of the locus coeruleus (LC, an orange point in Fig.2B) bilaterally increased extensor muscle tone (Fig.2Bd). Generally the locomotion evoking sites (blue circles in Fig.2D), i.e. the midbrain locomotor region (MLR), were located in the CNF, while the inhibitory region was located in the PPN (red circles in in Fig.2C). Neurons between these regions may be involved in both locomotion and muscular atonia. As show in Fig.2D, cholinergic neurons were abundantly distributed in the area corresponding to the inhibitory region, indicating that an activation of cholinergic neurons requires muscle tone suppression (Takakusaki et al., 2003a).

Our current perception of neuronal mechanisms of controlling postural muscle tone and locomotion is shown in Fig.3A on the basis of previous studies (Grillner 1981; Mori 1987; Rossignol 1996; Takakusaki et al., 2004b, 2006). Three locomotor regions are identified. They are the MLR, the subthalamic locomotor region (SLR) and the cerebellar locomotor region (CLR). Signals from the MLR may activate "muscle tone excitatory system" and "locomotor system or rhythm generating system". The former is composed of monoaminergic descending pathways such as the coerulospinal and raphespinal tracts, and excitatory reticulospinal tract arising from the ventromedial medullary reticular formation (v-MRF) which approximately corresponds to the nucleus reticularis magnocellularis. The latter is composed of the excitatory reticulospinal tract and central pattern generators (CPG) in the spinal cord. Cortical projections to the MLR have not yet been identified. It is possibly mediated by connections via the SLR (Rossignol, 1996). If decerebration was made at precollicular-premammillary level (y in Fig.2A), the cat spontaneously walked without stimulation. Thus the SLR exists between two decerebrate levels, and mostly corresponds to the lateral hypothalamus, and it may contribute to emotional behaviors (Griller et al. 1997). Signals from the SLR activate the locomotor system either directly or indirectly via the MLR (Grillner et al., 1997). The CLR corresponds to the mid-part of cerebellar white matter which contains massive fibers connecting bilateral fastigial nuclei. (Mori et al., 1999).

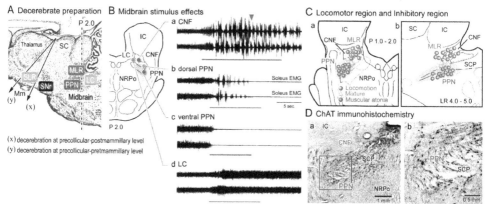

Fig. 2. Midbrain control of locomotion and muscle tone in decerebrate cat preparation

A. Two decerebrate levels (x and y) in parasagittal plane of the cat brainstem. B. Stimulus sites on coronal plane of the mesopontine tegmentum, which is indicated by dashed line in (A; at P 2.0). (a) - (d) Locomotion (a, b) and muscle tone alteration (b, c, d) induced by repetitive stimuli (30 μA, 50 Hz) applied to each site. Stimulus period is indicated under each record. C. Effective sites where stimulation evoked locomotion (blue circles), muscular atonia (red circles) and a mixture of both (green triangles) on coronal (a) and parasagittal (b) planes of the brainstem. D. Microphotographic presentation of cholinergic neurons identified by choline-acetyltransferase (ChAT) immunohistochemistry with lower (a) and higher (b) magnification of the mesopontine tegmentum. Abbreviations, EMG; electromyograms, IC; inferior colliculus, LDT; laterodorsal tegmental nucleus, LR; left and right, MLR; midbrain locomotor region, Mm; mammillary body, NRPo; nucleus reticularis pontis oralis, PPN; pedunculopontine tegmental nucleus, SC; superior colliculus, SCP; superior cerebellar peduncle, SLR; subthalamic locomotor region, SNr; substantia nigra pars reticulata.

Muscle tone control regions also exist in the brainstem. One is muscle tone inhibitory region in the PPN (Figs.2 and 3A). Cholinergic neurons in the PPN may activate "muscle tone inhibitory system", which is composed of cholinoceptive pontine reticular formation (PRF) neurons (Takakusaki et al., 2003a), reticulospinal neurons arising from the dorsomedial MRF corresponding to the nucleus reticularis gigantocellularis, and spinal inhibitory interneurons in the lamina VII of Rexed (Takakusaki et al., 1994, 2003b). This system then inhibits α- and γ-motoneurons innervating extensor and flexor muscles in parallel to interneurons mediating reflex pathways (Takakusaki et al., 2001). Because CPG is composed of spinal interneuronal circuits, an activation of the inhibitory system can simultaneously

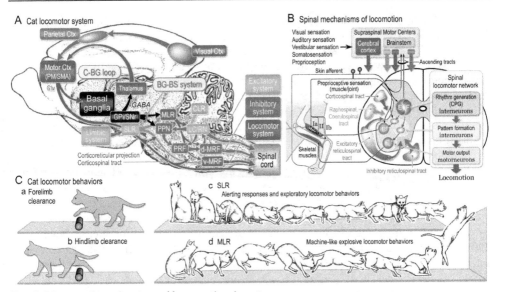

Fig. 3. Neuronal mechanism of locomotion in cats

A. Cat locomotor system. Signals from the MLR activate muscle tone excitatory system and locomotor system. Locomotor system is composed of excitatory reticulospinal tract from the ventromedial medullary reticular formation (v-MRF) and central pattern generator (CPG) in spinal cord. The excitatory reticulospinal tract also operates as the muscle tone excitatory system as well as the coerulospinal tract from the LC and raphespinal tract from the raphe nuclei (RN). Signals from the SLR and the cerebellar locomotor region (CLR) act on these systems to evoke locomotion. Cholinergic neurons in the PPN activate muscle tone inhibitory system, which arises from the pontine reticular formation (PRF) neurons and inhibitory reticulospinal tract neurons in the dorsomedial MRF (d-MRF). GABAergic output from the SNr to the MLR/PPN controls locomotion and muscle tone. Output from the basal ganglia to the thalamocortical neurons controls intentional and volitional gait behaviors. Visuospatial information from the visual cortex (Ctx) to motor Ctx via the parietal Ctx requires for programing accurate postural-gait synergy. B. Central and peripheral inputs to spinal locomotor network. Locomotor rhythm and pattern are generated by spinal interneurons. Activity of spinal neurons is modified by corticospinal tract, locomotor system (excitatory reticulospinal system) and muscle tone control systems (raphespinal, coerulospinal and inhibitory reticulospinal tracts). C. Obstacle clearance by forelimb (a) and hindlimb (b) during locomotion. Locomotor behaviors elicited by stimulating the SLR (c) and MLR (d) in cats with chronically implanted stimulating electrodes. Each picture was depicted at 0.5 sec and 0.1 sec intervals in (c) and (d), respectively. A and B are modified Takakusaki et al., 2008. (c) and (d) in C are modified Mori et al. 1989.

suppress postural muscle tone and locomotor rhythm (Takakusaki et al., 2003b). This inhibitory system is also thought to induce muscular atonia during the rapid eye movement (REM) sleep (Chase & Morales 1990; Takakusaki et al., 1993). There are serotonergic projections to the PPN (Honda & Semba, 1994) and to the cholinoceptive area of the PRF (Semba, 1993). Serotonergic projections to the PPN likely inhibit cholinergic neurons

(Leonald & Llinás, 1994), and those to the PRF may reduce activity of the inhibitory system (Takakusaki et al., 1994). In contrast, the inhibitory system suppresses the activity of the coerulospinal tract (Mileykovskiy et al., 2000). Accordingly muscle tone can be regulated by a counterbalance between the inhibitory and the excitatory systems (Takakusaki et al., 2006). It was reported that a patient with a lesion in the dorsolateral mesopontine tegmentum did not lose muscle tone during REM sleep ("REM without atonia") (Boeve et al., 2007; Culebras & Moore 1989). Also, a patient with a lesion in the dorsal part of mesopontine tegmentum could not stand and walk (Masdeu et al., 1994). These clinical case reports suggest that both a muscle tone inhibitory region and a MLR are realities in the mesopontine tegmentum of the human.

Spinal mechanisms of locomotor control are schematically illustrated in Fig.3B. Signals from the cerebral cortex and the brainstem, and those from peripheral sensory afferents are integrated at spinal cord to achieve appropriate locomotor control. Various combinations of spinal reflexes operate during locomotion. Those mediating flexion reflex and crossed extension reflex undertake major roles in the generation of locomotor rhythm (Rossignol 1996; Rossignol et al., 2006; Takakusaki et al., 2001, 2003b; McCrea & Rybak, 2008). Spinal interneurons that constitute CPG generate detailed locomotor rhythm. The locomotor rhythm is then translated to next order interneuronal groups which shape "locomotor pattern". Finally signals are sent to last-order interneurons, including reciprocal Ia interneurons, Ib interneurons and Renshaw cells. They are located in lamina IV-VII of Rexed and project to target motoneurons. Lamina VIII interneurons project to the contralateral side of spinal cord and may control alternating limb movements (Matsuyama & Takakusaki, 2008). Signals generated by spinal locomotor network are then transmitted back to the cerebral cortex, the brainstem and the cerebellum so that they monitor events in the spinal cord (Fig.3B).

2.3 Initiation of movements by the forebrain structures
2.3.1 Cortical control of locomotor behaviors

Drew et al. (1996) demonstrated, in cats with chronically implanted electrodes in the cerebral cortex, that a majority of motor cortical neurons exhibited simple rhythmic firing in relation to step cycles during steady-state locomotion. However their discharge rates considerably increased when the cats initiated to walk and had to accurately step over obstacles. Thus, commitment of cortical processing seems unnecessary during the automatic locomotor movements. On the other hand, stepping movements that accompany accurate foot placement resemble to the forelimb reaching of higher primates (Drew et al., 2004; Georgopoulos & Grillner, 1989). Such an accurate movement requires visuomotor cognitive processes (Fig.3A), which are controlled by neural circuits involving the cerebral cortex, basal ganglia, and cerebellum (Middleton & Strick, 2000). Subjects are aware of the locations of obstacles around them, and they are able to alter their stepping patterns even without available visual information of the location of the obstacles relative to the body (Fig.3C). McVea & Pearson (2007) reported that perturbing walking cats in a consistent manner evoked lasting changes to the walking pattern that were expressed only in the context in which walking was disturbed. Moreover, cats that had stepped over an obstacle by forelimb (Fig.3Ca) remembered the location of the obstacle and could use working memory to guide stepping for the hindlimb (Fig.3Cb). Therefore, sensory inputs that signal context –the surrounding visual and auditory environment– play an important role in shaping the basic pattern of locomotion. Lajoie & Drew (2007) observed, after unilateral lesion of area 5 of the posterior parietal cortex, that cats frequently hit the obstacle as they stepped over it. They also frequently hit the obstacle with their hindlimbs even when the forelimbs negotiated the obstacle successfully. These findings suggest an important role for the posterior parietal cortex in the coordination of the forelimbs and hindlimbs and in the planning and programming of visually-guided gait modification (Fig.3C). Neuroanatomical studies indicate that the posterior parietal cortex sends selected projections to the motor cortical areas from layer III, while those to the lateral cerebellum via the pontine nuclei arise from layer V (Andujar & Drew, 2007). Neurons in the primary motor cortex and those in the premotor/supplementary motor areas (PM/SMA) mainly project to the spinal cord and the reticular formation via corticospinal and corticoreticular projections, respectively (Matsuyama & Drew 1997).

2.3.2 Emotional locomotor behaviors

The MLR was initially established as a functional region involved in the initiation of locomotion on the basis of its connections with limbic structures and the basal ganglia (Armstrong, 1986; Megensen et al., 1991). Regardless of the nature of emotional stimuli, they usually elicit alert responses that produce stereotyped movements such as increased postural muscle tone and/or locomotion that accompanies autonomic sympathetic responses. The limbic-hypothalamic systems play crucial roles in these processes. Sinnamon (1993) proposed the following three types of locomotor systems that function in different behavioral or motivational contexts; an appetitive system, a primary defensive system, and an exploratory system. In cats with chronically implanted electrodes, stimulation of the SLR elicited alerting responses followed by exploratory (searching) or defensive behaviors (Fig.3Cc; Mori et al., 1989). Signals from the SLR are mediated by dense fibers in the medial forebrain bundle projecting to the midbrain (Rossignol, 1996). On the other hand, stimulation of the MLR abruptly elicited machine-like explosive locomotion (Fig.3Cd). Neural circuits connecting the nucleus accumbens (the oldest part of the striatum), the hippocampus, and the amygdala, are involved in emotional memory, and projections from the nucleus accumbens to the MLR may contribute to the expression of exploratory behaviors (Mogenson, 1991). In addition, projections from the lateral and the medial hypothalamic areas to the MLR are thought to operate as defensive and appetitive systems, respectively (Grillner et al., 1997; Jordan, 1998). The orexin-containing neurons located in the prefornical lateral hypothalamic area are considered to control appetite, energy balance, and vigilance states via projections to various areas in the nervous system (Peyron et al., 1998; Sakurai, 2002; Siegel, 2004). The orexinergic projections to the MLR facilitated the activity of the locomotor system (Takakusaki et al., 2005), indicating that the hypothalamic orexinergic system contributes to appetitive behaviors.

3. Basal ganglia control of movements and motor disturbances by the basal ganglia dysfunction

It is established that the C-BG loop is required for volitional movement (Delong & Wichmann, 2007; Middleton & Strick, 2000). Neural circuits between the prefrontal cortex and the caudate nucleus (cognitive loop) are involved in the regulation of complex, visually-guided limb movements and the planning and programming those movements. Neural circuits between motor cortical areas, including the primary motor cortex, PM and SMA, and the putamen (motor loop) contribute to the regulation of voluntary, discrete, ipsilateral limb movements. In addition the BG-BS system may control automatic and steady-state locomotor movements. This section first refers how the BG-BS system controls posture and locomotion and then considers how BG-BS contributes to pathophysiological mechanisms of motor disturbances in PD.

3.1 BG-BS system controls postural muscle tone and locomotion

How do the basal ganglia control locomotion and muscle tone via the BG-BS system? To answer this question, we employed decerebrate cat preparation where only the substantia nigra was preserved, whereas most basal ganglia structures were removed (Fig.4A). Then we examined how GABAergic output from the basal ganglia to the brainstem modulated the PPN/MLR-activated movements by manipulating the activity of neurons in the substantia nigra pars reticulata (SNr). Repetitive stimuli applied to the ventrolateral part of the PPN (red circles in Fig.4Ac) abolished muscle tone (Fig.4Ba). While stimulation of the lateral part of the SNr (filled squares in Fig.4Ab) alone did not alter muscle tone, it completely blocked the PPN-effects (Fig.4Bb). Stimulation of the MLR (blue circles in Fig.4Ac) increased muscle tone and evoked stepping movements on stationary surface (Fig.4Ca). But stimulation of the medial part of the SNr, indicated by filled squares in Fig.4Ab, arrested the MLR-activated locomotion (Fig.4Cb). It was re-established after termination of the SNr stimulation. In immobilized decerebrate preparation, MLR stimulation first depolarized the membrane potential and then generated rhythmic membrane oscillations associating with bursting firing, which corresponded to step cycles, in hindlimb motoneurons (fictive locomotion). During SNr stimulation, the rhythmic oscillation was arrested, and membrane potential was maintained at the depolarizing state in both extensor and flexor motoneurons, indicating that SNr stimulation co-contracts agonistic and antagonistic muscles, leading to disturbing rhythmic limb movements. Because these effects by SNr stimulation were blocked by injections of bicuculline (a GABA$_A$-receptor antagonist) into the PPN/MLR, the SNr stimulus effects can be mediated by GABAergic projections to these areas. These findings suggest that the BG-BS system controls steady state (e.g., rhythmic limb movements) and dynamic state (e.g., initiation and termination) of locomotion. It should be noted that the effects of SNr stimulation was depend on stimulus parameters. Step cycles and onset of MLR-activated locomotion was prolonged by increasing SNr stimulus intensity (Fig.4Da). However frequency more than 140 Hz was less effective while frequencies between 50 and 100 Hz were prominently inhibited locomotor activity (Takakusaki et al., 2003a). Similar findings were observed in the nigral control of muscle tone (Takakusaki et al., 2004c). Frequency between 50-100 Hz is almost the same as the spontaneous firing rates SNr neurons in alert monkey (Hikosaka & Wurtz, 1985). A frequency within this range can be a critical determinant in the control of muscle tone, locomotion and saccadic eye movements (Hikosaka et al., 2000).

Next we injected muscimol, a GABA$_A$ receptor agonist, into the SNr in order to inhibit neuronal activity. It was observed that muscimol injections into the lateral part of the SNr suppressed postural muscle tone (Fig.4Bc) and those into the medial part of the SNr evoked locomotion (Fig.4Cc). Judging from the relationship between effective stimulus sites in the SNr (Fig.4Ab) and those in the mesopontine tegmentum (Fig.4Ac), there exist functional topography in the nigrotegmental projections; lateral SNr controls muscle tone and the medial SNr controls locomotion. It follows that the BG-BS system can control locomotion and postural muscle tone independently.

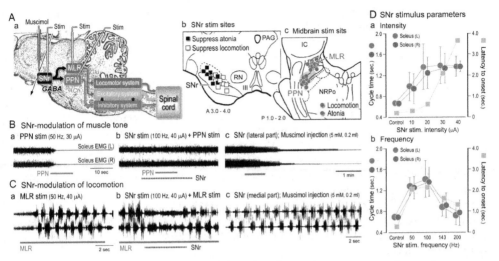

Fig. 4. Nigral stimulus effects on PPN/MLR-induced muscle tone suppression and locomotion in decerebrate cats

A. (a) Experimental design in decerebrate cat preparation. (b) Effective stimulus sites in the SNr for inhibition of the PPN (filled squares) and the MLR (open squares) effects. (c) Effective stimulus sites for evoking muscular atonia (PPN; red circles) and locomotion (MLR; blue circles) in the mesopontine tegmentum. B. (a) PPN-induced muscular atonia. (b) Inhibition of the PPN-induced atonia by SNr stimulation. (c) Muscular atonia induced by an injection of muscimol into the lateral part of the SNr. C. (a) MLR-activated stepping movements. (b) Inhibition of MLR-activated stepping by SNr stimulation. (c) Locomotion induced by an injection of muscimol into the medial part of the SNr. D. Changes in step cycles and gait onset of the MLR-activated locomotion following changes in stimulus intensity (a) and frequency (b) applied to the SNr. Abbreviations, III; oculomotor nerve, PAG; periaqueductal grey, RN; red nucleus.

3.2 Role of the C-BG loop and BG-BS system in relation to the gait control

As illustrated in Fig.5A, output from the SNr and the internal segment of globus pallidus (GPi) is regulated by hyper-direct, direct and indirect pathways in the basal ganglia circuits (Delong & Wichmann, 2007; Hikosaka et al., 2000; Numbu, 2004). Neurons in the GPi/SNr inhibit target neurons in the thalamus and brainstem with their tonic, high background activity, thus preventing unnecessary movements. To initiate movements, motor commands from the motor cortices first increase the basal ganglia output by an activation of the hyper-direct pathway to the subthalamic nucleus (STN) so that the excitability of target systems would be further reduced (Fig.5Ba). Signals via the direct pathway from the striatum to the GPi/SNr remove this sustained inhibition, resulting in a disinhibition of the target systems (Fig.5Bb). The phasic activity of GABAergic output neurons in the striatum, which are mostly silent, interrupts the tonic GPi/SNr inhibition, and movements are allowed to occur. Finally, signals through the indirect pathway, involving the external segment of the globus pallidus (GPe) and the STN, can further re-enhance the inhibition of the target systems (Fig.5Bc). This sequential information processing, an enhancement of tonic inhibition and disinhibition, would enhance the temporal contrast of the excitability of the target systems so that only the selected motor program could be initiated, executed and terminated at the appropriate timing, whereas other competing programs can be cancelled (Hikosaka et al., 2000; Numbu, 2004). This is the "first key mechanism" of movement control by the basal ganglia.

The above mechanisms may act on brainstem networks, including the locomotor system and muscle tone control systems (Fig.5A, lower right). Therefore the brainstem networks could be combined with basal ganglia motor circuits. In this "hybrid model", output of the basal ganglia controls the MLR for locomotion and the PPN for muscle tone via GABAergic projection. When locomotor movement is being prepared, tonic activity of SNr neurons would continuously inhibit both systems. When a trigger signal occurred, the hyper-direct pathway would enhance the inhibition. Then the direct pathway would release the activity of these systems, resulting in an initiation of locomotion that would be followed by a smooth reduction of the level of muscle tone. To terminate the locomotion, the direct pathway would inhibit each system, resulting in a cessation of rhythmic locomotor movements and an accompanying increase in the level of muscle tone (muscle co-contraction). A parallel organization from the SNr to the MLR/PPN would be therefore assist regulation of the level of muscle tone which was appropriate for the initiation and termination of locomotion.

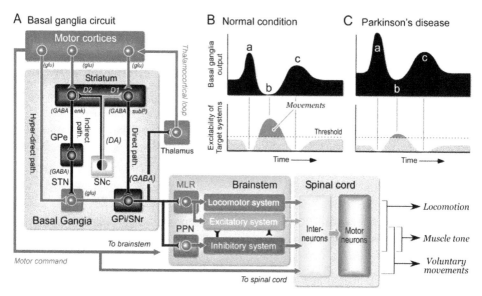

Fig. 5. Hybrid model of C-BG loop and BG-BS system
A. Left; basal ganglia motor circuits. Lower right; BG-BS system for controlling locomotion and muscle tone. B and C. Changes in the basal ganglia output and in the excitability of target systems following sequential information processing of hyper-direct (a), direct (b) and indirect (c) pathways. When excitability of target systems goes beyond the threshold, movements occur. Excitability of direct and indirect pathways is modified by dopaminergic projections from the SNc to the striatum. B. Normal condition. C. Parkinson's disease. Abbreviations, D1 and D2; D1 and D2-dopamine receptors, DA; dopamine, enk; enkephaline, Glu; glutamate, GPe; external segment of globus pallidus subP; substance P, STN; subthalamic nucleus

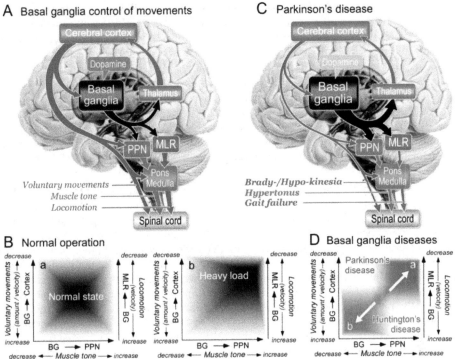

Fig. 6. Hypothetical models for movement control by the basal ganglia
A. GABAergic basal ganglia projections to the thalamocortical neurons are involved in the volitional control of movements, while those to the MLR and the PPN may be responsible for the automatic control of locomotion and muscle tone. B. Normal operation of the basal ganglia control of voluntary movements, locomotion and muscle tone. C. Pathophysiological changes in the activities of the cortico-BG loop and BG-BS system in PD. Loss of dopamine results in an increase in the basal ganglia output to the cerebral cortex, the limbic system and the brainstem. Consequently, voluntary and cognitive activities of the cerebral cortex and emotional expression can be reduced. Reduced cortical output results in bradykinesia and hypokinesia. Reduced activity in the MLR-locomotor system may induce gait failure. Inhibition of the PPN-muscle tone inhibitory system may induce hypertonus. D. Motor disturbances in basal ganglia disorders. (a) Parkinson disease. (b) Huntington's disease. Regardless of whether an increase or a decrease in the basal ganglia output, degree of freedom of movements may be restricted.

Given the above consideration, we propose a hypothetical model in Fig.6A for the basal ganglia control of movements. The motor cortical neurons that receive basal ganglia output may control the velocity and the amount of voluntary movement (Turner & Anderson, 1997), which is indicated in the ordinate on the left of the graph in Fig.6Ba. The GABAergic basal ganglia output to the MLR reduced the drive from the MLR, resulting in disruption of the activity of CPGs in the spinal cord. Basal ganglia efferents to the MLR may therefore control the locomotor pattern (ordinate on the right in Fig.6Ba). In addition, basal ganglia efferents to the PPN may determine the level of muscle tone via the muscle tone control systems (abscissa). Because the basal ganglia output is variable in a normal condition (Fig.6Ba), the degree of freedom for the amount and the velocity of movement, the locomotor velocity, and the muscle tone, can be large. Each parameter can take any of the coordinates within the frame in Fig.6Ba. For example, when a subject needs to adapt to a heavy load during walking, the subject may unconsciously select an appropriate gait pattern which is associated with a higher level of muscle tone and slower walking speed. Such a gait pattern could be realized by an increase in sustained SNr output to the PPN and the MLR. This would result in a decrease in the excitabilities of the inhibitory system and locomotor system (Fig.6Bb). Consequently, a sustained basal ganglia output may control the degree of freedom of the excitability of the target systems during movements. This can be the "second key mechanism" of motor control by the basal ganglia.

3.3 Pathophysiological mechanisms of motor disturbances in basal ganglia disorders
Gait disturbances and postural instability are observed in PD patients (Morris et al., 1994; Murray et al., 1978). These are delays in gait onset including freezing of gait (FOG), an increase in the stance phase in locomotor cycles, tiny steps and a decrease in gait velocity. Neurodegeneration of dopamine neurons in PD patients leads to higher activity in the hyper-direct and indirect pathways (Fig.5Ca and Cc) and lower activity of the direct pathway (Fig.5Cb). Therefore the GABAergic basal ganglia output is thought to be overactive in PD (Fig.6C). Excessive inhibitory actions on the target systems can consequently produce motor disturbances. For example, the excessive inhibition upon thalamocortical neurons may suppress cortical information processing (dysfunction of C-BG loop). A decrease in the output from the primary motor cortex reduces the amount (hypokinesia) and the velocity of movement (bradykinesia), leading to tiny step with a decrease in gait velocity. Moreover, reduced activities in the prefrontal cortex and PM/SMA may disturb planning and motor programming, respectively (Hanakawa et al. 1999). This may further disturb intentional gait control (gait initiation, precise hoot placement and obstacle avoidance), resulting in FOG. In the brainstem, the excessive inhibition of the MLR together with a decrease in cortical excitation of the reticular formation may decrease the activity of locomotor system and then disturb automatic aspect of steady-state gait control (rhythmic limb movements). Similarly, an increase in basal ganglia inhibition together with a decrease in cortical excitation of the PPN may reduce the activity of inhibitory system, which, in turn, facilitates excitatory systems. As a result, muscle tone would be increased (hypertonus). Therefore muscular rigidity, one of the most prominent symptoms of PD, can be the result of inhibition of the muscle tone inhibitory system that reduces the inhibition to α- and γ-motoneurons. As shown in Fig.4C, MLR-activated locomotion was arrested but the muscle tone was maintained at higher level during the period of SNr stimulation, indicating that muscle rigidity is a cause of gait disturbances. We postulate that dysfunction of the BG-BS system can be the primary basis for gait impairments of PD.

In contrast, an output from the basal ganglia is decreased in Huntington's disease (HD) because of increased activity of the direct pathway. This may extremely facilitate cortical information processing, thus unnecessary motor programs cannot be cancelled, resulting in hyperkinesia and involuntary movements (Chorea). The decrease in the basal ganglia output to the PPN may reduce muscle tone (hypotonus). It should be noted, regardless of PD or HD, the degree of freedom of movements would be reduced and restricted. The frame moves to the upper right for PD (Fig.6Da) and to lower left for HD (Fig.6Db). From these considerations, the reduction of the degree of freedom of movements could exist in the background of PD and HD. Consequently, dysfunction of the BG-BS system together with that of the C-BG loop may underlie the pathogenesis of the motor disturbances in these basal ganglia diseases.

Dystonia is a syndrome characterized by abnormal postures, muscle spasms and tremor, due to involuntary muscle co-contractions. Some dystonia are task specific, and patients only develop muscular co-contraction when performing skilled movements such as writing (Van der Kamp et al. 1989). By using positron emission tomography an inappropriate over-activity of the basal ganglia projections to the premotor and dorsal prefrontal cortex has been observed (Brooks 1995). However the activity of the primary sensorimotor and caudal premotor cortices is rather attenuated (Hutchins et al. 1988). Although alterations of noradrenaline and DA levels in brainstem structures have been reported in two cases (Hornykiewicz et al., 1986), most studies, by contrast, have not found abnormalities in the brainstem. This evidence suggests that the activity of the BG-BS system and that of the C-BG loop are controlled separately in dystonia.

Recently PPN/MLR area became one of targets of deep brain stimulation (DBS) for neurosurgical therapy for PD (PPN-DBS) (Stefani et al., 2007; Pierantozzi et al., 2008; Alessandro et al., 2010). Low frequency stimulation (~25Hz) applied to the above area ameliorated postural disturbance and gait failure. On the other hand, DBS applied to the SNr (SNr-DBS) with high frequency (135-190 Hz), which possibly intervened to the output from the SNr, also ameliorated axial symptoms such as gait akinesia and postural disturbances (Chasetan et al. 2009). Although evidence of the PPN-DBS and the SNr-DBS is still limited, these clinical findings agree well with our results suggesting that the BG-BS system contributes to the postural and locomotor synergies in human.

4. Disturbances of non-motor functions in Parkinson's disease

Disturbances in cognitive and psychotic processes have been observed in patients with degenerative disorders that involve primarily the basal ganglia such as PD (Mellers et al., 1995; Taylor et al., 1986) and HD (McHugh & Folsten, 1975). Awake-sleep states were also impaired in PD (Bliwise et al., 2000; Eisensehr et al., 2001). It is also reported that PD is preceded and accompanied by daytime sleep attacks, nocturnal insomnia, REM sleep behavior disorder, hallucinations and depression, symptoms which are frequently as troublesome as the motor symptoms of this disease. All these symptoms are present in narcolepsy (Thannical et al., 2007). These clinical evidences corroborate that the basal ganglia and their connections with the brainstem are also involved in the expression of non-motor function. In this section, we focus on the roles played by the BG-BS system in the regulation of vigilance states, arousal state, attention and cognition in relation to non-motor symptoms in PD.

4.1 Does output of the basal ganglia modulate sleep?

Cholinergic neurons in the PPN and laterodorsal tegmental nucleus are thought to be involved in not only the maintenance of arousal state but also generation of REM sleep (Datta and Siwek, 2002; Koyama & Sakai, 2000; Maloney et al., 1999). Therefore, we elucidated how GABAergic SNr-PPN projection altered the activities of the REM generator and the muscle tone inhibitory system (Takakusaki et al., 2004c). Summary of the results are shown in Fig.7. Stimulation of inhibitory region of the PPN induced REM which was associated with muscular atonia in decerebrate cats (REM and atonia; Fig.7Ba). Conditioning stimuli applied to the lateral part of the SNr (blue circles in Fig.7C) completely abolished the PPN-induced REM with atonia (Fig.7Bb). On the other hand, stimulation of the SNr, denoted by black squares in Fig.7C, only inhibited REM (Fig.7Bd). It was also observed that stimuli applied to the sites which were indicated by red circles in Fig.7C did not block REM but attenuated the muscular atonia (Fig.7Bc), i.e., REM without atonia (Sanford, 1994), which is considered to be relevant to RBD in human (Culebras & Moore, 1989), was evoked. These findings indicate that neurons in the PPN that are responsible for generation of REM sleep are affected by GABAergic projections from the SNr.

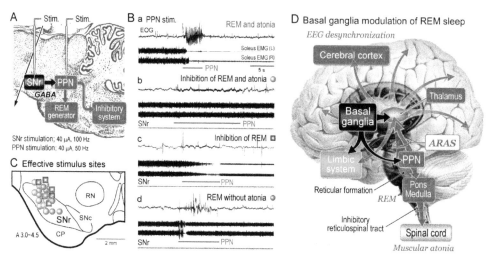

Fig. 7. Possible mechanisms of basal ganglia modulation of REM sleep
A. Experimental design in decerebrate cats. B. (a) Stimulation of the PPN induced REM and atonia. (b) ~ (d) Effects of stimuli applied to various sites of the SNr on the PPN-induced REM and atonia. (b) Stimulation of the sites indicated by blue circles in C inhibited both REM and atonia. (c) Stimulation of the sites indicated by black squares in C. only inhibited REM. (d) Stimulation of the sites indicated by red circles in C inhibited atonia but not REM (REM without atonia). C. Effective sites for modulating the eye movements and muscular atonia were located in the lateral part of the SNr. D. Possible mechanisms of basal ganglia modulation of REM sleep. Abbreviations, ARAS; ascending reticular activating system, REM; rapid eye movement.

4.2 Possible mechanisms of sleep disturbances in Parkinson's disease
4.2.1 Disturbance of REM sleep (REM sleep behavior disorder; RBD)
Sleep disturbance is one of early signs of PD (Askenasy, 2001; Ferini-Strambi & Zucconi, 2000; Larsen & Tandberg, 2001). There are several reports suggesting that nearly half number of PD patients who were diagnosed as idiopathic RBD but free of neurodegenerative diseases had developed PD (Boeve, 2007; Iranzo, 2006; Schenck, 1996). Postuma et al. (2010) conclude that severity of REM atonia loss in idiopathic RBD predicts PD. Neuronal loss in the PPN was reported in PD (Hirsch et al., 1987; Jellinger, 1988; Zweig et al., 1989), and loss of cholinergic neurons in the PPN is possibly related to disability of PD patients (Rinne et al., 2008).

Several mechanisms are postulated in relation to the basal ganglia regulation of sleep. On one hand, recent brain imaging studies revealed that damage of brainstem, particularly the reticular formation, is critically involved in the pathogenesis of RBD (Unger et al., 2010). The brainstem damage could also explain some non-motor symptoms in this disease, which often precede diagnosis, such as autonomic dysfunction and sleep disorders. On the other hand, roles of dopaminergic influence on the basal ganglia in the control of sleep-wake behavior are suggested (Mena-Segovia J et al., 2008). It is also possible that basal ganglia efferents to the non-specific thalamic nuclei may affect awake-sleep states by modulating the activity of ascending reticular activating system (ARAS). Since the classical study of Moruzzi and Magoun (1949), the pontomesencephalic reticular formation has been known to comprise the ARAS. The PPN has been considered as a part of the ARAS (Garcia-Rill, 1991; Inglis & Winn, 1995; Jones, 1991).

The SNr has a direct projection to the thalamic nuclei (Parent et al., 1983; Pare' et al., 1990) in addition to the PPN (Fig.7D). Because PPN has dense projections to the midbrain dopaminergic neurons, activity of the PPN neurons may affect awake-sleep states by modulating dopaminergic systems projecting to the basal ganglia and extra-basal ganglia areas. Consequently, our idea is that basal ganglia output from the SNr may affect awake-sleep cycles by modulating the activity of the ARAS through dual mechanisms (Fig.7D). One is through direct nigro-thalamic projection, and the other, which is considered in this study, is though indirect connections via the PPN (Takakusaki et al. 2004c, 2006).

4.2.2 Narcolepsy-like symptoms

The presence in PD patients of narcolepsy-like features, such as daytime REM sleep intrusions associated with visual hallucinations, has led some authors to suggest that a mechanism similar to that of narcolepsy might underlie excessive daytime sleepiness (EDS) in PD (Arnulf et al., 2000). Thannickal et al. (2007) demonstrated that a massive loss of orexin neurons was found in PD patients and suggested that it was a cause of the narcolepsy-like symptoms. However, Compta et al. (2009) showed that orexin-A level was normal in the cerebrospinal fluid and it was unrelated to severity of sleepiness or the cognitive status of PD patients. Therefore alternative mechanisms other than dysfunction of orexin neurons might be responsible for EDS and the disturbance of sleep architecture in PD. In animal experiments, midbrain strucutes, including the SNr, the PPN and the MLR, receive orexinergic efferents from the perifornical lateral hypothalams (Nambu et al., 1999; Peyron et al., 1998). Therefore it is interesting to elucidate how orexinergic projections to the midbrain are involved in alteration of sleep-awake states. Then we examined effects of injections of orexin-A into the MLR, PPN and the SNr upon motor behaviors in decerebrate cats (Takakusaki et al., 2005). Microinjections of orexin into the MLR facilitated locomotion, while those into either the PPN or the SNr suppressed PPN-induced muscular atonia. The latter effects were reversed by subsequent injection of bicuculline into the PPN. Thus the excitability seems to be higher in the locomotor system than in the atonia system in the presence of orexin. On the contrary the excitability of the muscle tone inhibitory system may be higher than that of the locomotor system in the absence of orexin. Accordingly GABAergic projection from the SNr to the PPN/MLR area (BG-BS system) may underlie orexin-mediated vigilance state regulation and its dysfunction may be one of pathophysiological mechanisms of narcolepsy-like features of PD (Takakusaki 2008).

4.3 Disturbances of arousal state, attention and cognition

Behavioral arousal requires an activation of dopaminergic projections arising from the SNc to the striatum and the ventral tegmental area (VTA) to the prefrontal cortex and the limbic system. The nigrostriatal projection is responsible for basal ganglia related motor functions. The mesocortical projection contributes to volitional expression and attention, and the mesolimbic projection is involved in emotional expression. On the other hand, ARAS plays a major role in the electroencephalographic arousal. An activation of the two arousal systems is required to maintain arousal state that enables alert, attention and cognition (Jones 1991). Because PPN has dense cholinergic and non-cholinergic excitatory connections with dopamine (DA) neurons in the SNc and other basal ganglia nuclei (Futami et al., 1994; Kitai, 1998; Takakusaki et al., 1996), these projections appear to play a role in more specific subcortical integration of motor and non-motor functions such as behavioral arousal, attention and reward (Kitai, 1998). For example, an injection of muscimol into the PPN reduced the speed and amount of arm movements and delayed the onset of movements but the accuracy was rather maintained (Matsumura and Kojima, 2001). Moreover, Kojima et al. (1997) demonstrated that kainic acid-induced lesion in the unilateral PPN induced hemiparkisonism which was observed in the contralateral side of the injection. From these findings they suggest that the PPN may thus facilitate the voluntary limb movements through its excitatory connections with the DA neurons.

Midbrain DA neurons are also involved in the predictive reward which is specifically linked with reinforcement behaviors. DA neurons are activated by rewarding events that are better than predicted, remain uninfluenced by events that are worse than predicted (Hikosaka et al., 2000; Schultz, 1998). Kobayashi et al. (2002) demonstrated that PPN neurons showed multi-modal activities during saccade tasks in alert monkey; their activities were related to the arousal levels, execution and preparation of movements, the level of task performance, and reward. Therefore the PPN may serve as an integrative interface between the various signals required for performing purposive behaviors (Kobayashi et al., 2004). We postulate that the PPN facilitates, possibly via dopaminergic systems, the central processes for motor command generation and extrinsic sensory processing by modulating arousal and attentive states.

In non-human primate, limited lesions of the striatum induce deficits in rule acquisition (Divac 1972), cognition (Taylor et al., 1990), working memory performance (Goldman-Rakic, 1987) and selected attention (Battig et al., 1962). Laplane et al. (1984) reported a patient with restricted bilateral pallidal lesions who was appeared apathetic and unconcerned or attention deficits, and his affect was flattened and emotional responses were blunted in the absence of any motor disorder or pure psychic akinesia. These symptoms were also described in progressive supranuclear palsy (PSP) in which major lesions were observed in the subcortical areas including the PPN. Because loss of cholinergic PPN neurons were observed not only in PSP (75-80%) but also PD (43-57%) (Hirsch et al., 1987; Jellinger, 1988; Zweig et al., 1987, 1989), the loss of cholinergic PPN neurons in both diseases could attribute to attentive and cognitive impairments and sleep deficiencies in these diseases (Scarnati & Florio, 1997).

Both neuroanatomical (von Krosigk et al., 1992; Smith & Bolam, 1990) and electrophysiological (Häusser & Yung, 1994; Saitoh et al., 2004; Paladini et al., 1999) studies demonstrated that dopaminergic neurons, as well as cholinergic neurons, receive GABAergic inhibitory effects from the basal ganglia, particularly from the SNr. Consequently a BG-BS system appears to involve the interdigitation of motor information with information relating to reward and reinforcement by modulating the excitability of both dopaminergic and cholinergic systems.

5. Concluding thoughts

The basal ganglia controls various function by acting on thalamocortical loop (C-BG loop) and the brainstem (BG-BS system). There are two key mechanisms for the operation by the basal ganglia circuit. One is sequential information processing, which would enhance the temporal contrast of the excitability of the target systems so that only the selected motor program could be appropriately executed, whereas other competing programs can be cancelled. The other is sustained output from the basal ganglia, which may control the degree of freedom of the excitability of the target systems during movements. We suggest that following roles can be played by the BG-BS system. First this system is involved in the automatic or unconscious control of movements that accompany voluntary movements. Second, the BG-BS systems may be involved in the maintenance of arousal and attentive states and in the regulation of REM sleep. Because output from the basal ganglia is thought to be overactive in PD, dysfunction of the BG-BS system in addition to that of C-BG loop can be seriously involved in motor and non-motor functions in this disease.

6. Acknowledgment

This work is supported by Grants-in-Aid for Challenging Exploratory Research (Project # 23650202) and Priority Areas "Emergence of Adaptive Motor Function through Interaction between Body, Brain and Environment (Area #454)" from the Japanese Ministry of Education, Culture, Sports, Science and Technology to K.T. We express sincere appreciation to Ms. Mihoko Ebisawa for preparation of this manuscript.

7. References

Aarsland, D., Bronnick, K., Williams-Gray, C., Weintraub, D., Marder, K., Kulisevsky, J., Burn, D., Barone, P., Pagonabarraga, J., Allcock, L., Santangelo, G., Foltynie, T., Janvin, C., Larsen, JP., Barker, RA. & Emre, M. (2010) Mild cognitive impairment in Parkinson disease: a multicenter pooled analysis. *Neurology*, Vol. 75, No.12,(September 21), pp. 1062-1069, ISSN 0028-3878.

Arnulf, I., Bonnet, AM., Damier, P., Bejjani, BP., Seilhean, D., Derenne, JP. & Agid, Y. (2000) Hallucinations, REM sleep, and Parkinson's disease: a medical hypothesis. *Neurology*, Vol. 55, No.2, (July 25), pp. 281-288, ISSN 0028-3878 .

Alessandro, S., Ceravolo, R., Brusa, L., Pierantozzi, M., Costa, A., Galati, S., Placidi, F., Romigi, A., Iani, C., Marzetti, F. & Peppe, A. (2010) Non-motor functions in parkinsonian patients implanted in the pedunculopontine nucleus: focus on sleep and cognitive domains. *J. Neurol. Sci.*, Vol. 289, No. 1-2, (Feb. 15) pp. 44-48, ISSN 0022-510X.

Andujar, J-E. & Drew, T. (2007) Organization of the projections from the posterior parietal cortex to the rostral and caudal regions of the motor cortex of the cat. *J. Comp. Neurol.* Vol. 504, No.1, (Sep. 1), pp. 17–41, ISSN 0092-7317.

Armstrong, DM. (1986) Supraspinal contribution to the initiation and control of locomotion in the cat. *Prog. Neurobiol.*, 26, (n.d.), pp. 273-361, ISSN 0301-0082.

Askenasy, JJ. (2001) Approaching disturbed sleep in late Parkinson's disease: first step toward a proposal for a revised UPDRS. *Parkinsonism Relat. Disord.*, Vol.8, No.2, (October) pp. 123–131, ISSN 1353-8020.

Battig, K., Rosvold, HE. & Mishkin, M. (1962) Comparison of the effects of frontal and caudate lesions on discrimination learning in monkeys. *J. Comp. Physiol. Psychol.*, Vol. 55, (August), pp. 458-463, ISSN 0021-9940.

Bliwise, DL., Willians, ML., Irbe, D., Ansari, FP. & Rye, DB. (2000) Inter-rater reliability for identification of REM sleep in Parkinson's disease. *Sleep*, Vol. 23, No 1, (August 1) pp. 671–676, ISSN 0161-8105.

Boeve, BF., Silber, MH., Saper, CB., Ferman, TJ., Dickson, DW., Parisi, JE., Benarroch, EE., Ahlskog, JE., Smith, GE., Caselli, RC., Tippman-Peikert, M., Olson, EJ., Lin S-C., Young, T., Wszolek, Z., Schenck, CH., Mahowald, MW., Castillo, PR., Del Tredici, K. & Braak, H. (2007) Pathophysiology of REM sleep behaviour disorder and relevance to neurodegenerative disease. *Brain*, Vol.130, Pt.11, (November), pp. 2770-2788, ISSN 0006-8950.

Brooks, DJ. (1995) The role of the basal ganglia in motor control: contributions from PET. *J. Neurol. Sci.*, Vol. 128, No. 1, (January), pp. 1-13, ISSN 0022-510X.

Chase, MH. & Morales, FR. (1990) The atonia and myoclonia of active (REM) sleep. *Annu. Rev. Psychol.*, Vol. 41, (n.d.), pp. 557–584, ISSN 0066-4308.

Chastan, N., Westby, GW., Yelnik, J., Bardinet, E., Do, MC., Agid, Y. & Welter, ML. (2009) Effects of nigral stimulation on locomotion and postural stability in patients with Parkinson's disease. *Brain*, 132, Pt.1, (January), pp. 172-184, ISSN 0006-8950.

Compta, Y., Santamaria, J., Ratti, L., Tolosa, E., Iranzo, A., Muñoz, E., Valldeoriola, F., Casamitjana, R., Ríos, J. & Marti, MJ. (2009) Cerebrospinal hypocretin, daytime sleepiness and sleep architecture in Parkinson's disease dementia. *Brain*, Vol. 132, Pt. 12, (December), pp. 3308-3317, ISSN 0006-8950.

Culebras, A, Moore, JT. (1989) Magnetic resonance findings in REM sleep behavior disorder. *Neurology*, Vol. 39, No. 11, (November), pp. 1519–1523, ISSN 0028-3878.

Datta, S. (2002). Evidence that REM sleep is controlled by the activation of brain stem pedunculopontine tegmental kainate receptor. *J. Neurophysiol.*, Vol. 87, No. 4, (April), pp. 1790–1978, ISSN 0022-3077.

Datta, S. & Siwek, DF. (2002) Single cell activity patterns of pedunculopontine tegmentum neurons across the sleep-wake cycle in the freely moving rats. *J. Neurosci. Res.*, Vol.70, No. 4, (November 15), pp. 611-621, ISSN 0168-0102.

DeLong, MR. & Wichmann, T. (2007) Circuits and circuit disorders of the basal ganglia. *Arch. Neurol.*, Vol. 64, No. 1, (January), pp. 20-24, ISSN 0003-9942.

Divac, I. (1972) Neostriatum and functions of the prefrontal cortex. *Acta Neurobiol. Exp.*, Vol. 32, No. 2, (n.d.), pp. 461-477,ISSN 0065-1400.

Drew, T., Jiang, W., Kably, B. & Lavoie, S. (1996) Role of the motor cortex in the control of visually triggered gait modifications. *Can J. Physiol. Pharmacol.*, Vol. 74, No. 4, (April), pp. 426-442, ISSN 0008-4212.

Drew, T., Prentice, S. & Schepens, B. (2004) Cortical and brainstem control of locomotion. Prog. Brain Res., Vol. 143, (n.d.), pp. 251-261, ISSN 0079-6123.

Eisensehr, I., Lindeiner, H., Jager, M. & Noachtar, S. (2001) REM sleep behavior disorder in sleep-disordered patients with versus without Parkinson's disease: is there a need for polysomnography? *J. Neurol. Sci.*, Vol. 186, No. 1-2, (May 1), pp. 7–11, ISSN 0022-510X.

Ferini-Strambi, L. & Zucconi, M. (2000) REM sleep behavior disorder. *Clin. Neurophysiol.*, Vol. 111, Suppl. 2, (September), S136-140, ISSN 1388-2457.

Futami, T., Takakusaki, K., Kitai, ST. (1995) Glutamatergic and cholinergic inputs from the pedunculopontine tegmental nucleus to dopamine neurons in the substantia nigra pars compacta. *Neurosci. Res.*, Vol. 21, No. 4, (February), pp. 331-342, ISSN 0168-0102.

Garcia-Rill, E. (1991) The pedunculopontine tegmental nucleus. *Prog. Neurobiol.*, Vol. 36, No. 5, (n.d.), pp. 363-389, ISSN 0301-0082.

Georgopoulos, AP. & Grillner, S. (1989) Visuomotor coordination in reaching and locomotion. *Science*, 245, pp.1209-1210, ISSN 0036-8075.

Goldman-Rakic, PS. (1987) Circuitry of primate prefrontal cortex and regulation of behavior by representational memory. In: *Handbook of Physiology*, the Nervous System V, F. Plum (Ed.), 273-416, ISBN 019-520662-2, American Physiological Society Press, Bethesda.

Grillner, S. (1981) Control of locomotion in bipeds, tetrapods, and fish. In: *Handbook of Physiology*, the Nervous System II, V.B. Brooks, (Ed.), 1179-1236, ISBN 10: 0195206592, ISBN 13: 9780195206593, (Published November 30, 1980), American Physiological Society Press, Bethesda.

Grillner, S., Georgopoulos, A.P. & Jordan L.M. (1997) Selection and initiation of motor behavior. In: *Neurons, Networks, and Motor Behavior*, P.S.G. Stein, S. Grillner, A.I. Selverson, D.G. Stuart, (Eds.), 3-19, ISBN-10: 0-262-19390-6, MIT Press.

Hanakawa, T., Katsumi, Y., Fukuyama, H., Honda, M., Hayashi, T., Kimura, J. & Shibasaki, H. (1999) Mechanisms underlying gait disturbance in Parkinson's disease: a single photon emission computed tomography study. *Brain*, Vol. 122, Pt.7, (July), pp. 1271-1282, ISSN 0006-8950.

Häusser, MA. & Yung, WH. (1994) Inhibitory synaptic potentials in guinea-pig substantia nigra dopamine neurones in vitro. *J. Physiol.*, Vol. 479, Pt.3, (September 15), pp. 401-422, ISSN 0022-3751.

Hikosaka, O., Takikawa, Y. & Kawgoe, R. (2000) Role of the basal ganglia in the control of purposive saccadic eye movements. *Physiol. Rev.*, Vol. 80, No. 3, (July), pp. 954–978, ISSN 00319333.

Hikosaka, O. & Wurtz, RH. (1985) Modification of saccadic eye movements by GABA-related substances: II. Effects of muscimol in monkey substantia nigra pars reticulata. *J. Neurophysiol.*, Vol. 53, No. 1, (January), pp. 292-308, ISSN 0022-3077.

Hirsch, EC., Graybiel, AM. ,Duyckaerts, C. & Javoy-Agid, F. (1987) Neuronal loss in the pedunculopontine tegmental nucleus in Parkinson disease and in progressive supranuclear palsy. *PNAS, USA*, Vol. 84, No. 16, (August), pp. 5976-5980, ISSN 0027-8424.

Honda, T. & Semba, K. (1994) Serotonergic synaptic input to cholinergic neurons in the rat mesopontine tegmentum. *Brain Res.*, Vol. 647, N0. 2, (Jun 6), pp. 299-306, ISSN 0006-8993.

Hornykiewicz, O., Kish, S.J., Becker, L.E., Farley, I. & Shannak, K. (1986) Brain neurotransmitters in dystonia musculorum deformans. *New Engl. J. Med.*, Vol. 315, No. 6. (August), pp. 347-353, ISSN 0028-4793.

Hutchins, KD., Martino, AM. & Strick, PL. (1988) Corticospinal projections from the medial wall of the hemisphere. *Exp. Brain Res.*, Vol. 71, No3, (n.d.), pp. 667-672, ISSN 0735-7044.

Inglis, WL. & Winn, P. (1995). The pedunculopontine tegmental nucleus: where the striatum meets the reticular formation. *Prog. Neurobiol.*, Vol. 47, No.1, (September), pp. 1-29, ISSN 0301-0082.

Iranzo, A., Molinuevo, JL., Santamaría, J., Serradell, M., Martí, MJ., Valldeoriola, F. & Tolosa, E. (2006) Rapid-eye movement sleep behaviour disorder as an early marker for a neurodegenerative disorder: a descriptive study. *Lancet Neurol.*, Vol. 5, No. 7, (July), pp. 572-577, ISSN 1474-4422.

Jellinger, K. (1988) The pedunculopontine nucleus in Parkinson's disease, progressive supranuclear palsy and Alzheimer's disease. *J. Neurol. Neurosurg. Psychiatry*, Vo. 51, No. 4, (April), pp. 540-543, ISSN 0022-3050.

Jones, BE. (1991) Paradoxical sleep and its chemical/structural substrates in the brain. *Neuroscience*, Vo. 40, No. 3, (n.d.) pp. 637–656, ISSN 0306-4522.

Jordan, LM. (1998). Initiation of locomotion in mammals. *Ann. NY. Acad. Sci.*, Vol. 860, (November 16), pp. 83-93, ISSN 0077-8923.

Kitai, ST. (1998) Afferent control of substantia nigra compacta dopamine neurons: anatomical perspective and role of glutamatergic and cholinergic inputs. *Advances in Pharmacology*, Vol. 42, (n.d.), pp. 700-702.

Kobayashi, Y., Inoue, Y. & Isa, T. (2004) Pedunculopontine control of visually guided saccades. *Prog. Brain Res.*, Vol. 143, (n.d.), pp. 439-145, ISSN 0079-6123.

Kobayashi, Y., Inoue, Y., Yamamoto, M., Isa, T. & Aizawa, H. (2002) Contribution of pedunculopontine tegmental nucleus neurons to performance of visually guided saccade tasks in monkeys. *J. Neurophysiol.*, Vol. 88, No. 2, (August), pp. 715-731, ISSN 0022-3077.

Kojima. J., Yamaji. Y., Matsumura. M., Nambu. A., Inase. M., Tokuno. H., Takada. M. & Imai. H. (1997) Excitotoxic lesions of the pedunculopontine tegmental nucleus produce contralateral hemiparkinsonism in the monkey. *Neurosci. Lett.*, Vol. 226, No.2, (April 25) pp. 111- 114, ISSN 0304-3940.

Koyama, Y. & Sakai, K. (2000) Modulation of presumed cholinergic mesopontine tegmental neurons by acetylcholine and monoamines applied iontophoretically in unanesthetized cats. *Neuroscience*, Vol. 96, No. 4, (n.d.) pp. 723-733, ISSN 0306-4522.

Lajoie, K. & Drew T. (2007) Lesions of area 5 of the posterior parietal cortex in the cat produce errors in the accuracy of paw placement during visually guided locomotion. *J. Neurophysiol.*, Vol. 97, No. 3, (March), pp. 2339-2354, ISSN 0022-3077.

Laplane, D., Baulac, M., Widlocher, D. & Dubois, B. (1984). Pure psychic akinesia with bilateral lesions of basal ganglia. *J. Neurol. Neurosurg. Psychiatry*, Vol. 47, No. 4, (April), pp. 377-385, ISSN 0022-3050.

Larsen, JP. & Tandberg, E. (2001) Sleep disorders in patients with Parkinson's disease: epidemiology and management. *CNS Drugs*, Vol. 15, No. 4, (n.d.), pp. 267-75, ISSN 1172-7047.

Lavoie, B. & Parent, A. (1994) Pedunculopontine nucleus in the squirrel monkey: projections to the basal ganglia as revealed by anterograde tract-tracing methods. *J. Comp. Neurol.*, Vol. 344, No. 2, (Jun 8), pp. 210-231, ISSN 0021-9967.

Leonald, CS. & Llinás, R. (1994) Serotonergic and cholinergic inhibition of mesopontine cholinergic neurons controlling REM sleep; an in vitro electrophysiological study. *Neuroscience* Vol. 59, No. 2, (March), pp. 309-330, ISSN 0306-4522.

Maloney, KJ., Mainville, L. & Jones, BE. (1999) Differential c-Fos expression cholinergic, monoaminergic and GABAergic cell groups of the pontomesencephalic tegmentum after paradoxical sleep deprivation and recovery. *J. Neurosci.*, Vol. 19, No. 8, (April 15), pp. 3057-3072, ISSN0306-4522.

Masdeu, JC., Alampur, U., Cavaliere, R. & Tavoulareas, G. (1994) Astasia and gait failure with damage of the pontomesencephalic locomotor region. *Ann. Neurol.*, Vo. 35, No.5, (May), pp. 619-621, ISSN 0364-5134.

Matsumura, M. & Kojima, J. (2001) The role of the pedunculopontine tegmental nucleus in experimental parkinsonism in primates. *Stereotactic and Functional Neurosurgery*, Vol. 77, No. 1-4, (n.d.), pp.108- 115, ISSN 1011-6125.

Matsumura, M., Nambu, A., Yamaji, Y., Watanabe, K., Imai, H., Inase, M., Tokuno, H. & Takada, M. (2000). Organization of somatic motor inputs from the frontal lobe to the pedunculopontine tegmental nucleus in the macaque monkey. *Neuroscience*, Vol. 98, No.1, (n.d.) pp. 97- 110, ISSN 0306-4522.

Matsuyama, K. & Drew, T. (1997) Organization of the projections from the pericruciate cortex to the pontomedullary brainstem of the cat: a study using the anterograde tracer Phaseolus vulgaris- leucoagglutinin. *J.Comp. Neurol.*, Vol. 389, No. 4, (December 29), pp. 617-641, ISSN 0021-9967.

Matsuyama, K. & Takakusaki, K. (2009) Organizing principles of axonal projections of the long descending reticulospinal pathway and its target spinal lamina VIII commissural neurons: with special reference to the locomotor function. In: *Handbook on White Matter: Structure, Function and Changes, Chapter XVIII*, T.B. Westland, R.N. Calton (eds). 335-356, (n.d.), Nova Science Publishing Co. New York, USA, ISBN: 978-1-61668-975-9.

McCrea, DA. & Rybak, IA. (2008) Organization of mammalian locomotor rhythm and pattern generation. *Brain Res. Rev.*, Vol. 57, No. 1, (January), pp. 134-146, ISSN 0165-0173.

McHugh, PR. & Folsten, MF. (1975) Psychiatric syndromes of Huntington's chorea: a clinical and phenomenologic study. In: *Psychiatric aspects of neurological disease. vol. 13*, F. Beston, D. Blumer (Eds.), 267-286, (n.d.), Grune & Stratton, New York. ISBN13: 978-0-19-530943-0, ISBN10: 0-19-530943-X

McVea, DA. & Pearson, KG. (2007) Long-lasting, context-dependent modification of stepping in the cat after repeated stumbling-corrective responses. *J. Neurophysiol.*, Vo. 97, No.1, (January), pp. 659-669, ISSN 0022-3077.

Mellers, JD., Quinn, NP. & Ron, MA. (1995) Psychotic and depressive symptoms in Parkinson's disease. A study of the growth hormone response to apomorphine. *Br. J. Psychiatry*, Vol. 167, No. 4, (October), pp. 522-526, ISSN 0007-1250.

Mena-Segovia, J., Winn, P. & Bolam, JP. (2008) Cholinergic modulation of midbrain dopaminergic systems. *Brain Res. Rev.*, Vol. 58, No. 2, (August), pp. 265–271, ISSN 0165-0173.

Middleton, FA. & Strick, PL (2000) Basal ganglia and cerebellar loops: motor and cognitive circuits. *Brain Res. Rev.*, Vol. 31, No. 2-3, (March), pp. 236–250, ISSN 0165-0173.

Mileykovskiy, BY., Kiyashchenko, LI., Kodama, T., Lai, YY. & Siegel, JM. (2000) Activation of pontine and medullary motor inhibitory regions reduces discharge in neurons located in the locus coeruleus and the anatomical equivalent of the midbrain locomotor region. *J. Neurosci.*, Vol. 20, No. 22, (November 15), pp. 8551-8558, ISSN 0270-6474.

Mogenson, GI. (1991) The role of mesolimbic dopamine projections to the ventral striatum in response initiation. In: *Neurobiological Basis of Human Locomotion*, M. Shimamura, S. Grillner, V.R. Edgarton (Eds.), 33-44, (October) Japan Scientific Press, Tokyo. ISBN 4762246468.

Mori, S. (1987) Integration of posture and locomotion in acute decerebrate cats and in awake, free moving cats. *Prog. Neurobiol.*, Vol. 28, No. 2, (n.d.), pp. 161-196, ISSN 0301-0082.

Mori, S., Matsui, T., Kuze, B., Asanome, M., Nakajima, K. & Matsuyama, K. (1999) Stimulation of a restricted region in the midline cerebellar white matter evokes coordinated quadrupedal locomotion in the decerebrate cat. *J. Neurophysiol.*, Vol. 82, No. 1, (July), pp. 290-300, ISSN 0022-3077.

Mori, S., Sakamoto, T., Ohta, Y., Takakusaki, K. and Matsuyama, K (1989) Site-specific postural and locomotor changes evoked in awake, freely moving intact cats by stimulating the brainstem. *Brain Res.*, Vol. 505, No. 1, (December 25), pp. 66-74, ISSN 0006-8993.

Morris, ME, Iansek R, Matyas, TA & Summers, JJ. (1994) The pathogenesis of gait hypokinesia in Parkinson's disease. *Brain,* Vol. 117, Pt. 5, (October), pp. 1169-1181, ISSN 0006-8950.

Moriizumi, T., Nakamura, Y., Tokuno, H., Kitao, Y. & Kudo, M. (1988) Topographic projections from the basal ganglia to the nucleus tegmenti pedunculopontinus pars compacta of the cat with special reference to pallidal projections. *Exp. Brain Res.*, Vol. 71, No. 2, (n.d.), pp. 298–306, ISSN 0932-4011.

Moruzzi, G. & Magoun, HW (1949) Brain stem reticular formation and activation of the EEG. *Clin. Neurophysiol.*, Vol. 1, No. 4, (November), 455-473, ISSN 1388-2457.

Murray, MP, Sepic, SB, Gardner, GM & Downs, WJ. (1978) Walking patterns of men with parkinsonism. *Am. J. Phys. Med.*, Vol. 57, No. 6, (December), pp. 278-294, ISSN 0002-9491.

Nambu A. (2004) A new dynamic model of the cortico-basal ganglia loop. *Prog. Brain Res.*, 143, (n.d.), pp. 461-466, ISSN 0079-6123.

Nambu, T., Sakurai, T., Mizukami, K., Hosoya, Y., Yanagisawa, M. & Goto, K. (1999) Distribution of orexin neurons in the adult rat brain. *Brain Res.*,Vol. 827, No. 1-2, (May 8), pp. 243-260, ISSN 0006-8993.

Pahapill, PA. & Lozano, AM. (2000) The pedunculopontine nucleus and Parkinson's disease. *Brain*, Vol. 123, Pt. 9, (September), pp. 1767-1783, ISSN 0006-8950.

Paladini, CA., Iribe, Y. & Tepper, JM. (1999). GABA$_A$ receptor stimulation blocks NMDA-induced bursting of dopaminergic neurons in vitro by decreasing input resistance. *Brain Res.*, Vol. 832, No. 1-2, (Jun 19), pp. 145-151, ISSN 0006-8993.

Paré, D., Curro-Dossi, R., Datta, S. & Steriade, M (1990) Brainstem genesis of reserpine - induced ponto-geniculo-occipital waves: an electrophysiological and morphological investigation. *Exp. Brain Res.*, Vol. 81, No. 3, (n.d.), pp. 533-544, ISSN 0932-4011.

Parent, A., Mackey, A., Smith, Y. & Boucher, R. (1983) The output organization of the substantia nigra in primate as revealed by a retrograde double labeling method. *Brain Res. Bull.*, Vol. 10, No. 4, (April), pp. 529-537, ISSN 0361-9230.

Peyron, C., Tighe, DK., van den Pol, AN., de Lecea, L., Heller, HC., Sutcliffe, JG. & Kilduff, TS. (1998) Neurons containing hypocretin (orexin) project to multiple neuronal systems. *J. Neurosci.*, Vol. 18, No. 23, (December 1), pp. 9996-10015, ISSN 0270-6474.

Pierantozzi, M., Palmieri, MG., Galati, S., Stanzione, P., Peppe, A., Tropepi, D., Brusa, L., Pisani, A., Moschella, V., Marciani. MG., Mazzone, P. & Stefani A. (2008) Pedunculopontine nucleus deep brain stimulation changes spinal cord excitability in Parkinson's disease patients. *J. Neural Transm.*, Vol. 115, No. 5, (May), pp. 731-735, ISSN 0300-9564.

Postuma, RB., Gagnon, JF., Rompré, S. & Montplaisir, JY. (2010) Severity of REM atonia loss in idiopathic REM sleep behavior disorder predicts Parkinson disease. *Neurology*, Vol. 74, No. 3, (January 19) pp. 239-244, ISSN 0028-3878.

Rinne, JO., Ma, SY., Lee, MS., Collan, Y. & Röyttä, M. (2008) Loss of cholinergic neurons in the pedunculopontine nucleus in Parkinson's disease is related to disability of the patients. *Parkinsonism Relat. Disord*, Vol. 14, No. 7, (November), pp. 553-557, ISSN 1353-8020.

Rossignol, S. (1996) Neural control of stereotypic limb movements. In: *Handbook of Physiology, sec. 12*, L.B. Rowell, J.T. Shepherd (Eds.), 173-216, (n.d.), New York: Oxford University Press, ISBN 019-509174-4

Rossignol, S , Dubuc, R. & Gossard, JP. (2006) Dynamic sensorimotor interactions in locomotion. *Physiological Reviews,* Vol. 86, No. 1, (January), pp. 89-154, ISSN 0031-9333.

Rye, DB (1997) Contributions of the pedunculopontine region to normal and altered REM sleep. *Sleep*, Vol. 20, No. 9, (September), pp. 757–788, ISSN 0161-8105.

Rye DB., Saper CB., Lee HJ. & Wainer, BH. (1987) Pedunculopontine tegmental nucleus of the rat: cytoarchitecture, cytochemistry, and some extrapyramidal connections of the mesopontine tegmentum. *J.Comp. Neurol.*, Vol. 259, No. 4, (May 22), pp. 483–528, ISSN 0028-3878.

Saitoh, K., Isa, T. & Takakusaki, K. (2004) Nigral GABAergic inhibition upon mesencephalic dopaminergic cell groups in rats. *Eur. J. Neurosci.*, Vol. 19, No. 9, (May), pp. 2399-2409, ISSN 0953-816X.

Sakurai, T. (2002) Roles of orexins in regulation of feeding and wakefulness. *Neuroreport*, Vol. 13, No. 8, (Jun 12), pp. 987–995, ISSN 0959-4965.

Sanford, RD., Morrison, AD., Mann, GL., Harris, JS., Yoo, L. & Ross, RJ. (1994) Sleep pattern and behaviour in cats with pontine lesions creating REM without atonia. *J. Sleep Res.*, Vol. 3, No. 4, (December), pp. 233–240, ISSN 0962-1105.

Scarnati, E. & Florio, T. (1997) The pedunculopontine nucleus and related structures. Functional organization. *Adv. Neurol.*, 74, (n.d.), pp. 97-110, ISSN 0091-3952.

Schenck, CH., Bundlie, SR. & Mahowald, MW. (1996) Delayed emergence of a parkinsonian disorder in 38% of 29 older men initially diagnosed with idiopathic rapid eye movement sleep behaviour disorder. *Neurology,* Vol. 46, No. 2, (February), pp.388 – 393, ISSN 0028-3878.

Schultz, W. (1998) Predictive reward signals of dopamine neurons. *J. Neurophysiol.*, Vol. 80, No. 1, (July), pp. 1-27, ISSN 0022-3077.

Semba, K. (1993) Aminergic and cholinergic afferents to REM sleep induction regions of the pontine reticular formation in the rat. *J. Comp. Neurol.*, Vol. 330, No. 4, (April 22), pp. 543–556, ISSN 0021-9967.

Siegel, JM. (2004) Hypocretin (orexn): Role in normal behavior and neuropathology. *Annu. Rev. Psychol.*, 55, (n.d.), pp. 125-148, ISSN 0066-4308.

Sinnamon, HM. (1993) Preoptic and hypothalamic neurons and initiation of locomotion in the anesthetized rat. *Prog. Neurobiol.*, Vol. 41, No. 3, (September), pp. 323-344, ISSN 0301-0082.

Smith, Y. & Bolam, JP. (1990) The output neurones and the dopaminergic neurones of the substantia nigra receive a GABA-containing input from the globus pallidus in the rat. *J. Comp. Neurol.*, Vol. 296, No. 1, (Jun 1), pp. 47-64, ISSN 0021-9967.

Spann, BM. & Grofova, I. (1991) Nigro-pedunculopontine projection in the rat: an anterograde tracing study with Phaseolus Vulgaris-Leucoagglutinin (PHA-L). *J. Comp. Neurol.*, Vol. 311, No.3, (September 15), pp. 375–388, ISSN 0021-9967.

Stefani, A., Lozano, AM., Peppe, A., Stanzione, P., Galati, S., Tropepi, D., Pierantozzi, M., Brusa, L., Scarnati, E. & Mazzone, P. (2007) Bilateral deep brain stimulation of the pedunculopontine and subthalamic nuclei in severe Parkinson's disease. *Brain,* Vol. 130, Pt. 6, (Jun), pp. 1596-1607, ISSN 0006-8950.

Takakusaki, K. (2008) Forebrain control of locomotor behaviors. *Brain Res. Rev.,* Vol. 57, No. 1, (January), pp. 192-198, ISSN 0165-0173.

Takakusaki, K., Habaguchi, T., Ohtinata-Sugimoto, J., Saitoh, K. & Sakamoto, T. (2003a) Basal ganglia efferents to the brainstem centers controlling postural muscle tone and locomotion; A new concept for understanding motor disorders in basal ganglia dysfunction. *Neuroscience,* Vol. 119, No. 1, (n.d.),pp. 293-308, ISSN 0306-4522.

Takakusaki, K., Habaguchi, T., Saitoh, K. & Kohyama, J. (2004a) Changes in the excitability of hindlimb motoneurons during muscular atonia induced by stimulating the pedunculopontine tegmental nucleus in cats. *Neuroscience,* Vol. 124, No. 2, (n.d.), pp. 467-480, ISSN 0306-4522.

Takakusaki, K., Kohyama, J. & Matsuyama, K. (2003b) Medullary reticulospinal tract mediating a generalized motor inhibition in cats: III. Functional organization of spinal interneurons in the lower lumbar segments. *Neuroscience,* Vol. 121, No. 3, (n.d.), pp. 731-746, ISSN 0306-4522.

Takakusaki, K., Kohyama, J., Matsuyama, K. & Mori, S. (1993) Synaptic mechanisms acting on lumbar motoneurons during postural augmentation induced by serotonin injection into the rostral pontine reticular formation in decerebrate cats. *Exp. Brain Res.,* Vol. 93, No. 3, (n.d.), pp. 471-82, ISSN 0932-4011.

Takakusaki, K., Kohyama, J., Matsuyama, K., Mori, S. (2001) Medullary reticulospinal tract mediating the generalized motor inhibition in cats: parallel inhibitory mechanisms acting on motoneurons and on interneuronal transmission in reflex pathways. *Neuroscience*, Vol. 103, No. 2, (n.d.), pp. 511–527, ISSN 0306-4522.

Takakusaki, K., Saitoh, K., Harada H. & Kashiwayanagi, M (2004b) Role of basal ganglia – brainstem pathways in the control of motor behaviors *Neurosci. Res.*, Vol. 50, No. 2, (October), pp. 137-151, ISSN 0168-0102.

Takakusaki, K., Saitoh, K., Harada, H., Okumura, T. & Sakamoto T. (2004c) Evidence for a role of basal ganglia in the regulation of rapid eye movement sleep by electrical and chemical stimulation for the pedunculopontine tegmental nucleus and the substantia nigra pars reticulata in decerebrate cats. *Neuroscience*, Vol. 124, No. 1, (n.d.), pp. 207-220, ISSN 0306-4522.

Takakusaki, K., Saitoh, K., Nonaka, S., Okumura, T., Miyokawa, N. & Koyama, Y. (2006) Neurobiological basis of state-dependent control of motor behavior. *Sleep and Biological Rhythms*, 4, (n.d.), pp. 87-104, ISSN 1446-9235.

Takakusaki, K., Shimoda, N., Matsuyama, K. & Mori, S. (1994) Discharge properties of medullary reticulospinal neurons during postural changes induced by intrapontine injections of carbachol, atropine and serotonin, and their functional linkages to hindlimb motoneurons in cats. *Exp. Brain Res.*, Vol. 99, No. 3, (n.d.), pp. 361–374, ISSN 0932-4011.

Takakusaki, K., Shiroyama, T., Yamamoto, T., Kitai, ST. (1996) Cholinergic and noncholinergic tegmental pedunculopontine projection neurons in rats revealed by intracellular labeling. *J. Comp. Neurol.*, Vol. 371, No. 3, (July 29), pp. 345-361, ISSN 0021-9967.

Takakusaki, K., Takahashi, K., Saitoh, K., Harada, H., Okumura, T., Kayama, Y. & Koyama, Y. (2005) Orexinergic projections to the cat midbrain mediate alternation of emotional behavioural states from locomotion to cataplexy. *J. Physiol.*, Vol. 568, Pt. 3, (November 1), pp. 1003–1020, ISSN 0022-3751.

Taylor, JR., Elsworth, JD., Roth, RH., Slodek, JR. & Redmond, DE. (1990) Cognitive and motor deficits in the acquisition of an object retrieval/detour task in MPTP-treated monkeys. *Brain*, Vol. 113, Pt. 3, (Jun), pp. 617-637, ISSN 0006-8950..

Taylor, JR., Saint-Cyr, JA. & Lang, AE. (1986) Frontal lobe dysfunction in Parkinson's disease. *Brain*, Vol. 109, Pt.5, (October), pp. 845-883, ISSN 0006-8950..

Thannickal, TC., Lai, YY. & Siegel, JM. (2007) Hypocretin (orexin) cell loss in Parkinson's disease. *Brain*, Vol. 130, Pt. 6, (Jun), pp. 1586-1595, ISSN 0006-8950.

Turner, RS. & Anderson, ME. (1997) Pallidal discharge related to the kinematics of reaching movements in two dimensions. *J. Neurophysiol.*, Vol. 77, No. 3, (March), pp. 1051-1074, ISSN 0022-3077.

Unger, MM., Belke, M., Menzler, K., Heverhagen, JT., Keil, B., Stiasny-Kolster, K., Rosenow, F., Diederich, NJ., Mayer, G., Möller, JC., Oertel, WH. & Knake S. (2010) Diffusion tensor imaging in idiopathic REM sleep behavior disorder reveals microstructural changes in the brainstem, substantia nigra, olfactory region, and other brain regions. *Sleep*, Vol. 33, No. 6, (Jun 1)pp. 767-773, ISSN 0161-8105.

Van der Kamp, W., Berardelli, A., Rothwell, JC., Thompson, PD., Day, BL. & Marsden, CD. (1989) Rapid elbow movements in patients with torsion dystonia. *J. Neurol., Neurosurg. Psychiatry*, Vol. 52, No. 9, (September), 1043-1049, ISSN 0022-3050.

von Krosigk, M., Smith, Y., Bolam, JP. & Smith, AD. (1992) Synaptic organization of GABAergic inputs from the striatum and the globus pallidus onto neurons in the substantia nigra and retrorubral field which project to the medullary reticular formation. *Neuroscience*, Vol. 50, No. 3, (October), pp. 531-549, ISSN 0306-4522.

Zweig, RM., Jankel, WR., Hedreen, JC., Mayeux, R. & Price, DL. (1989) The pedunculopontine nucleus in Parkinson's disease. *Ann. Neurol.*, Vol. 26, No. 1, (July)pp. 41-46, ISSN 0364-5134.

Zweig, RM., Whitehouse, PJ., Casanova, MF., Walker, LC., Jankel, WR. & Price, DL. (1987) Loss of pedunculopontine neurons in progressive supranuclear palsy. *Ann. Neurol.*, Vol. 22, No. 1SN 0364-5134.

8

Physiological and Biomechanical Analyses of Rigidity in Parkinson's Disease

Ruiping Xia
Department of Physical Therapy, Creighton University, Omaha, Nebraska
USA

1. Introduction

Parkinson's disease is one of the most common movement disorders characterized by bradykinesia, rigidity, resting tremor and postural instability (Fahn, 2003). It affects nearly five million elderly people worldwide (de Lau & Breteler, 2006). As the population ages, the incidence and prevalence of Parkinson's disease are expected to increase dramatically (Dorsey et al., 2007; Tanner & Goldman, 1996; Tanner & Ben-Shlomo, 1999). Rigidity is one of the clinical hallmark symptoms that characterize and define Parkinson's disease. Rigidity is one form of the increased muscle tone, which is defined as a resistance to a passive movement. Rigidity is clinically characterized by an increase in muscle tone, and is felt as a constant and uniform resistance to the passive movement of a limb persisting throughout its range (Bantam, 2000; Fung & Thompson, 2002; Hallett, 2003). There are two types of rigidity: plastic or lead-pipe rigidity, in which resistance remains uniform, constant and smooth, such as experienced when bending a piece of lead; and cogwheel rigidity, in which tremor is superimposed on increased tone, giving rise to the perception of intermittent fluctuation in muscle tone. The latter is principally attributable to the combination of plastic rigidity and tremor.

In addition to being a key element of parkinsonian rigidity, increased muscle tone also characterizes spasticity which is a common motor symptom in a few other neurological disorders, such as multiple sclerosis, stroke and cerebral palsy. Spasticity is clinically described as an increased resistance to passive movement due to hyperexcitability of stretch reflex (Lance, 1980; Rymer & Katz, 1994). Rigidity and spasticity share the characteristic feature of the increased muscle tone to a passive movement. However, the unique lead-pipe resistance can distinguish the increased muscle tone in rigidity from that associated with spasticity. In particular, the differentiation between rigidity and spasticity is not straightforward in a clinical scenario (Fung & Thompson, 2002).

Rigidity generally responds well to dopaminergic medication and surgical intervention. Thus, it is used as a diagnostic criterion and to evaluate the efficacy of therapeutic interventions (Prochazka et al., 1997). Clinical examination and assessment of rigidity is determined by an examiner's perception of resistance while rotating the limb at major joints, based upon the Unified Parkinson Disease Rating Scale (Fahn & Elton, 1987; Goetz et al., 2008). A better understanding of the physiological and biomechanical characteristics of rigidity merits scientific significance and clinical implication. In this chapter, studies on elucidation of the physiological mechanisms and biomechanical quantification of parkinsonian rigidity will be reviewed and the latest research on this topic will be presented.

2. Physiological studies of parkinsonian rigidity

2.1 Reflex responses to passive stretch

The history of studying the pathophysiology of rigidity can be traced back to nearly a century ago. Forester's observation (1921) that parkinsonian rigidity is reduced by the dorsal root section suggested that rigidity could be of reflex origin, although other equally plausible explanations are possible. The most widespread view was that rigidity arose from the increased response of muscle receptors to externally imposed stretch. This view was supported by earlier experiments (Pollock & Davis, 1930; Rushworth, 1960), demonstrating that rigidity was substantially reduced by dorsal root section or local anesthetic block. However, illustration by microneurographic recordings from muscle nerves has provided evidence that increased muscle afferent discharge (due to increased fusimotor drive) was not sufficient to explain the presence of rigidity (Burke et al., 1977). Recent studies using electrophysiological techniques demonstrated that monosynaptic segmental stretch reflexes showed no significant differences between individuals with Parkinson's disease and healthy controls (Bergui et al., 1992; Delwaide, 1985; Delwaide et al., 1986; Meara and Cody, 1993; Rothwell et al., 1983). Numerous studies on stretch reflexes have also shown that most reflexes (H-reflex, tendon jerks and tonic vibration reflex), considered to be principally mediated by Ia afferents and to be spinal in origin, appear normal in Parkinson's disease (Burke et al., 1972a; Dietrichson, 1971; Lance et al., 1973). In brief, there is no evidence that Ia muscle afferent pathway might explain the pathophysiological basis of parkinsonian rigidity.

If the response of the spinal machinery to muscle primary spindle afferent input is intact in Parkinson's disease, supraspinally mediated reflexes might well play a role in the pathophysiology of rigidity. Lee and Tatton (1975) were the first to demonstrate that long-latency stretch reflexes in forearm muscles were exaggerated in patients with Parkinson's disease. This observation was subsequently confirmed by several other investigators who studied rigidity in the same or different muscle groups (Berardelli et al., 1983; Cody et al., 1986; Mortimer & Webster, 1979; Rothwell et al., 1983). Some studies found a quantitative association between the degree of increase in long-latency stretch reflex and the clinically assessed degree of rigidity (Mortimer & Webster, 1979; Berardelli et al., 1983), whereas others found that no correlation existed between the two based on a larger number of patients (Cody et al., 1986; Rothwell et al., 1983). The lack of a consistent correlation might be because rigidity is often assessed using a sustained static stretch whereas long-latency stretch reflexes is elicited by transient and brisk muscle stretches (Marsden, 1990). However, it is certain that patients with parkinsonian rigidity show a marked increase in long-latency stretch reflexes, compared with healthy controls (Marsden, 1990; Fung & Thompson, 2002), though there is no universal agreement as to the origin of the long-latency stretch reflexes (Matthews, 1991). In addition, the tonic muscle response to slow and sustained stretch is reported to be exaggerated in Parkinson's disease (Dietrichson, 1971; Andrews et al., 1972).

Findings obtained from the aforementioned studies provide partial explanations for increased resistance, *i.e.*, one of the two elements defining parkinsonian rigidity. However, they cannot account for the constancy and uniformity of resistance which is uniquely associated with rigidity. Recent studies have shed light on the underlying mechanism of the uniform nature of parkinsonian rigidity (Xia & Rymer, 2004; Xia et al., 2011). Evidence indicates that shortening reaction and stretch-induced inhibition play pivotal roles in the genesis of lead-pipe characteristics of rigidity.

2.2 Responses to passive shortening – Shortening reaction

Besides abnormal muscle responses to stretch, anomalous reactions in the shortened muscles during a passive joint motion have also been described in Parkinson's disease. More than a century ago, Westphal (1877, 1880) observed muscular contraction in the passively shortened skeletal muscles. Before he observed this phenomenon, he had already studied the muscular contraction in lengthening or stretched muscles. Thus, he named it 'paradoxer Muskel-contraction'. At that time, he also described enhanced activation of tibialis anterior corresponding to the shortening phase in patients who had great difficulty in passively aiding imposed movement. The phenomenon he observed is often referred to as "Westphal's phenomenon". Later, Sherrington (1909) described analogous findings in both the spinal dog and the decerebrate cat under the name "shortening reaction'. This term has been used since then.

Application of electromyographic (EMG) recording method has demonstrated that inappropriate activation of shortened muscles occurs widely in basal ganglia disorders (Rondot & Metral, 1973), and most prominently in Parkinson's disease (Andrews et al., 1972; Angel, 1983; Berardelli & Hallett, 1984; Rondot & Metral, 1973; Xia & Rymer, 2004). An example of shortening reaction is illustrated in Fig. 1B (Xia et al., 2011). During the passive wrist flexion movement, flexor muscles were progressively shortened. There occurred strong muscle activations in the wrist flexor muscles. Shortening reaction has been reported to be manifested in both upper and lower limb muscles. Some investigators suggested that shortening reaction plays an important role in the pathophysiology of rigidity (Angel, 1983; Rondot & Metral, 1973), given that it represents a reflex action that agonistically assists with a passive movement in contrast to antagonistic opposition of a motion caused by stretch reflex. Correlational analysis showed that there was no direct relationship between shortening reaction and changes in muscle tone (Berardelli & Hallett, 1984).

Nevertheless, the neural mechanism of the shortening reaction was virtually unknown. Since shortening reaction was first reported a century ago, very little attention has been paid to exploring its underlying physiology. Shortening reaction is the opposite of stretch reflex, a topic that has been extensively studied for a long period of time. In contrast, only a limited number of studies were conducted to understand and characterize shortening reaction, and these previous studies simply monitored muscle electromyographic activity (Andrews et al. 1972; Angel, 1983; Berardelli et al. 1983; Berardelli and Hallett, 1984; Rondot and Metral, 1973). The importance of shortening reaction in the pathophysiology of parkinsonian rigidity is undoubtedly underestimated. Utilization of both EMG recording and joint torque measure has provided us with useful information to reveal the role of shortening reaction in mediating rigidity in Parkinson's disease (Xia & Rymer, 2004; Xia et al., 2011). A parallel mechanism responsible for mediating parkinsonian rigidity is stretch-induced inhibition which will be discussed in the next section.

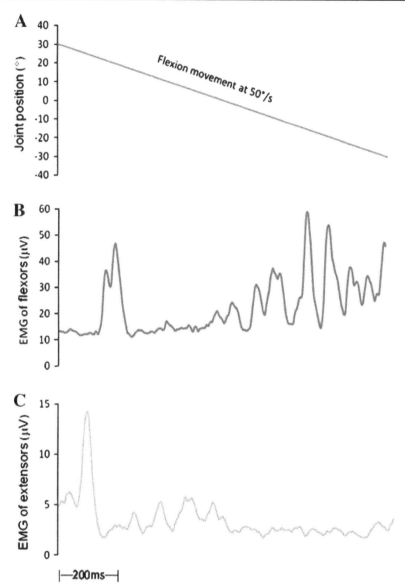

Fig. 1. Kinematic and EMG recordings during passive flexion movement obtained from a patient after an overnight withdrawal of medication (Off-medication). **A.** Wrist joint position during the passive flexion movement; the subject's wrist joint was externally rotated from 30 degree to -30 degree at 50°/s. **B.** Shortening reaction was recorded in shortened flexors in the Off-medication state in a parkinsonian subject. There was an increased EMG activation in passively shortened muscles. **C.** Stretch-induced inhibition was observed in the stretched extensor muscles during the same movement. There was an EMG reduction, when the stretch exceeded the neutral position and the muscle length was elongated [from Xia et al. (2011) with permission].

2.3 Lengthening reaction or stretch-induced inhibition

In addition to shortening reaction, Sherrington (1909) also observed in the above-noted animal preparations that "... *when an examiner bent the knee against the knee-extensor's contraction, the examiner felt the opposition offered by the extensor gave away almost abruptly at a certain pressure; the knee could then be flexed without opposition ...*". He named this phenomenon "lengthening reaction". Lengthening reaction was demonstrated in both spinal dog and in decerebrate rigidity of the cat, yet the reaction was recognized to have differential features in the two preparations. In his monograph, he also pointed out that muscles, exhibiting shortening reaction and lengthening reaction, were all extensor muscles. The distinction of the flexor and extensor muscle groups has been documented in parkinsonian rigidity (Mera et al., 2009; Xia et al., 2006).

The well-know clasp-knife phenomenon associated with human spasticity, appears to be the equivalent of the lengthening reaction (Burke et al., 1970, 1971). The clasp-knife reflex is characterized by an abrupt decline in muscle force that occurs when a spastic limb is moved beyond a certain joint angle. There is a common ground between lengthening reaction in animal preparations (Burke et al., 1972b; Rymer et al., 1979) and clasp-knife reflex in human spasticity in that the essential feature of both phenomena is the sudden release of the resistance due to continuous stretch of the elongated muscle, hence also referred to as "stretch-induced inhibition" (Rymer et al., 1979). The physiological framework previously established or explored in the context of the lengthening reaction or stretch-induced inhibition has recently been investigated in parkinsonian rigidity (Xia & Rymer, 2004; Xia et al., 2011).

Fig. 1C illustrates a stretch-induced inhibition recorded from a parkinsonian patient in the Off-medication state. During the passive flexion movement (Fig. 1A), there was a large initial stretch reflex in the wrist extensor muscles. The initial stretch reflex was followed by a period of sustained activity and curtailed by an evident decline when the progressive movement approached at almost the neutral position and the muscle length of the extensors was elongated, demonstrating the stretch-induced inhibition (Fig. 1C). It is noted that both shortening reaction and stretch-induced inhibition occur during the same movement phase (Fig. 1). The importance and functional role stretch-induced inhibition and the above described shortening reaction may have played in parkinsonian rigidity will be explained and discussed in Section 3.

3. Pathophysiological mechanisms of lead-pipe rigidity

This session will begin with an overview of the basic principles of muscle mechanics. When an active muscle is stretched, the muscle force output increases proportionally with the increasing muscle length. The dependence of muscle force on muscle length gives rise to a "spring-like" behavior (Gordon et al., 1966; Matthews, 1959; Rack & Westbury, 1969). This spring-like property of skeletal muscle has been shown to play a key role in the maintenance of posture and control of movement. A limb's posture is maintained when the forces exerted by agonist and antagonist muscle groups are equal and opposite.

Rotational movements about human joints are promoted by a resultant torque which is a summation of the individual contributions of agonist muscles minus contributions of antagonist muscles, where a single torque is mathematically defined as the product of force times the moment arm for each muscle. The corresponding measure of rotational position is the joint angle, which determines the length of each muscle acting on the joint. Ultimately, it is the torque-angle relationship that serves to characterize the musculature of the joint as a whole (Feldman, 1966). Given the phenomenon that individual muscles are characterized by the length-tension relationship or spring-like property, thus the net torque-angle relation, arising from the summation of the stretched muscles and shortening muscles in normal subjects, manifests a steep curve. Fig. 2A shows that the net torque-angle characteristics of the joint arising from the summation of the spring-like properties of the stretched flexor muscle and shortening extensor muscle display spring-like behavior in healthy subjects, which is characterized by a steep torque-angle curve.

However, the natural spring-like property can be altered, generating a relatively flat torque-angle relationship that is equivalent to a plastic sensation perceived in parkinsonian rigidity. Such a flattened torque-angle relationship can be resulted from either the impact of a shortening reaction or a stretch-induced inhibition or a combination of the two. In the case of parkinsonian rigidity (Figs. 2B-2D), the torque produced by the stretched muscles (i.e., wrist flexors in this example) is increased due to the exaggerated long-latency stretch reflexes (Lee & Tatton, 1975) and enhanced tonic muscle responses (Dietrichson, 1971). There are two ways in which a joint could generate relatively constant torque with the changing joint position. Firstly, if there is an inappropriate shortening reaction in parkinsonian rigidity, the increasing force generated by the stretched flexor is offset by increasing activation of the shortening extensor. This muscle interaction could lead to a flat net torque-angle relationship, and promote the perception of the constant rigidity. Fig. 2B shows the potential interactions between stretched and activated shortening muscle in the presence of a shortening reaction. Another possibility, shown in Fig. 2C, is that a reduction in activation of stretched muscle at an elongated muscle length counteracts the otherwise gradual increase in muscle force (i.e., spring-like or elastic-like muscle force) as the muscle length of the stretched flexors is elongated throughout the stretch. Due to this counteracting effect, the net torque is relatively constant throughout the rotation of the limb. During the passive flexion or extension movement, one group of muscles is shortened whereas the other group is stretched. Both shortening reaction and stretch-induced inhibition have counteracting effects within a specified movement, generating the promotion of constant rigidity (uniformity) as defined in rigidity. Fig. 2D schematically illustrates the net torque resulting from a combined effect of the two mechanisms.

During passive movements, one group of muscles is shortened whereas the other group of muscles is stretched. Thus, the two mechanisms are potentially generating counteracting effects on the net torque resistance simultaneously. However, a dissociation of the two mechanisms is not readily available and technically challenging. Application of a biomechanical model (Holzbaur et al., 2005) implemented through the Software for Interactive Musculoskeletal Modeling (Delp & Loan, 1995) made it possible to quantify the torque generated by shortening muscles and by stretched muscles, separately, and to identify which mechanism predominates. Our findings obtained through the biomechanical modeling approach indicate that both shortening reaction and stretch-induced inhibition contribute significantly to the lead-pipe nature of parkinsonian rigidity (Xia et al., 2011). During the passive flexion movement, shortening reaction plays a predominant role in the genesis of lead-pipe rigidity, whereas stretch-induced inhibition is a primary contributor to the manifestation of lead-pipe rigidity during the passive extension movement. The knowledge gained from these studies provides new insights into the biomechanical and physiological underpinnings of this common symptom in patients with Parkinson's disease. The use of this approach may offer a means of assessing the efficacy of rehabilitation programs and therapeutic interventions. Efficacy of anti-Parkinson medication on the biomechanical and physiological characteristics associated with parkinsonian rigidity will be discussed in later section of this Chapter.

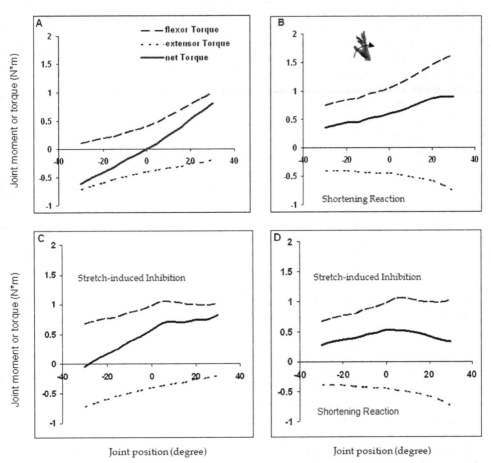

Fig. 2. Schematics of the net (solid line) torque-angle relationship showing four possible types of interactions between stretched and shortening muscles during extension of a right wrist. **A**: torque-angle relationship characterizing spring-like property of the stretched flexor and shortening extensor muscles in healthy subjects; **B**: the potential impact of a shortening reaction in the extensor muscles (contributing to extensor torque), inducing a flattened net torque-angle relation and promoting the perception of the constant rigidity; **C**: the effect of a stretch-induced inhibition in flexor muscles, causing spring-like force generated by a muscle stretch to decline as the muscle length increases. **D**: The combined effect of shortening reaction and stretch-induced inhibition on the net torque. The units and torque curves are arbitrary.

4. Non-neural factor responsible for parkinsonian rigidity

Evidence has indicated that in addition to neural-mediated abnormal muscle reflex responses, the non-neural component also contributes to parkinsonian rigidity (Dietz, 1987; Dietz et al., 1981; Watts et al., 1986). The non-neural component includes visco-elastic (i.e., mechanical) properties of muscle fiber and passive connective tissues. Dietz et al. (1981) examined ten patients with parkinsonian rigidity aiming to identify the physiological mechanism with respect to altered muscle activity to account for impaired gait pattern in Parkinson's disease. Compared to healthy control subjects, parkinsonian patients exhibited significantly stronger EMG activity in tibialis anterior during the swing phase of gait, while the strength and timing of EMG activity recorded from triceps surae were similar in two groups of participants. The authors stated that the increased muscle tone in parkinsonian rigidity cannot be explained by the electrical activity of the antagonist muscle groups of the limb, since there was no co-contraction of tibialis anterior and triceps surae muscles. It was concluded that the altered mechanical properties of muscle fibers were mainly responsible for the increased muscle tone in rigidity. This conclusion was also drawn by Watts et al. (1986) who examined elbow joint of patients with Parkinson's disease and normal controls by using a torque motor. Even in patients with relatively mild symptoms, the upper limb was stiffer than controls in the totally relaxed state with no EMG activity present. The study findings suggested that changes in the passive mechanical properties of the upper limb likely accounted for greater passive stiffness. Using the torque motor, natural progression of the disease can be quantified and followed.

Evidence indicates that neural and non-neural mechanisms operate in parallel, both contributing to parkinsonian rigidity. However, there is no simple and easy solution in differentiation and quantification of the neural and non-neural components because clinical measures of rigidity consist of the two parallel components. Using advanced technology and computational algorithm, a few sophisticated approaches have been developed to segregate the two responsible factors and quantify the individual component contributing to the overall joint stiffness (Kearney et al., 1997; Meinders et al., 1996; Sinkjaer et al., 1993; Sinkjaer & Magnussen, 1994; Zhang & Rymer, 1997). One approach, termed as parallel-cascaded system identification technique, was initially applied to separate the overall stiffness into neural reflex stiffness and non-neural mechanical stiffness at ankle joint in normal healthy adults (Kearney et al., 1997; Mirbagheri et al., 2000). Subsequently, the system identification approach has been applied to characterize the dynamic joint stiffness and to quantify the neural and non-neural contribution to the abnormal muscle tone in spasticity associated with upper motor neuron syndromes, such as stroke and spinal cord injury (Alibiglou et al., 2008; Galiana et al., 2005; Mirbagheri et al., 2001, 2009, 2010). The validity of this method has been demonstrated as well as its efficiency, accuracy and advantages by Mirbagheri et al. (2000) and Alibiglou et al. (2008).

More recently, we have applied the parallel-cascaded system identification technique to make a distinction between the neural and non-neural contributions to rigidity in patients with Parkinson's disease (Xia et al., 2010). Patients participated in the protocol under two medication states: initially under a temporary overnight withdrawal of dopaminergic medication and then after the resumption of medication. The results have shown that both neural and non-neural components contributed to parkinsonian rigidity, with the neural component being predominating over the non-neural to the overall rigidity. Medication therapy caused a reduction of torque resistance in the neural reflex torque, but did not decrease the non-neural mechanical torque. This observation appears to be attributed to the mechanism of anti-Parkinson medication therapy.

5. Biomechanical quantification of parkinsonian rigidity

In clinic, parkinsonian rigidity is examined and assessed using a numerical rating scale which is known as the Unified Parkinson Disease Rating Scale (Fahn & Elton, 1987; Goetz et al., 2008). However, the nature of this assessment tool is highly qualitative and subjective because it is largely dependent on examiners' individual interpretation and experience (Patrick et al., 2001; Prochazka et al., 1997). When the actual change in rigidity resulting from treatment is small, it may be challenging for the examiners to detect. This can limit ability for evaluation of treatment effectiveness especially in large multi-center clinical drug trials in which a large number of investigators are involved, because differences can exist between different examiners (i.e., inter-rater) and between assessments performed on different visits by a given examiner (i.e., intra-rater) with respect to the efficacy of treatment. Reliability studies have demonstrated varying degrees of inter-rater reliability with respect to rigidity component of clinical rating tools, ranging from low, moderate, very good to excellent (Martinez-Martin, 1993; Rabey et al., 1997; Richards et al., 1994; Van Dillen & Roach, 1988). A need for more accurate evaluations has been expressed to improve the management of symptoms in patients with Parkinson's disease (Obeso et al., 1996; Ondo et al., 1998; Ward et al., 1983).

During the past several decades, considerable efforts have been made aiming to quantify assessment of parkinsonian rigidity by means of biomechanical measures. A variety of quantitative methods have been developed to measure the dynamics of joint stiffness associated with rigidity (Lee et al., 2002; Prochazka et al., 1997; Teräväinen et al., 1989; Watts et al., 1986; Wiegner & Watts, 1986). The underlying approach is to measure the amount of imposed force resistance to externally generated passive movement about the examined joint. The passive movements applied in earlier studies were induced either by a torque motor (Fung et al., 2000; Mak et al., 2007; Shapiro et al., 2007; Watts et al., 1986; Xia et al., 2006) or generated by an examiner to closely resemble a clinical setting (Caligiuri, 1994; Endo et al., 2009; Patrick et al., 2001; Prochazka et al., 1997; Sepehri et al., 2007). Variables described in these previous studies included peak torque (Mak et al., 2007), impulse (i.e., an integral of torque with respect to time; Fung et al., 2000), work score which is calculated as a torque integral with respect to joint angular position (see Fig. 3; Fung et al., 2000; Mak et al., 2007; Shapiro et al., 2007; Teräväinen et al., 1989; Xia et al., 2006, 2009), elastic coefficient (Endo et al., 2009), and mechanical impedance calculated based on the force imposed and displacement of the movement (Patrick et al., 2001; Prochazka et al., 1997).

There are a few advantages of quantification by force or torque measures over quantification by EMG. Torque-based assessment of rigidity is more objective and reliable than EMG-derived evaluation. However, there are limitations in estimation of using surface EMGs as its measures are susceptible to the placement of electrodes, condition of soft tissues and concerns of cross-talk. Biomechanical measures using torque can avoid the limitations inherent in EMG measures. In addition, non-neural contribution to parkinsonian rigidity is also included in torque measures but is not reflected in EMG recordings. Previous studies have shown that correlation is relatively weak between clinical degree of rigidity and EMG quantification of rigidity while correlation is found to be much stronger between clinical degree of rigidity and torque quantification of rigidity (Endo et al., 2009; Levin et al., 2009;

Park et al., 2010; Teräväinen et al., 1989). Evidence indicates that torque measure has proven to be a more objective and robust way for assessing rigidity, compared to EMG evaluation of rigidity.

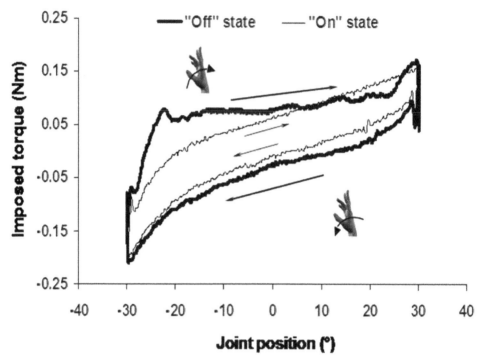

Fig. 3. Torque-angle relationship in a parkinsonian subject in the Off-medication (thicker line) and On-medication (thinner line) states. The subject's more affected side was tested. The upper traces represent imposed extension movements and the lower traces flexion movements. The wrist joint was externally rotated at 50 °/s between 30° flexion and 30° extension shown as a loop. The subject was instructed to remain relaxed. The work, used to quantify the degree of rigidity, was equivalent to the areas inside the loop of torque-angle plots in the respective medication states [from Xia et al. (2006) with permission].

Application of biomechanical measures has also enabled us to investigate more profoundly some of the characteristics associated with parkinsonian rigidity, thus further increasing our understanding of this motor symptom. Firstly, only through the measures of torque resistance and joint position, can lead-pipe nature of rigidity be examined and revealed (Mera et al., 2009; Xia & Rymer, 2004; Xia et al., 2006, 2011). The slope of torque-angle curve was used to quantify the degree of lead-pipe property. The smaller slopes represent higher degrees of constant and uniform resistance through the range of passive movement. The torque-angle slopes are smaller when patients were tested in the untreated conditions, and become greater in the treated conditions (Xia & Rymer, 2004; Xia et al., 2006).

Secondly, rigidity has been thought to be plastic with respect to direction of the movement (Berardelli et al., 1983; Delwaide, 2001). However, recent studies employing the biomechanical measures have demonstrated that rigidity associated with extension movement is more evident as compared to rigidity during flexion movement in the upper limb including the wrist and elbow (Mera et al., 2009; Park et al., 2010; Xia et al., 2006). These authors used mechanical parameters, such as work, torque-angle slope and visco-elastic parameter, to evaluate the difference and distinction between the passive flexion and extension movements.

Thirdly, parkinsonian rigidity has traditionally been considered to be independent of velocity in contrast to spasticity which is highly velocity-dependent (Lance, 1980). The notion of velocity-independency of rigidity might be anecdotal. As such, this view has been examined by a few recent studies. Lee et al. (2002) studied hypertonia at the elbow joint in patients with Parkinson's disease and patients with hemiparesis as compared to control subjects. Four different stretching velocities were applied, ranging from 40 to 160 °/s. The authors concluded that both rigidity and spasticity have approximately equal velocity-dependent property. Quantitative measure of trunk rigidity in patients with Parkinson's disease also revealed a velocity-dependent feature (Mak et al., 2007). Our results on the effect of movement velocity on rigidity concurred with those reports. Velocity-dependency of rigidity was also demonstrated at the wrist joint of patients with Parkinson's disease (Xia et al., 2009) in which both slow velocity at 50 degree/second and fast speed at 280 °/s were applied. The results showed that the work done during the fast movement was significantly larger than the work associated with the slower movement. The accumulating evidence has pointed out the velocity-dependency of parkinsonian rigidity.

Fourthly, compared to the effect of movement velocity on quantitative analysis of parkinsonian rigidity, effect of displacement amplitude on rigidity has thus far sparsely been investigated, except for one study by Terävänäinen et al. (1989). To determine the optimal angular velocity and displacement amplitude for detecting abnormal muscle tone, four movement amplitudes or central ranges of motion, ranging from ±15, ±20, ±25 to ±30 degrees, were applied to examine rigidity at the wrist joint in 29 patients with Parkinson's disease. The results showed that the larger movement amplitudes were more sensitive for detecting parkinsonian rigidity and had stronger correlation with the clinical scores of rigidity. Given the situation that some clinicians rotate the limb back and forth rapidly in the mid-range whereas others focus on the extremes of range of motion or the entire range of motion with slow stretches (Prochazka et al., 1997), it is important and significant to explore the influence of displacement amplitude on objective measurements of rigidity. We recently conducted a study aiming to examine the effect of displacement amplitude. Twenty four patients participated in the experiment under treated (On-medication) and untreated (Off-medication) conditions, with the more affected side of the wrist joint tested. Passive movements of wrist flexion and extension were imposed with two displacement amplitudes, ±30 degree and ±45 degree, respectively, at either 50 °/s or 280 °/s, and the order of movement pattern was presented in a random fashion. Figure 4 depicts and compares the torque-angle plots associated with two ranges of motion: 60 degree (Fig. 4A) and 90 degree (Fig. 4B), in a parkinsonian subject under the two medication conditions. The work score was calculated to quantify rigidity, and was normalized to the range of motion to validate the comparison. Clearly, there is a difference in the area of the torque-angle loop between the two displacement amplitudes or the ranges of motion. Figure 4B shows that the extreme joint position, the larger displacement amplitude, caused increase in rigidity work score.

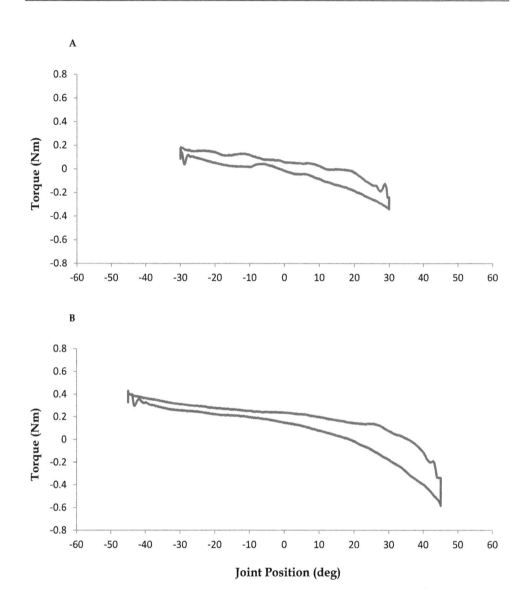

Fig. 4. Comparison of torque-position traces of passive flexion and extension movements of two ranges of motion: 60° (A) and 90° (B) at angular velocity of 50° /s from a subject with Parkinson's disease tested in the Off-medication state. The rigidity score, quantified by the integral of the torque with respect to angular position (Nm-deg), increased in response to the greater range of motion. Upper traces are associated with extension movements while lower traces are associated with flexion movements [from Powell et al. (in press) with permission].

Finally, the phenomenon that rigidity can be reinforced by a concurrent ipsi- or contra-lateral voluntary activation has recently been further quantified using biomechanical measures (Hong et al., 2007; Powell et al., 2011). Figure 5 illustrates torque-angle traces of the entire cycle of flexion and extension movements when a subject with PD was tested in the Off-medication condition. Torque resistance was elevated by the presence of contra-lateral activation (Active condition) as compared to the Passive condition. There is an obvious difference in the contained area of torque-angle plots between the Passive and Active conditions. These studies aimed to provide quantitative data and objective evaluation of clinical assessment of rigidity as a component of the Unified Parkinson Disease Rating Scale (Fahn & Elton, 1987; Goetz et al., 2008). The type of voluntary activations applied in clinical examinations include a variety of motor acts such as tapping fingers, fist opening–closing or heel tapping. The use of reinforcing maneuvers was originated and first investigated by Jules Froment, a French neurologist, in the 1920's (Broussolle et al., 2007). Froment studied muscle tone at the wrist joint while the subject was in different positions, at rest in a sitting position, and standing in stable and unstable postures. In addition to clinical examination, Fremont also conducted experiments recording activity of forearm extensors using a myograph. He described an increased resistance to passive movements of a limb about a joint during the presence of a voluntary action of a contralateral body part. Due to his contributions to the study of parkinsonian rigidity, the activation or facilitation test has been referred to as the "Froment maneuver". The impact of facilitation test is significant as it has been formalized in the motor scale of the Unified Parkinson Disease Rating Scale. The maneuver is particularly used to detect increased muscle tone at an early stage of the disease when rigidity is not otherwise manifested during the examination.

6. Effect of anti-Parkinson medication on physiological and biomechanical measures of rigidity

Rigidity generally responds well to anti-Parkinson medication. Several studies have examined the changes in muscle activation, joint torque resistance and torque-angle slope associated with rigidity reduction as a result of medication therapy (Kirollos et al., 1996; Mera et al., 2009; Powell et al., 2011; Xia & Rymer, 2004; Xia et al., 2006, 2009). Following a standard protocol, patients are tested initially in the Off-medication state, i.e., 12 hours after the last dose of medication when the majority of the beneficial effects of medication therapy are eliminated (Defer et al., 1999). Twelve-hour overnight withdrawal of medication has been broadly used to examine the effect of medication on motor performance and on basal ganglia function (Brown & Marsden, 1999; Corcos et al., 1996; Jahanshahi et al., 2010; Robichaud et al., 2004; Tunik et al., 2004). After the initial tests are completed, patients are retested approximately one hour after taking their regular dose of medication in the On-medication state. These studies have demonstrated that stretch-reflex and shortening reaction are diminished following the treatment (Powell et al., 2011; Xia & Rymer, 2004). The same effects are observed in the changes associated with torque resistance (Kirollos et al., 1996; Mera et al., 2009; Xia et al., 2006, 2009). Further, torque-angle curves associated with the On-medication test become steeper, manifesting the spring-like feature and the typical length-tension relationship (Gordon et al., 1966; Matthews, 1959; Rack & Westbury, 1969; Xia et al., 2006, see Fig. 2).

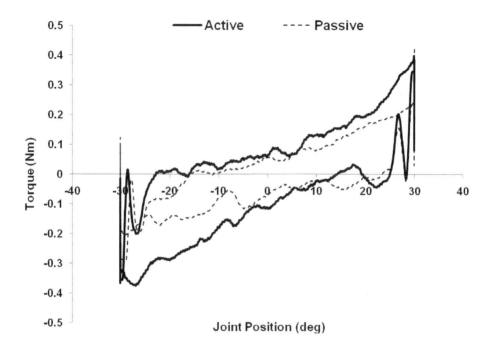

Fig. 5. Comparison of torque-angle traces between the Passive (dashed) and Active (solid) conditions recorded in a subject with Parkinson's disease under the Off-Medication condition. Under the Active condition, passive movement of the wrist joint was concurrent with a contra-lateral hand gripping activation at 20% of maximal voluntary contraction. Rigidity score, calculated as the integral of the torque with respect to position for the entire cycle of flexion and extension movements, was enhanced under the Active condition. Upper traces are associated with the passive extension movement and the lower ones with the flexion movement [from Powell et al. (2011) with permission].

Effects of deep brain stimulation of the subthalamic nucleus in conjunction with medication have also been evaluated on the work rigidity and clinical rigidity scores in patients with Parkinson's disease (Shapiro et al., 2007). Subjects' elbow joints were tested under four experimental conditions determined by various combinations of medication (Off vs. On) and deep brain stimulation (Off vs. On) status. Treatment by deep brain stimulation reduced rigidity as indicated by work score and by rigidity score on the Unified Parkinson Disease Rating Scale. The results suggested that the surgical treatment may be more effective in alleviating rigidity in the upper limb of parkinsonian patients than medications administered at pre-surgery dosage level.

7. Interaction of rigidity with other motor symptoms

Parkinson's disease is characterized by both motor and non-motor related symptoms. Motor symptoms, often referred to as cardinal symptoms, include bradykinesia (slowness and decreased amplitude of movement), muscle rigidity, tremor-at-rest, and postural instability.

According to the diagnostic criteria, clinical diagnosis is based on two cardinal features of the disease (Fahn & Sulzer, 2004; Lang & Lozano, 1998). Parkinson's disease is a heterogeneous disease both across different patients and during the natural progression of the same patient. The heterogeneity of the disease among different patients is reflected by multiple sub-types of Parkinson's disease, i.e., akinetic-rigid type, tremor-predominant type, and postural instability gait difficulty sub-type (Burn et al., 2006; Hallett, 2003; Jankovic et al., 1990). Bradykinesia is labeled as a negative symptom due to its describing the poverty and slowing of voluntary movement, whereas rigidity and tremor are referred to as positive motor symptoms.

Many clinical studies have indicated that the distinctions are significant among the hallmark motor symptoms although they share similarities and common origins (Elias et al., 2008). The distinctive nature has also been revealed by Temperli and coauthors (2003) who studied the reappearance of the clinical signs of Parkinson's disease when subthalamic nucleus deep brain stimulation was switched off in 35 patients treated with implanted deep brain stimulators. Authors reported that a sequential pattern of return of motor signs was observed, with a fast worsening of tremor within 10 to 15 minutes, followed by a smoother, slower worsening of bradykinesia and rigidity over half an hour to an hour, and finally a slow and steady worsening of axial signs over three to four hours. When switching the stimulation "on" again, all motor signs improved with a similar pattern. It was concluded that the four major parkinsonian signs may respond to brain stimulation by different mechanisms.

8. Clinical interventions of Parkinson's disease

Our knowledge and understanding of Parkinson's disease have dramatically increased over the past years, consequently shifting the descriptions of this disease. Parkinson's disease, previously considered to be characterized by only motor symptoms (bradykinesia, rigidity, resting tremor and postural instability), is now viewed as a disease affected by both motor symptoms and a range of non-motor symptoms such as depression, disturbed sleeping patterns, fatigue, hallucination, cognitive impairments, changes in ability to taste or smell and a few other domains. Only during the last couple of decades or so, non-motor related symptoms have begun receiving attention in medical and research communities. As a result, a number of clinical rating tools have been developed to target specific or general non-motor symptoms (Brown et al., 2005; Chaudhuri et al., 2007).

Rigidity is treated as part of parkinsonian motor symptoms. Among the motor symptoms of Parkinson's disease, bradykinesia and rigidity are the signs that are most responsive to medication and surgical treatments. A variety of pharmacological and surgical interventions are available for the management of Parkinson's disease. Levodopa was the first major breakthrough in the treatment of Parkinson's disease, and still remains the "gold standard" in the management of symptoms. Levodopa is converted in the brain into dopamine to replenish the brain's dwindling supply in patients with Parkinson's disease. The introduction of dopamine agonists was a milestone in the treatment of parkinsonian symptoms. In contrast to levodopa, dopamine agonists act directly on dopamine receptors in the brain, and thus can help alleviate the symptoms of Parkinson's disease. Based on preclinical observation, there is an increasingly popular theory known as continuous dopamine agonist stimulation that helps to prevent the occurrence of long-term complications.

However, with the treatment of medication on advanced stage of this progressive disease, many patients experience motor complications, which is broadly classified as "wearing off reactions", "On-Off reactions", dyskinesia, confusion, sleepiness, hallucination, and low blood pressure when standing (Stacy, 2009). In patients who are severely affected or in those who fail to respond satisfactorily to pharmacological therapy, surgical treatments have reportedly been effective in reducing symptoms and improving function. These include pallidotomy, thalamotomy and subthalamotomy, and high frequency deep brain stimulation via electrodes implanted in the globus pallidus, thalamus (a "relay station" deep in brain), or subthalamic nucleus. Rigidity can be specifically improved by subthalamic nucleus deep brain stimulation (Temperli et al., 2003).

9. Conclusion

Evidence has indicated that no single mechanism can account for parkinsonian rigidity, which is influenced by a multitude of physiological phenomena and biomechanical features. Treatment of rigidity primarily involves an administration of dopaminergic medication. However, serious side effects usually occur after a few years' drug treatment. Therefore, rehabilitative programs are highly desirable for patients with Parkinson's disease. A better understanding of the comprehensive characteristics of parkinsonian rigidity is crucial for designing effective evidence-based exercise program and physical therapy intervention. An objective assessment of rigidity is essential for evaluating the efficacy of therapeutic interventions, especially in large clinical studies in which trials are conducted across multiple centers.

10. Acknowledgments

The author would like to acknowledge support of the National Institutes of Health, Nebraska Tobacco Settlement Biomedical Research Development Fund, Health Future Foundation of Creighton University, and Faculty Development Fund of School of Pharmacy and Health Professions, Creighton University in Omaha Nebraska, USA.

11. References

Alibiglou, L.; Rymer, WZ.; Harvey, RL. & Mirbagheri MM. (2008). The relation between Ashworth scores and neuromechanical measurements of spasticity following stroke. *J Neuroeng Rehabil*, Vol.5, pp. 18-31.

Andrews, CJ.; Burke, D. & Lance, JW. (1972). The response to muscle stretch and shortening in Parkinsonian rigidity. *Brain*, Vol.95, pp. 795-812.

Angel, RW. (1983). Muscular contractions elicited by passive shortening. *Adv Neurol*, Vol.39, pp. 555-563.

Bantam Medical Dictionary (2000). 3rd edition, New York, USA: Bantam Books, Incorporated.

Berardelli, A. & Hallett, M. (1984). Shortening reaction of human tibialis anterior. *Neurology*, Vol. 34, pp. 242-246.

Berardelli, A.; Sabra, AF. & Hallett, M. (1983). Physiological mechanisms of rigidity in Parkinson's disease. *J Neurol Neurosurg Psychiatry*, Vol.46, pp. 45-53.

Broussolle, E.; Krack, P.; Thobois, S.; Xie-Brustolin, J.; Pollak, P. & Goetz, C.G. (2007). Contribution of Jules Froment to the study of parkinsonian rigidity. *Mov Disord*, Vol.22, pp. 909-14.

Brown, R.G.; Dittner, A.; Findley, L. & Wessely, S.C. (2005). The Parkinson fatigue scale. *Parkinsonism Relat Disord*, Vol. 11, pp. 49–55.

Brown, P. & Marsden, CD. (1999). Bradykinesia and impairment of EEG desynchronization in Parkinson's disease. *Mov Disord*, Vol.14, pp.423-429.

Bergui, M.; Lopiano, L.; Paglia, G.; Quattrocolo, G.; Scarzella, L. & Bergamasco, B. (1992). Stretch reflex of quadriceps femoris and its relation to rigidity in Parkinson's disease. *Acta Neurol Scand*, Vol. 86, pp. 226-229.

Burke, D.; Andrews, CJ. & Lance JW. (1972a). Tonic vibration reflex in spasticity, Parkinson's disease, and normal subjects. *J Neurol Neurosurg Psychiatry*, Vol.35, pp. 477-486.

Burke, D.; Gillies, JD. & Lance, JW. (1970). The quadriceps stretch reflex in human spasticity. *Journal of Neurology, Neurosurgery and Psychiatry*, Vol. 33, pp. 216-223.

Burke, D.; Hagbarth, KE. & Wallin, BG. (1977). Reflex mechanisms in Parkinsonian rigidity. *Scand J Rehabil Med.*, Vol.9, pp. 15-23.

Burke, D.; Knowles, L.; Andrews, C. & Ashby, P. (1972b). Spasticity, decerebrate rigidity and the clasp-knife phenomenon: an experimental study in the cat. *Brain*, Vol. 95, pp. 31-48.

Burn, DJ.; Rowan, EN.; Allan, LM.; Molloy, S.; O'Brien, JT. & McKeith, IG. (2006). Motor subtype and cognitive decline in Parkinson's disease, Parkinson's disease with dementia, and dementia with Lewy bodies. *J Neurol Neurosurg Psychiatry*, Vol. 77, pp.585-9.

Caligiuri, M.P. (1994). Portable device for quantifying parkinsonian wrist rigidity. *Mov Disord*, Vol. 9(1), pp. 57-63.

Chaudhuri KR, Martinez-Martin P, Brown RG, Sethi K, Stocchi F, Odin P, Ondo W, Abe K, Macphee G, Macmahon D, Barone P, Rabey M, Forbes A, Breen K, Tluk S, Naidu Y, Olanow W, Williams AJ, Thomas S, Rye D, Tsuboi Y, Hand A, Schapira AH 2007. The metric properties of a novel non-motor symptoms scale for Parkinson's disease: Results from an international pilot study. *Mov Disord*. Oct 15;22(13):1901-11.

Cody, FWJ.; MacDermott, N.; Matthews, PBC. & Richardson, HC. (1986). Observations on the genesis of the stretch reflex in Parkinson's disease. *Brain*, Vol.109, pp. 229-249.

Corcos, DM.; Chen, CM.; Quinn, NP.; McAuley, J. & Rothwell, JC. (1996). Strength in Parkinson's disease: relationship to rate of force generation and clinical status. *Ann Neurol*, Vol.39, pp.79-88.

De Lau, LM. & Breteler, MM. (2006). Epidemiology of Parkinson's disease. *Lancet Neurol*, Vol.5, pp. 525-535.

Defer, GL.; Widner, H.; Marié, RM.; Rémy, P. & Levivier, M. (1999). Core assessment program for surgical interventional therapies in Parkinson's disease (CAPSIT-PD). *Mov Disord*, Vol.14, pp.572-84.

Delp, SL. & Loan, JP. (1995) A graphics-based software system to develop and analyze models of musculoskeletal structures. *Comput Biol Med*, Vol. 25, pp. 21–34.

Delwaide, PJ. (1985). Are there modifications in spinal cord functions of parkinsonian patients? In: *Clinical Neurophysiology in Parkinsonism*, P.J. Delwaide, A. Agnoli, (Ed.) pp. 19- 32, Elsevier, New York, USA.

Delwaide, P.J. (2001). Parkinsonian rigidity. *Funct Neurol* Vol. 16(2), pp. 147-56.

Delwaide, PJ.; Sabbatino, M. & Delwaide, C. (1986). Some pathophysiological aspects of the parkinsonian rigidity. *J Neural Transm Suppl*, Vol.22, pp.129-39.

Dietrichson, P. (1971). Phasic ankle reflex in spasticity and Parkinsonian rigidity. The role of the fusimotor system. *Acta Neurol Scand*, Vol.47, pp. 22-51.

Dietz, V. (1987). Changes of inherent muscle stiffness in Parkinson's disease. *J Neurol Neurosurg Psychiatry*, Vol. 50, pp. 944.

Dietz, V.; Quintern, J. & Berger, W. (1981). Electrophysiological studies of gait in spasticity and rigidity. Evidence that altered mechanical properties of muscle contribute to hypertonia. *Brain*, Vol.104, pp. 431-449.

Dorsey, E.R.; Constantinescu, R.; Thompson, JP.; Biglan, KM.; Holloway, RG.; Kieburtz, K.; Marshall, FJ.; Ravina, BM.; Schifitto, G.; Siderowf, A. & Tanner, CM. (2007). Projected number of people with Parkinson disease in the most populous nations, 2005 through 2030. *Neurol*, Vol. 68(5), pp.384-6.

Elias, S.; Israel, Z. & Bergman, H. (2008). Physiology of Parkinson's disease. In: *Therapeutics of Parkinson's Disease and Other Movement Disorders*, M. Hallett, W. Poewe, (Ed). 25-36, John Wiley & Sons Ltd., ISBN 978-0-470-06648-5, West Sussex, UK.

Endo, T.; Okuno, R.; Yokoe, M.; Akazawa, K. & Sakoda, S. (2009). A novel method for systematic analysis of rigidity in Parkinson's disease. *Mov Disord*, Vol.24, pp. 2218-2224.

Fahn, S. & Elton, RL. (1987) Members of the UPDRS development committee. Unified parkinson's disease rating scale, In: *Recent developments in Parkinson's disease*, S. Fahn, D. C. Marsden, P. Jenner, P. Teychenne, (Ed). 153-164, Macmillian Healthcare, ISBN 978-088-1671-32-2, Florham, New Jersey, USA.

Fahn, S. (2003). Description of Parkinson's disease as a clinical syndrome. *Ann NY Acad Sci*, Vol.991, pp. 1-14.

Fahn, S. & Sulzer, D. (2004). Neurodegeneration and neuroprotection in Parkinson disease. *NeuroRx*, Vol. 1, pp.139-54.

Feldman, AG. (1966). Functional tuning of the nervous system on control of movement or maintenance of a steadyposture. II. Controllable parameters of the muscle. *Biophysics*, Vol.11, pp. 565-578.

Forester, O. (1921). Zur Analyse und Pathophysiologie der striaten Bewegungsstörungen. *Z Ges Neurol Psychiat*, Vol.73, pp. 1-169

Fung, VS. & Thompson, PD. (2002). Rigidity and spasticity, In: *Parkinson's disease and Movement Disorders*, J. J. Jankovic, E. Tolosa (4th. Ed.), 473-482, Lippincott Williams & Wilkins, ISBN: 0-7817-7881-6, Philadelphia, USA.

Fung, VS.; Burne, JA. & Morris, JG. (2000). Objective quantification of resting and activated parkinsonian rigidity: a comparison of angular impulse and work scores. *Mov Disord*, Vol.15, pp. 48-55

Galiana, L.; Fung, J. & Kearney, R. (2005). Identification of intrinsic and reflex ankle stiffness components in stroke patients. *Exp Brain Res*, Vol.165, pp. 422-434.

Goetz, CG.; Tilley, BC.; Shaftman, SR.; Stebbins, GT.; Fahn, S.; Martinez-Martin, P.; Poewe, W.; Sampaio, C.; Stern, MB.; Dodel, R.; Dubois, B.; Holloway, R.; Jankovic, J.; Kulisevsky, J; Lang, AE.; Lees, A.; Leurgans, S.; LeWitt, PA.; Nyenhuis, D.; Olanow, CW.; Rascol, O.; Schrag, A.; Teresi, JA.; van Hilten, JJ. & LaPelle, N. (2008). Movement Disorder Society-sponsored revision of the Unified Parkinson's Disease Rating Scale (MDS-UPDRS): scale presentation and clinimetric testing results. *Mov Disord*, Vol.23, pp. 2129-2170

Gordon, AM.; Huxley, AF. & Julian, FJ. (1966). The variation in isometric tension with sarcomere length in vertebrate muscle fibres. *J Physiol*, Vol. 184, pp. 170-192.

Hallett, M. (2003). Parkinson revisited: pathophysiology of motor signs. *Adv Neurol*, Vol.91, pp. 19-28.

Holzbaur, KR.; Murray, WM. & Delp, SL. (2005) A model of the upper extremity for simulating musculoskeletal surgery and analyzing neuromuscular control. *Ann Biomed Eng*, Vol.33. pp. 829–840.

Hong, M.; Perlmutter, J.S. & Earhart, G.M. (2007). Enhancement of rigidity in Parkinson's disease with activation. *Mov Disord*, Vol. 22, pp. 1164-8.

Jahanshahi, M.; Jones, CR.; Zijlmans, J.; Katzenschlager, R.; Lee, L.; Quinn, N.; Frith, CD. & Lees AJ. (2010). Dopaminergic modulation of striato-frontal connectivity during motor timing in Parkinson's disease. *Brain*, Vol. 133, pp.727-745.

Jankovic, J.; McDermott, M.; Carter, J.; Gauthier, S.; Goetz, C.; Golbe, L.; Huber, S.; Koller, W.; Olanow, C.; Shoulson, I. et al. (1990). Variable expression of Parkinson's disease: a base-line analysis of the DATATOP cohort. The Parkinson Study Group. *Neurol*, Vol. 40, pp.1529-34.

Kearney, RE.; Stein, RB. & Parameswaran, L. (1997). Identification of intrinsic and reflex contributions to human ankle stiffness dynamics. *IEEE Trans Biomed Eng*, Vol.44, pp. 493-504.

Kirollos, C.; Charlett, A.; O'Neill, CJ.; Kosik, R.; Mozol, K.; Purkiss, AG.; Bowes, SG.; Nicholson, PW.; Hunt, WB.; Weller, C.; Dobbs, SM. & Dobbs, RJ. (1996). Objective measurement of activation of rigidity: diagnostic, pathogenetic and therapeutic implications in parkinsonism. *Br J Clin Pharmaco*, Vol. 41, pp.557-64.

Lance, JW. (1980). Pathophysiology of spasticity and clinical experience with baclofen, In: *Spasticity: disordered motor control*, R. G. Feldman, R. R. Young, W. P. Koella, (Ed). 185-203, ISBN – 978-081-5132-40-0, Year Book Medical Publishers, Chicago, Illinois, USA.

Lance, JW.; Burke, D. & Andrews, CJ. (1973). The reflex effects of muscle vibration. In: *New Developments in Electromyography and Clinical Neurophysiology*, J. E. Desmedt (Ed), 3:44-462, ISBN 978-380-5514-09-5 Basel: Karger, Switzerland

Lang, A.E. & Lozano, A.M. (1998). Parkinson's disease. First of two parts. *N Engl J Med*, 339:1044-53.

Lee, HM.; Huang, YZ.; Chen, JJ. & Hwang, IS. (2002). Quantitative analysis of the velocity related pathophysiology of spasticity and rigidity in the elbow flexors. *J Neurol Neurosurg Psychiatry*, Vol.72, pp. 621–9.

Lee, RG. & Tatton, WG. (1975). Motor responses to sudden limb displacements in primates with specific CNS lesions and in human patients with motor system disorders. *Can J Neurol Sci*, Vol.2, pp. 285-293.

Levin, J.; Krafczyk, S.; Valkovic, P.; Eggert, T.; Claassen, J. & Bötzel, K. (2009). Objective measurement of muscle rigidity in Parkinsonian patients treated with subthalamic stimulation. *Mov Disord*, Vol.24(1), pp. 57-63.

Mak, MK.; Wong, EC. & Hui-Chan, CW. (2007). Quantitative measurement of trunk rigidity in Parkinsonian patients. *J Neurol*, Vol.254, pp. 202–209.

Martinez-Martin, P. (1993). "Rating sales in Parkinson's disease," In: *Parkinson's Disease and Movement Disorders*, 2nd ed, J. Jankovic, E. Tolosa, (Eds.), 281-292, Williams & Wilkins, Baltimore, MD, USA.

Marsden, CD. (1990). Neurophysiology. In: *Parkinson's disease*, G. Stern, (Ed.), 57-98, Johns Hopkins University Press, Baltimore, MD, USA.

Matthews, PBC. (1959). The dependence of tension upon extension in the stretch reflex of the soleus muscle of the decerebrate cat. *J Physiol*, Vol.147, pp.521-546

Matthews, PBC. (1991). The human stretch reflex and the motor cortex. *Trends Neurosci*, Vol.14, pp. 87-91

Meara, RJ. & Cody, FWJ. (1993). Stretch reflexes of individual parkinsonian patients studied during changes in clinical rigidity following medication. *Electroencephalogr Clin Neurophysiol*, Vol.89, pp. 261-268

Mera, T.O.; Johnson, M.D.; Rothe, D.; Zhang, J.; Xu, W.; Ghosh, D.; Vitek, J. & Alberts, J.L. (2009). Objective quantification of arm rigidity in MPTP-treated primates. *J Neurosci Methods*. Vol.177(1):20-29.

Meinders, M.; Price, R.; Lehmann, JF. & Questad, KA (1996). The stretch reflex response in the normal and spastic ankle: effect of ankle position. *Arch Phys Med Rehabil*, Vol. 77(5), pp. 487-92.

Mirbagheri, MM.; Barbeau, H.; Ladouceur, M. & Kearney, RE. (2001). Intrinsic and reflex stiffness in normal and spastic, spinal cord injured subjects. *Exp Brain Res*, Vol.141, pp. 446-459.

Mirbagheri, MM.; Chen, D. & Rymer W.Z. (2010). Quantification of the effects of an alpha-2 adrenergic agonist on reflex properties in spinal cord injury using a system identification technique. *J Neuroeng Rehabil*, Vol.7, pp. 29-35.

Mirbagheri, M.M.; Tsao, C. & Rymer, W.Z. (2009). Natural history of neuromuscular properties after stroke: a longitudinal study. *J Neurol Neurosurg Psychiatry*, Vol. 80, pp. 1212-1217.

Mortimer, JA. & Webster, DD. (1979). Evidence for a quantitative association between EMG stretch responses and Parkinsonian rigidity. *Brain Res.*, Vol.162, pp. 169-173.

Obeso, JA.; Linazasoro, G.; Rothwell, JC.; Jahanshahi, M. & Brown, R. (1996). Assessing the effects of pallidotomy in Parkinson's disease. *The Lancet*, Vol. 347(9013), pp. 1490

Ondo, WG.; Jankovic, J.; Lai, EC.; Sankhla, C.; Khan, M.; Ben-Arie, L.; Schwartz, K.; Grossman, RG. & Krauss, JK. (1998). Assessment of motor function after stereotactic pallidotomy. *Neurology*, Vol.50(1), pp. 266-70

Park, B.K.; Kwon, Y.; Kim, J.W.; Lee, J.H.; Eom, G.M.; Koh, S.B.; Jun, J.H. & Hong, J. (2010). Analysis of viscoelastic properties of wrist joint for quantification of Parkinsonian rigidity. *IEEE T Neur Sys Reh*, Vol.99, ISSN: 1534-4320

Patrick, S.K.; Denington, A.A.; Gauthier, M.J.; Gillard, D.M. & Prochazka, A. (2001). Quantification of the UPDRS Rigidity Scale. *IEEE Trans Neural Syst Rehabil Eng.*, Vol. 9, pp. 31-41.

Pollock. LJ. & Davis, L. (1930). Muscle tone in Parkinsonian states. *Arch Neurol Psychiatry*, Vol.23, Pp. 303- 319

Powell, D.; Hanson, N.; Threlkeld, AJ.; Fang, X. & Xia, R. (2011). Enhancement of parkinsonian rigidity with contralateral hand activation. *Clin Neurophysiol* Vol.122, pp. 1595-1601.

Powell, D.; Threlkeld, AJ.; Fang, X.; Muthumani, A. & Xia, R. Amplitude- and velocity-dependency of rigidity measured at the wrist in Parkinson's disease. *Clin Neurophysiol (in press)*.

Prochazka, A.; Bennett, DJ.; Stephens. MJ.; Patrick, SK.; Sears-Duru, R.; Roberts, T, & Jhamandas, JH. (1997). Measurement of rigidity in Parkinson's disease. *Mov Disord*, Vol.12, pp. 24-32

Rabey, JM.; Bass, H.; Bonuccelli, U.; Brooks, D.; Klotz, P.; Korczyn, AD.; Kraus, P.; Martinez-Martin, P.; Morrish, P.; Van Sauten, W. & Van Hilten, B. (1997). Evaluation of the Short Parkinson's Evaluation Scale: a new friendly scale for the evaluation of Parkinson's disease in clinical drug trials. *J Neuropharmacol*, Vol.20(4), pp. 322-37.

Rack, PM. & Westbury, DR. (1969). The effects of length and stimulus rate on tension in the isometric cat soleus muscle. *J Physiol*, Vol. 204, pp. 443-460.

Richards, M.; Marder, K.; Cote, L. & Mayeux, R. (1994). Interrater reliability of the Unified Parkinson's Disease Rating Scale motor examination. *Mov Disord*, Vol.9(1), pp. 89-91.

Robichaud, JA.; Pfann, KD.; Comella, CL.; Brandabur, M. & Corcos DM. (2004). Greater impairment of extension movements as compared to flexion movements in Parkinson's disease. *Exp Brain Res*, Vol. 156, pp.240-254.

Rondot, P. & Metral, S. (1973). Analysis of the shortening reaction in man. In: *New Developments in Electromyography and Clinical Neurophysiology*, J.E. Desmedt, (Ed), 3:629-634, ISBN 978-380-5514-09-5, Basel: Karger, Switzerland

Rothwell, JC.; Obeso, JA.; Traub, MM. & Marsden, CD. (1983). The behaviour of the long-latency stretch reflex in patients with Parkinson's disease. *J Neurol Neurosurg Psychiatry*, Vol.46, pp. 35-44

Rushworth, G. (1960). Spasticity and rigidity: An experimental study and review. *J Neurol Neurosurg Psychiatry*, Vol.23, pp. 99-118

Rymer, WZ. & Katz, RT. (1994). Mechanisms of spastic hypertonia. *Phys Med Rehabil: State of the Art Reviews*, Vol.8, pp. 441-454.

Rymer, WZ.; Houk. JC. & Crago, PE. (1979). Mechanisms of the clasp-knife reflex studied in an animal model. *Exp Brain Res*, Vol.37, pp. 93-113.

Sepehri, B.; Esteki, A.; Ebrahimi-Takamjani, E.; Shahidi, GA.; Khamseh, F. & Moinodin, M. (2007). Quantification of rigidity in Parkinson's disease. *Ann Biomed Eng*, Vol.35(12), pp. 2196-203.

Shapiro, MB.; Vaillancourt, DE.; Sturman, MM.; Metman, LV.; Bakay, RA. & Corcos, DM. (2007). Effects of STN DBS on rigidity in Parkinson's disease. *IEEE Trans Neural Syst Rehabil Eng*. Vol.15, pp. 173-181.

Sherrington, CS. (1909). On plastic tonus and proprioceptive reflexes. *Q J Exp Physiol* , Vol.2, pp. 109- 156.

Sinkjaer, T. & Magnussen, I. (1994). Passive, intrinsic and reflex-mediated stiffness in the ankle extensors of hemiparetic patients. *Brain*, Vol.117, pp. 355–363.

Sinkjaer, T.; Toft, E.; Larsen, K.; Andreassen, S. & Hansen, HJ. (1993). Non-reflex and reflex mediated ankle joint stiffness in in multiple sclerosis patients with spasticity. *Muscle Nerve*, Vol.16, pp. 69–76.

Tanner, CM. & Ben-Shlomo, Y. (1999). Epidemiology of Parkinson's disease. *Adv Neurol* Vol.80, pp.153-159.

Tanner, CM. & Goldman, SM. (1996). Epidemiology of Parkinson's disease. *Neurol Clin*, Vol.14, pp.317-335.

Temperli, P.; Ghika, J.; Villemure, J.G.; Burkhard, P.R.; Bogousslavsky, J. & Vingerhoets, F.J. (2003). How do parkinsonian signs return after discontinuation of subthalamic DBS? *Neurology*, Vol.60, pp. 78-81.

Teräväinen, H.; Tsui, JKC.; Mak, E., & Calne, DB. (1989). Optimal indices for testing parkinsonian rigidity. *Can. J. Neurol Sci.*, Vol.16, pp. 180-183.

Tunik, E.; Poizner, H.; Adamovich, SV.; Levin, MF. & Feldman, AG. (2004). Deficits in adaptive upper limb control in response to trunk perturbations in Parkinson's disease. *Exp Brain Res*, Vol.159, pp.23-32.

Van Dillen, LR. & Roach, KE. (1988). Interrater reliability of a clinical scale of rigidity. *Phys Ther*, Vol.68(11), pp. 1679-81.

Ward, CD.; Sanes, JN.; Dambrosia, JM. & Calne, DB. (1983). Methods for evaluating treatment in Parkinson's disease. *Adv Neurol*, Vol. 37, pp. 1-7.

Watts, RL.; Wiegner, AW. & Young, RR. (1986). Elastic properties of muscles measured at the elbow in man: II. Patients with parkinsonian rigidity. *J Neurol Neurosurg Psychiatry*, Vol.49, pp. 1177-1181.

Westphal, C. (1877). Unterschenkelphänomen und Nervendehnung. *Archiv Fur Psychiatrie Und Nervenkrankheiten*, Vol. 7, pp. 666-670.

Westphal, C. (1880). Über eine Art paradoxer Muskel-contraction. *Archiv Fur Psychiatrie Und Nervenkrankheiten*, Vol.10, pp. 243-248.

Wiegner, AW. & Watts, RL. (1986). Elastic properties of muscles measured at the elbow in man: I. Normal controls. *J Neurol Neurosurg Psychiatry*, Vol.49(10), pp. 1171-6.

Xia, R. & Rymer, WZ. (2004). The role of shortening reaction in mediating rigidity in Parkinson's disease. *Exp Brain Res*, Vol.156, pp. 524-528.

Xia, R.; Markopoulou, K.; Puumala, SE. & Rymer, WZ. (2006). A comparison of the effects of imposed extension and flexion movements on Parkinsonian rigidity. *Clin Neurophysiol*, Vol.117, pp. 2302-2307.

Xia, R.; Powell, D.; Rymer, WZ.; Hanson, N.; Fang, X. & Threlkeld, AJ. (2011). Differentiation of contributions between shortening reaction and stretch-induced inhibition in Parkinson's disease. *Exp Brain Res'*, Vol.209, pp.609–618 DOI 10.1007/s00221-011-2594-2.

Xia, R.; Radovic, M.; Mao, ZH. & Threlkeld, AJ. (2010). System identification and modeling approach to characterizing rigidity in Parkinson's disease: neural and non-neural contributions. *Proceedings of the 4th International Conference on Bioinformatics and Biomedical Engineering* (iCBBE 2010), Paper No. 40046 (4 pages), doi: 10.1109/ICBBE.2010.5514861

Xia, R.; Sun, J. & Threlkeld. AJ, (2009). Analysis of interactive effect of stretch reflex and shortening reaction on rigidity in Parkinson's disease. *Clin Neurophysiol*, Vol.120, pp. 1400-1407.

Zhang, LQ. & Rymer, WZ. (1997). Simultaneous and nonlinear identification of mechanical and reflex properties of human elbow joint muscles. *IEEE Trans Biomed Eng*, Vol. 44(12), pp. 1192-209.

9

Pathophysiology of Non-Dopaminergic Monoamine Systems in Parkinson's Disease: Implications for Mood Dysfunction

Nirmal Bhide and Christopher Bishop
Department of Psychology, Binghamton University, Binghamton, NY
USA

1. Introduction

Parkinson's disease (PD) is a neurodegenerative disorder affecting millions worldwide and is one of the most common diseases affecting the aging population (Delau et al., 2006). Clinical hallmarks of PD feature severe motor deficits characterized by bradykinesia, tremor, rigidity and postural instability. Though less recognized, PD symptoms also include psychiatric complications such as depression, anxiety and psychosis that deleteriously influence quality of life. While the origin of motor deficits is the progressive degeneration of nigrostriatal dopamine (DA) neurons, other monoamine neurons within the serotonin (5-HT) and norepinephrine (NE) system also degenerate, likely contributing to mood dysfunction. In this chapter the pathophysiology of non-dopaminergic monoamine systems, their contribution to PD-related mood dysfunction, and therapeutics targeting them will be discussed.

2. Norepinephrine system

In PD, the cardinal cell death of the dopaminergic substantia nigra pars compacta (SNpc) neurons is accompanied by deficits in other monoamine neurotransmitter systems. Of these, NE appears most most consistently affected. Numerous studies, both neuroanatomical and biochemical, have documented severe loss of NE neurons, originating from the locus coeruleus (LC), concomitant with or even preceding the loss of DA neurons (Mann and Yates, 1983; Marien et al., 2004; Schapira et al., 2006). The precise anatomical relationship between the LC and the SNpc and the striatum remains to be elucidated; however, evidence exists for a functional relationship between these brain regions (Fornai et al., 2007). Most notable, loss of NE may exacerbate damage to the DA nigrostriatal system, as NE is postulated to play a neuroprotective and neuromodulator role in the progression of PD (Rommelfanger and Weinshenker, 2007). The following sections will focus on the pathophysiology of NE, its relative contribution to the development of psychiatric symptoms of PD, and the treatment of these symptoms using noradrenergic drugs.

2.1 CNS pathophysiology of NE system in PD
2.1.1 Neuroanatomical evidence in PD patients
As early as 1917, noradrenergic neurons originating from the LC were reported to be severely deteriorated in patients suffering from PD (Tretiakoff et al., 1917; Fornai et al.,

2007). In a landmark study by Hornykiewicz et al., (1960), direct biochemical evidence supported these initial findings, by showing the loss of both NE neurons and NE content in several brain regions in PD, including the caudate nucleus and putamen (Ehringer and Hornykiewicz, 1960).

Neuropathological evidence in post-mortem tissue of PD patients ranges from observation of Lewy bodies (LB) within single NE cells and cytoplasmic neurofibrillary tangles (NT) to a loss of neurons in the LC (Mann, 1983). Patt and Gerhard (1993), using a variant of the Golgi method, found that medium-sized LC neurons containing neuromelanin granules were most affected in PD patients (Patt and Gerhard, 1993) correlating with loss of synaptic spines, a reduction in dendritic length, swollen perikarya and apoptosis. Bertrand et al., (1997) reported the presence of glial proliferation along with extracellular neuromelanin granules around dying NE neurons. Post-mortem studies carried out in PD patients have established a loss of approximately 70% of NE neurons when compared to age-matched controls (Bertrand et al., 1997; Zarow et al., 2003). Interestingly, the NE neuronal loss was greater in the LC compared to cholinergic loss in the nucleus basalis and dopaminergic loss in the SNpc in Alzheimer and PD patients, respectively (Zarow et al., 2003). Of note, the loss of LC neurons observed in PD patients is not homogenous as there appears to be a disease specific and regional pattern to degeneration in the LC. For example, German and co-workers (1992) observed that in PD patients with no dementia complications, the degeneration was consistent throughout the rostral and caudal portion of the LC, whereas, in PD patients with dementia, the cell loss occurred more severely in the rostral portion of the LC nucleus. These findings have led to the postulation that LC degeneration patterns could be used to classify and differentiate between various sub-groups of PD patients. Comprehensive evidence by Braak and colleagues have found that, in PD patients, the degeneration of NE neurons progressed from lower brain stem regions, like the LC, to more rostral areas, like the SNpc (Braak and Braak, 2000; Braak et al., 2003).

Biochemical evidence obtained from post-mortem and ante-mortem studies in PD patients suggests that NE levels in multiple brain regions, including the motor cortex, hippocampus, striatum, substantia nigra and hypothalamus, are significantly decreased (Gesi et al., 2000). Interestingly, brain regions that are innervated by NE nuclei other than LC are relatively spared from NE loss.

Accumulating evidence strongly suggests that the loss of NE neurons originating from the LC is a very important aspect of the pathophysiology of PD and contributes to the progression of PD, deleteriously affecting the survival of DA neurons. For example, various experimental studies have demonstrated that prior loss of NE innervation increases the vulnerability of the DA neurons to a further neurotoxic insult (Fornai et al., 1995; Mavridis et al., 1991). Conversely, it has been established that increased NE stimulation is neuroprotective against 1-methyl-4-phenyl-1,2,3,6-tetrahydropyridine (MPTP)-induced induced neurotoxicity (Kilbourn et al., 1998; Rommelfanger et al., 2004). Thus, it appears that NE may play a neurotrophic role acting as a neuroprotective mechanism for DA neurons. This was corroborated by Tong and colleagues (2006) who found an inverse relationship between intact NE innervation and DA loss in PD patients. Collectively, these findings suggest that the loss of LC neurons precedes and facilitates the subsequent damage to nigrostriatal DA neurons.

Therefore, since NE is known to act as a modulator of the dopaminergic system in various brain regions, the loss of NE appears to be a very critical event in the timeline of PD.

2.1.2 Mechanism(s) of NE loss

The mechanisms underlying NE loss like DA neurodegeneration remain to be elucidated. However, NE neurons are susceptible to the same insults that affect DA neurons such as oxidative stress, neuroinflammation, protein misfolding and neurotoxin-induced cell death. For example, Yavich et al. (2006) demonstrated that mice expressing a pathogenic mutation of α-synuclein have abnormal compartmentalization and metabolism of both DA and NE. In addition, it is well known that monoamines have a tendency to auto-oxidize leading to oxidative stress and neuronal cell loss (Chiueh et al., 2000; Maker et al., 1986); and the aforementioned abnormal compartmentalization of NE may make LC neurons vulnerable to oxidative stress. Genetic mutations in Parkin, a genotype found in PD, also make LC neurons vulnerable to cell death. Studies in mice have demonstrated that Parkin mutations lead to loss of LC neurons (Von Coelln et al., 2004) likely via protein misfolding and dysregulation of the ubiquitous-proteasome system. This is a compelling finding since alterations in the expression of proteasome activators have been shown to correlate with neuronal loss in SNpc and the LC. Poor expression of proteasome activators correlated with neuronal cell loss in the LC and regions expressing normal levels of the proteasome activators did not suffer from neuronal degeneration (McNaught et al., 2010). Finally, NE neurons are also susceptible to neurotoxin-induced apoptosis. For example, in the experimental 6-hydroxydopamine (6-OHDA) model of PD, administration of desipramine, a NE transporter (NET) inhibitor, infers protection to NE neurons. Since DA and NE transporters share homology in structure and display common affinity for several substrates, it is likely that NET takes up the same neurotoxins that affect DA neurons in sporadic PD. Collectively these factors could make the LC neurons vulnerable to damage in both genetic and sporadic models of PD. More studies that shed light on the neurodegenerative processes in the LC are necessary to better understand the progression of PD. Moreover, neuroprotective strategies directed toward LC neurons may be warranted since loss of LC neurons makes the DA neurons more vulnerable to neurodegeneration.

2.2 Non-motor symptoms

2.2.1 NE loss and non-motor symptoms

Although motor symptoms of PD are widely acknowledged hallmarks of this neurodegenerative disease, there exists compelling evidence for the presence of psychiatric complications, such as depression, anxiety and psychotic symptoms (Bosboom et al., 2004). Loss of dopaminergic and noradrenergic innervation has been associated with psychiatric complications such as depression (Remy et al., 2005) and anxiety (Stein et al., 1990; Lauterbach et al., 2003). Cognitive and mood dysfunction has been reported in >50% of PD patients. In patients with early PD, depression (40%), apathy (27%), and anxiety (27%) are widely reported (Aarsland et al., 2009) and it is notable that these non-motor symptoms are identified as the most important and devastating feature contributing towards poverty of quality of life (McKinlay et al., 2008; Schrag, 2006). Moreover, the incidence of depression and anxiety in PD exceeds not only rates within the normal population but also other neurological disorders (Weintraub et al., 2003), with anxiety disorders, such as off-period panic attacks and specific phobias, have been reported in nearly 40% of PD patients (Lauterbach, 2005). Collectively these findings lead to the important observation that depression and anxiety are likely a result of neuropathological processes rather than as a result of motor impairments.

The exact pathophysiology underlying these mood dysfunctions are unknown though given the role of NE in several of these symptoms, it is likely that NE loss in PD plays a critical role. As discussed earlier, neurodegeneration of LC neurons in PD is a well established phenomenon that precedes DA neuronal loss (Braak et al., 2003). It has been postulated that a compromised LC produces significant changes in NE receptors and transporters that may lead to the development or exacerbation of depression/anxiety (Eskow Jaunarajs et al., 2010). Additionally, Remy et al. (2005) have reported reduced binding for the DA/NE transporter, suggesting a loss of terminals, in the LC of PD patients suffering from anxiety and depression (Remy et al., 2005). In a rodent model of PD, alterations in DA and NE systems in the striatum have been reported to produce anxiety (Tadaiesky et al., 2008), consistent with findings in naïve rats that NE regulates anxiety behavior. Experimental studies have reported depression and anxiety-like behaviors in a 6-OHDA lesion model of PD (Branchi et al., 2010; Eskow Jaunarajs et al., 2010; Tadaiesky et al., 2008). Additionally, concomitant depletion of NE, 5-HT and DA in a unilateral rodent model of PD produced symptoms of depression, suggesting that loss of all three systems contribute to PD-like depression (Delaville et al., 2010). In an interesting study, Taylor et al. (2009) used a vesicular monoamine transporter-2 (VMAT-2) deficient mouse model to induce severe NE and DA loss thereby mimicking PD. VMAT-2 deficient mice exhibited severe depression and anxiety-like symptoms that worsened with advancing age (Taylor et al., 2009) highlighting a possible interplay between DA and NE. Histological studies have highlighted the fact that LC neuron morphology is more severely affected in PD with depression than in PD without depressio (Chan-Palay and Asan, 1989). While most of the evidence in clinical and experimental models correlating NE deficit with mood dysfunction is indirect, there exists evidence that noradrenergic drugs might provide relief in the treatment of these mood disorders.

2.2.2 Treatment of non-motor symptoms with NE drugs

The role for the NE system in affective disorders such as anxiety and depression has been partially implicated by the effectiveness of drugs that enhance NE levels. Reboxetine, a NET inhibitor, has been proven to be effective in the treatment of depression associated with PD (Pintor et al., 2006). In one of the largest Randomized Clinical Trials (RCT) to date Menza and colleagues (2009) found that Nortryptaline, a tricyclic antidepressant (TCA), with preferential actions as a NET inhibitor, was proven to be more effective in treating depression in PD patients compared to selective 5-HT reuptake inhibitors (SSRIs: Menza et al., 2009). In a similar placebo controlled study in PD patients, Desipramine, a NET inhibitor, was found to be effective in treating depression; however, these improvements were accompanied with mild adverse side effects (Devos et al., 2008). These therapeutic findings suggest a more prominent role for NE in the development of depression in PD. The few drugs that seem to be effective in treating depression likely act to elevate extracellular NE levels in the brain, by blocking NET (Dziedzicka-Wasylewska et al., 2006). Therefore, it seems feasible that drugs that mimic NE or elevate NE levels in the brain would be effective in treating NE-related non-motor symptoms in PD.

3. Serotonin system

The 5-HT system like the NE system undergoes significant, though more variable, neurodegeneration as PD progresses; a finding documented in various studies, both post-

and ante-mortem (Miyawaki et al., 1997; Scatton et al., 1983). Since the 5-HT system ubiquitously innervates and modulates basal ganglia nuclei, 5-HT loss likely affects both motor symptoms of PD and l-DOPA related side effects. In addition, given the role of 5-HT in mood, such alterations may also correlate with the preponderance of depression and anxiety seen in PD. Therefore, various treatment strategies have been developed that modulate the 5-HT system. In the following sections, we review the neuropathology of the 5-HT system in PD, the consequences of a damaged 5-HT system on non-motor aspects, and the line of experimental and clinical treatments targeting the 5-HT system to provide symptomatic relief for the PD patient.

3.1 CNS pathophysiology of 5-HT system in PD
3.1.1 Neuroanatomical evidence in PD patients
Even though degeneration of DA neurons in the SNpc remains the best identified neuropathological hallmark in PD, there exists increasing evidence suggesting PD-related pathology in the principle 5-HT cell bodies, the raphe nuclei and other regions innervated by raphe neurons (Braak et al., 2003).

Multiple studies have reported the presence of LB in the caudal group of raphe nuclei, like the raphe magnus and raphe pallidus, in early PD, sometimes occurring even before the onset of motor symptoms (Braak et al., 2003; Del Tredici et al., 2002; Parkkinen et al., 2008). It is interesting to note that these caudal raphe nuclei contain 5-HT neurons associated with functions like pain perception, and gastrointestinal motility that are manifest as early symptoms in PD patients prior to motor complaints (Chaudhuri and Schapira, 2009). The rostral raphe nuclei consisting of dorsal and medial raphe nuclei are equally affected in PD and according to Braak staging, are affected before the SNpc but after the caudal raphe nuclei (Braak et al., 2003).

Despite reports of raphe LB formation, evidence for the degeneration of 5-HT neurons in the rostral raphe nuclei is variable; post-mortem analysis of PD brains by Paulus and Jellinger (1991) revealed a profound loss of 5-HT neurons, however, other studies have not (Halliday et al., 1990; Mann and Yates, 1983). Several studies have employed transcranial sonography to study the midbrain raphe nuclei. This work has revealed abnormal pathology in the form of hypoechogenicity or an absence of sonographic signals in PD vs. control subjects. Interestingly, PD patients in one study also suffered from higher incidence of depression, reflecting a direct relationship between raphe nuclei loss and PD-related depression (Becker et al., 1997; Berg and Gaenslen, 2010; Walter et al., 2007b). MRI imaging studies carried out in depressed PD patients have also demonstrated a loss of homogeneity in the midbrain raphe consistent with neuronal compromise and/or cell loss (Berg et al., 1999).

PD-related pathology of the 5-HT system is not limited to the cell bodies of the raphe nuclei. Convincing evidence exists for damaged 5-HT projections and terminals as well. For example, post-mortem studies in PD patients have described significant loss of 5-HT markers, such as brain 5-HT concentrations. In cortical and the basal ganglia regions 5-HT content has been reported to be reduced by as much as 50% compared to controls (Birkmayer and Birkmayer, 1987). Kish and colleagues (2008) investigated the integrity of the forebrain 5-HT system. In contrast to DA loss, which was preferential to the putamen, 5-HT loss was more prominent in the caudate for all 5-HT markers including 5-HT (-66%), the 5-HT metabolite 5-HIAA (-42%), 5-HT transporter (SERT), (-56%) and the rate limiting enzyme in 5-HT synthesis tryptophan hydroxylase (-59%). These corroborated ante-mortem observations in PD patients that examined levels of 5-HIAA in cerebrospinal fluid and have found significant reductions when compared to control patients. Interestingly, the deficits in cerebrospinal fluid 5-HIAA levels were more pronounced in PD patients with depression in comparison to non-depressed PD patients, again supporting a relationship between decreased 5-HT function and depression in PD (Mayeux et al., 1984; Mayeux et al., 1986). Development of additional imaging technologies, like PET and SPECT, has facilitated the measurement of SERT and thus the evaluation of the integrity of the 5-HT terminal (Meyer et al., 2007). In vivo SPECT studies, using non-specific ligands for SERT, found decreased binding in the cortex and hypothalamus of PD patients (Berding et al., 2003a; Berding et al., 2003b). However, these findings have been contradicted by studies that did not find any changes in the mid-brain but rather reduction in the thalamic nuclei of PD patients (Caretti et al., 2008; Kim et al., 2003; Roselli et al., 2010). Decreased SERT binding has been observed by use of PET imaging using more specific ligands. Under these circumstances reduced SERT was observed in the striatum, frontal cortex, caudate nucleus, putamen and the mid-brain raphe region of patients with PD (Albin et al., 2008; Guttman et al., 2007; Kerenyi et al., 2003). SERT binding is also labile, changing as PD progresses. For example, in the early stages of PD, SERT binding has been shown to be reduced in only in the striatum, thalamus and cingulate cortex. In later symptomatic stages of PD these alterations appear to extend to the prefrontal cortex and the raphe nuclei (Haapaniemi et al., 2001; Politis et al., 2010). Such findings suggest that a progressive reduction in SERT binding may serve as good a bio-marker for the diagnosis and development of treatment strategies for PD patients.

In addition to neuronal integrity, 5-HT receptors are also affected in PD. Modification of pre- and post-synaptic 5-HT receptors has been observed in various animal and human studies of PD. While it is not clear whether these compensatory changes are due to lost 5-HT input, DA innervation, or DA replacement, it is established that dopaminergic tone regulates the expression of several 5-HT receptors. 5-HT_{1A} receptor binding is not consistently affected in the 6-OHDA model of PD; however, studies in MPTP-treated macaques suggest increases in striatal and cortical binding (Frechilla et al., 2001; Huot et al., 2010b). 5-HT_{1B} receptor binding is significantly increased in the striatum (54%) and the globus pallidus (33%). Intranigral lesions have also been reported to increase 5-HT_4 receptor density in the caudate and the globus pallidus (Di Matteo et al., 2008). Studies using in situ hybridization and autoradiographic radioligand binding have revealed few changes in 5-HT_{1A} and 5-HT_{2B} receptor binding (Numan et al., 1995; Zhang et al., 2008); however, 5-HT_{2A} receptors have been shown to increase in the striatum (Zhang et al., 2008). The possibility exists that striatal 5-HT_{2A} and 5-HT_{2C} receptor are differentially regulated in 6-OHDA-lesioned animals and the changes observed in these receptors could be a reflection of the compensatory changes in the PD-afflicted brain. Some of the changes in 5-HT receptor binding are reversible after treatment with l-DOPA, Zhang and colleagues (2008) reported a reversal of increased striatal 5-HT_{2A} receptor mRNA in a 6-OHDA rodent model of PD after l-DOPA treatment. Interestingly, l-DOPA did not alter the changes in striatal 5-HT_{2C} receptor mRNA levels. It appears that changes in regulation of the 5-HT_{2A} receptor are dependent on striatal DA levels and the 5-HT_{2C} loss could be due to nigrostriatal loss, thus reflecting a difference in regulation between the two receptor sub-types. The 5-HT receptor changes seen in PD patients are partly similar to changes in the experimental PD models. Similar increases were seen in the density of 5-HT_{2A} and 5-HT_{2C} receptor in the striatum as well as other regions (Fox and Brotchie, 2000; Huot et al., 2010c; Radja et al., 1993). It is important to note that these changes may not be direct evidence of 5-HT neuropathology but definitely provide an insight into neuroplasticity of the 5-HT system that may unravel potential targets for therapeutic strategies in the treatment of PD.

An indirect marker for 5-HT alterations in PD is the assessment of responses to 5-HT challenge tests. Of these, the most common is the endocrine response to the 5-HT releasing agent, Fenfluramine. In normal subjects Fenfluramine produces robust increases in prolactin and corticosterone levels. However, in PD patients it was found that this endocrine response was impaired (Kostic et al., 1996; Volpi et al., 1997). Such effects may also correlate with non-motor symptoms since PD patients suffering from depression also displayed blunted prolactin responses in comparison to non-depressed PD patients (Kostic et al., 1996). Collectively these findings provide substantial evidence for neurochemical, neuroanatomical and functional alterations of the 5-HT system.

3.2 Non-motor symptoms
3.2.1 5-HT loss and non-motor symptoms
As previously mentioned depression and anxiety are some of the most common non-motor symptoms in PD and are even associated with an elevated risk towards the development of PD (Leentjens et al., 2003; Schuurman et al., 2002; Shiba et al., 2000). The underlying pathophysiological mechanisms remain to be completely understood; however, it is well established that 5-HT dysfunction plays an important role in several mood-disorders in non-PD patients (Michelsen et al., 2008). Depression not only reduces the quality of life for PD patients but has a negative effect on caregivers as well (Schrag et al., 2000; 2004).

During the progression of PD it has been observed that brain regions, like rostral raphe, thalamus and cortex, that mediate mood disturbances in PD are severely affected by the presence of Lewy bodies (Braak and Del Tredici, 2008). Currently, most evidence linking abnormal serotonergic neurotransmission to mood disturbances in PD is corroborative but points to a role for 5-HT pathology. For example, depressed PD patients display reduced brainstem raphe echogenicity, in comparison to non-depressed PD patients (Walter et al., 2007a). Post-mortem comparisons of neuronal density in the dorsal raphe nucleus between depressed and non-depressed PD patients found lower neuronal density in depressed PD patients (Paulus and Jellinger, 1991). In vivo studies measuring cerebrospinal fluid levels found lower levels of 5-HIAA in depressed PD patients indicating reduced 5-HT metabolism (Mayeux et al., 1986). Imaging studies have been less conclusive and have found either no change in SERT uptake (Kim et al., 2003) or reported elevated 5-HT receptor binding in depressed PD patients when compared to non-depressed PD patients (Boileau et al., 2008). Interestingly, acute tryptophan depletion in a small group of PD patients did not produce depression or anxiety in these patients (Leentjens et al., 2006). Another major non-motor symptom affecting PD patients is the development of psychosis that may lead to development of paranoid delusions in some PD patients (Ravina et al., 2007). The underlying cause remains to be elucidated and some investigators have postulated that there may be a serotonergic involvement. $5-HT_2$ receptors, responsible for hallucinations and psychosis, are relatively intact or may even be upregulated in the cortex of PD patients suffering from psychosis compared to PD patients free from any psychotic disorder (Cheng et al., 1991; Huot et al., 2010a).

3.2.2 Treatment of non-motor symptoms with serotonergic drugs

Drugs acting on the serotonergic system are currently the standard of care for the treatment and management of psychiatric dysfunction, like anxiety, depression and psychosis in PD, despite causal evidence or 5-HT dysfunction in PD-related mood disorders. Most of the SSRIs currently used act by elevating the extracellular 5-HT levels and thus act indirectly on various post-synaptic 5-HT receptors, many of which have been implicated in mood disorders (Dobkin et al., 2011; Dobkin et al., 2010; Fox et al., 2009; Menza et al., 2009; Weintraub et al., 2006). The other potential side effects such as postural hypotension, sedation and 5-HT syndrome, due to 5-HT$_1$ receptor stimulation, continue to limit the use of these antidepressants in PD patients (Veazey et al., 2005). It is important to note that many PD patients suffer from orthostatic hypotension and tremors and these could get exacerbated. Nefazodone, a 5-HT$_2$ receptor antagonist/re-uptake inhibitor has been used as an antidepressant and to reduce extrapyramidal symptoms in PD patients (Avila et al., 2003).

Psychotic complications usually treated with drugs that have an anti-dopaminergic profile are not ideal for the PD patient since it can lead to worsening of motor symptoms. Therefore, atypical antipsychotics, like Clozapine and Quetiapine, have been found to be effective in treating psychosis in PD patients (Kurlan et al., 2007), an effect attributed to their 5-HT$_2$ receptor antagonistic properties. Another non-selective 5-HT$_2$ receptor antagonist Mianserin has been demonstrated to reduce visual hallucinations in a small group of PD patients without affecting the parkinsonian motor symptoms. Preliminary findings from a Phase II study evaluating Pimavanserin, a 5-HT2A receptor inverse agonist, are encouraging and show a trend in improving psychosis without affecting PD motor scores (Meltzer et al., 2010).

It is of interest to note that l-DOPA therapy has been traditionally assumed to improve affective symptoms, like depression and anxiety; however, emerging evidence suggests that chronic use of l-DOPA may aggravate mood problems (Eskow Jaunarajs et al., 2011). Preclinical investigations have reported that 6-OHDA-lesioned rats chronically treated with l-DOPA exhibit reduced 5-HT and 5-HIAA levels (Carta et al., 2007; Eskow Jaunarajs et al., 2011). Studies employing in vivo microdialysis have confirmed reductions in 5-HT levels, after acute l-DOPA, in the 6-OHDA-lesioned striatum as well as in non-motor affective sites (Navailles et al., 2010). Chronic l-DOPA treatment has been demonstrated to reduce expression of tryptophan hydroxylase within the dorsal raphe nucleus, which may lead to reduced 5-HT synthesis and release in efferent structures (Eskow Jaunarajs et al., 2011). l-DOPA uptake and release of DA by 5-HT terminals into the striatum may compete with native 5-HT function leading to an aggravation of affective disorders like depression and anxiety in PD patients undergoing chronic l-DOPA therapy (Eskow Jaunarajs et al., 2011) .

In sum, drugs acting on the serotonergic system provide some symptomatic relief for PD patients. However, l-DOPA therapy by itself has the potential to exacerbate mood disorders.

4. Conclusion

In conclusion, there exists convincing evidence that both 5-HT and NE systems are severely affected in PD and that they contribute towards PD progression and symptoms. Therapeutics targeting these systems appear beneficial; however, more research is necessary to develop more efficacious therapeutic targets and strategies.

5. References

Aarsland, D., Marsh, L., Schrag, A., 2009. Neuropsychiatric symptoms in Parkinson's disease. Movement disorders : official journal of the Movement Disorder Society. 24, 2175-86.

Albin, R.L., Koeppe, R.A., Bohnen, N.I., Wernette, K., Kilbourn, M.A., Frey, K.A., 2008. Spared caudal brainstem SERT binding in early Parkinson's disease. Journal of cerebral blood flow and metabolism : official journal of the International Society of Cerebral Blood Flow and Metabolism. 28, 441-4.

Avila, A., Cardona, X., Martin-Baranera, M., Maho, P., Sastre, F., Bello, J., 2003. Does nefazodone improve both depression and Parkinson disease? A pilot randomized trial. Journal of clinical psychopharmacology. 23, 509-13.

Becker, T., Becker, G., Seufert, J., Hofmann, E., Lange, K.W., Naumann, M., Lindner, A., Reichmann, H., Riederer, P., Beckmann, H., Reiners, K., 1997. Parkinson's disease and depression: evidence for an alteration of the basal limbic system detected by transcranial sonography. Journal of neurology, neurosurgery, and psychiatry. 63, 590-6.

Berding, G., Brucke, T., Odin, P., Brooks, D.J., Kolbe, H., Gielow, P., Harke, H., Knoop, B.O., Dengler, R., Knapp, W.H., 2003a. [[123I]beta-CIT SPECT imaging of dopamine and serotonin transporters in Parkinson's disease and multiple system atrophy. Nuklearmedizin. Nuclear medicine. 42, 31-8.

Berding, G., Schrader, C.H., Peschel, T., van den Hoff, J., Kolbe, H., Meyer, G.J., Dengler, R., Knapp, W.H., 2003b. [N-methyl 11C]meta-Hydroxyephedrine positron emission tomography in Parkinson's disease and multiple system atrophy. European journal of nuclear medicine and molecular imaging. 30, 127-31.

Berg, D., Supprian, T., Hofmann, E., Zeiler, B., Jager, A., Lange, K.W., Reiners, K., Becker, T., Becker, G., 1999. Depression in Parkinson's disease: brainstem midline alteration on transcranial sonography and magnetic resonance imaging. Journal of neurology. 246, 1186-93.

Berg, D., Gaenslen, A., 2010. Place value of transcranial sonography in early diagnosis of Parkinson's disease. Neuro-degenerative diseases. 7, 291-9.

Bertrand, E., Lechowicz, W., Szpak, G.M., Dymecki, J., 1997. Qualitative and quantitative analysis of locus coeruleus neurons in Parkinson's disease. Folia neuropathologica / Association of Polish Neuropathologists and Medical Research Centre, Polish Academy of Sciences. 35, 80-6.

Birkmayer, J.G., Birkmayer, W., 1987. Improvement of disability and akinesia of patients with Parkinson's disease by intravenous iron substitution. Annals of clinical and laboratory science. 17, 32-5.

Bosboom, J.L., Stoffers, D., Wolters, E., 2004. Cognitive dysfunction and dementia in Parkinson's disease. Journal of neural transmission. 111, 1303-15.

Braak, H., Braak, E., 2000. Pathoanatomy of Parkinson's disease. Journal of neurology. 247 Suppl 2, II3-10.

Braak, H., Del Tredici, K., Rub, U., de Vos, R.A., Jansen Steur, E.N., Braak, E., 2003. Staging of brain pathology related to sporadic Parkinson's disease. Neurobiology of aging. 24, 197-211.

Braak, H., Del Tredici, K., 2008. Invited Article: Nervous system pathology in sporadic Parkinson disease. Neurology. 70, 1916-25.

Branchi, I., D'Andrea, I., Armida, M., Carnevale, D., Ajmone-Cat, M.A., Pezzola, A., Potenza, R.L., Morgese, M.G., Cassano, T., Minghetti, L., Popoli, P., Alleva, E., 2010. Striatal 6-OHDA lesion in mice: Investigating early neurochemical changes underlying Parkinson's disease. Behavioural brain research. 208, 137-43.

Caretti, V., Stoffers, D., Winogrodzka, A., Isaias, I.U., Costantino, G., Pezzoli, G., Ferrarese, C., Antonini, A., Wolters, E.C., Booij, J., 2008. Loss of thalamic serotonin transporters in early drug-naive Parkinson's disease patients is associated with tremor: an [(123)I]beta-CIT SPECT study. Journal of neural transmission. 115, 721-9.

Carta, M., Carlsson, T., Kirik, D., Bjorklund, A., 2007. Dopamine released from 5-HT terminals is the cause of L-DOPA-induced dyskinesia in parkinsonian rats. Brain : a journal of neurology. 130, 1819-33.

Chaudhuri, K.R., Schapira, A.H., 2009. Non-motor symptoms of Parkinson's disease: dopaminergic pathophysiology and treatment. Lancet neurology. 8, 464-74.

Chaudhuri, K.R., Schapira, A.H., 2009. Non-motor symptoms of Parkinson's disease: dopaminergic pathophysiology and treatment. Lancet neurology. 8, 464-74.

Chan-Palay, V.,Asan, E., 1989. Alterations in catecholamine neurons of the locus coeruleus in senile dementia of the Alzheimer type and in Parkinson's disease with and without dementia and depression. Journal of comparative neurology. 287, 373-392.

Chiueh, C.C., Andoh, T., Lai, A.R., Lai, E., Krishna, G., 2000. Neuroprotective strategies in Parkinson's disease: protection against progressive nigral damage induced by free radicals. Neurotoxicity research. 2, 293-310.

Del Tredici, K., Rub, U., De Vos, R.A., Bohl, J.R., Braak, H., 2002. Where does parkinson disease pathology begin in the brain? Journal of neuropathology and experimental neurology. 61, 413-26.

Delaville, C., Chetrit, J., Abdallah, K., Morin, S., Cardoit, L., De Deurwaerdere, P., Benzazzouz, A. 2010. Involvement of monoamine deficiency in motor and nonmotor disabilities in Parkinson's disease: behavioral, bicochemical and electrophysiological studies. International Basal Ganglia Society abstract

Di Matteo, V., Pierucci, M., Esposito, E., Crescimanno, G., Benigno, A., Di Giovanni, G., 2008. Serotonin modulation of the basal ganglia circuitry: therapeutic implication for Parkinson's disease and other motor disorders. Progress in brain research. 172, 423-63.

Dobkin, R.D., Menza, M. Bienfait, K.L., Gara, M., Marin, H., Mark, M.H., Dicke, A., Troster, A. 2010. The impact of antidepressant treatment on cognitive functioning in depressed patients with Parkinson's disease. Joural of neuropsychiatry and neurological sciences. 22(2), 188-95.

Dobkin, R.D., Menza, M. Bienfait, K.L., Gara, M., Marin, H., Mark, M.H., Dicke, A., Friedman,J. 2011. Depression in Parkinson's disease: symptom improvement and residual symptoms after acute pharmacologic management. American joural of Geriatric Psychiatry. 19(3), 222-9.

Devos,D., Dujordin, K., Poirot, I., Moreau, C., Cottencin, O., Thomas, P., Destee, A., Bordet, R., Defebvre, L. 2008. Comparison of desipramine and citalopram treatments for depression in Parkinson's disease: a double-blind, randomized, placebo-controlled study. Movement Disorders.23 (6), 850-857.

Ehringer, H., Hornykiewicz, O., 1960. [Distribution of noradrenaline and dopamine (3-hydroxytyramine) in the human brain and their behavior in diseases of the extrapyramidal system]. Klinische Wochenschrift. 38, 1236-9.

Eskow Jaunarajs, K.L., Dupre, K.B., Ostock, C.Y., Button, T., Deak, T., Bishop, C., 2010. Behavioral and neurochemical effects of chronic L-DOPA treatment on nonmotor sequelae in the hemiparkinsonian rat. Behavioural pharmacology. 21, 627-37.

Eskow Jaunarajs, K.L., Angoa-Perez, M., Kuhn, D.M., Bishop, C., 2011. Potential mechanisms underlying anxiety and depression in Parkinson's disease: consequences of l-DOPA treatment. Neuroscience and biobehavioral reviews. 35, 556-64.

Fornai, F., Bassi, L., Torracca, M.T., Scalori, V., Corsini, G.U., 1995. Norepinephrine loss exacerbates methamphetamine-induced striatal dopamine depletion in mice. European journal of pharmacology. 283, 99-102.

Fornai, F., di Poggio, A.B., Pellegrini, A., Ruggieri, S., Paparelli, A., 2007. Noradrenaline in Parkinson's disease: from disease progression to current therapeutics. Current medicinal chemistry. 14, 2330-4.

Fox, S.H., Brotchie, J.M., 2000. 5-HT2C receptor binding is increased in the substantia nigra pars reticulata in Parkinson's disease. Movement disorders : official journal of the Movement Disorder Society. 15, 1064-9.

Fox, S.H., Chuang, R., Brotchie, J.M., 2009. Serotonin and Parkinson's disease: On movement, mood, and madness. Movement disorders : official journal of the Movement Disorder Society. 24, 1255-66.

Frechilla, D., Cobreros, A., Saldise, L., Moratalla, R., Insausti, R., Luquin, M., Del Rio, J., 2001. Serotonin 5-HT(1A) receptor expression is selectively enhanced in the striosomal compartment of chronic parkinsonian monkeys. Synapse. 39, 288-96.

German, D.C., Manaye, K.F., White, C.L., 3rd, Woodward, D.J., McIntire, D.D., Smith, W.K., Kalaria, R.N., Mann, D.M., 1992. Disease-specific patterns of locus coeruleus cell loss. Annals of neurology. 32, 667-76.

Gesi, M., Soldani, P., Giorgi, F.S., Santinami, A., Bonaccorsi, I., Fornai, F., 2000. The role of the locus coeruleus in the development of Parkinson's disease. Neuroscience and biobehavioral reviews. 24, 655-68.

Guttman, M., Boileau, I., Warsh, J., Saint-Cyr, J.A., Ginovart, N., McCluskey, T., Houle, S., Wilson, A., Mundo, E., Rusjan, P., Meyer, J., Kish, S.J., 2007. Brain serotonin transporter binding in non-depressed patients with Parkinson's disease. European journal of neurology : the official journal of the European Federation of Neurological Societies. 14, 523-8.

Haapaniemi, T.H., Ahonen, A., Torniainen, P., Sotaniemi, K.A., Myllyla, V.V., 2001. [123I]beta-CIT SPECT demonstrates decreased brain dopamine and serotonin transporter levels in untreated parkinsonian patients. Movement disorders : official journal of the Movement Disorder Society. 16, 124-30.

Halliday, G.M., Li, Y.W., Blumbergs, P.C., Joh, T.H., Cotton, R.G., Howe, P.R., Blessing, W.W., Geffen, L.B., 1990. Neuropathology of immunohistochemically identified brainstem neurons in Parkinson's disease. Annals of neurology. 27, 373-85.

Hein, L., Altman, J.D., Kobilka, B.K., 1999. Two functionally distinct alpha2-adrenergic receptors regulate sympathetic neurotransmission. Nature. 402, 181-4.

Huot, P., Johnston, T.H., Darr, T., Hazrati, L.N., Visanji, N.P., Pires, D., Brotchie, J.M., Fox, S.H., 2010a. Increased 5-HT(2A) receptors in the temporal cortex of parkinsonian patients with visual hallucinations. Movement disorders.25(10), 1399-1408.

Huot, P., Johnston, T.H., Koprich, J.B., Winkelmolen, L., Fox, S.H., Brotchie, J.M., 2010b. Regulation of cortical and striatal 5-HT(1A) receptors in the MPTP-lesioned macaque. Neurobiology of aging.

Huot, P., Johnston, T.H., Winkelmolen, L., Fox, S.H., Brotchie, J.M., 2010c. 5-HT(2A) receptor levels increase in MPTP-lesioned macaques treated chronically with L-DOPA. Neurobiology of aging.

Jackson, M.J., Al-Barghouthy, G., Pearce, R.K., Smith, L., Hagan, J.J., Jenner, P., 2004. Effect of 5-HT1B/D receptor agonist and antagonist administration on motor function in haloperidol and MPTP-treated common marmosets. Pharmacology, biochemistry, and behavior. 79, 391-400.

Kerenyi, L., Ricaurte, G.A., Schretlen, D.J., McCann, U., Varga, J., Mathews, W.B., Ravert, H.T., Dannals, R.F., Hilton, J., Wong, D.F., Szabo, Z., 2003. Positron emission tomography of striatal serotonin transporters in Parkinson disease. Archives of neurology. 60, 1223-9.

Kilbourn, M.R., Sherman, P., Abbott, L.C., 1998. Reduced MPTP neurotoxicity in striatum of the mutant mouse tottering. Synapse. 30, 205-10.

Kim, S.E., Choi, J.Y., Choe, Y.S., Choi, Y., Lee, W.Y., 2003. Serotonin transporters in the midbrain of Parkinson's disease patients: a study with 123I-beta-CIT SPECT. Journal of nuclear medicine : official publication, Society of Nuclear Medicine. 44, 870-6.

Kish, S.J., Tong, J., Hornykiewicz, O., Rajput, A., Chang, L.J., Guttman, M., Furukawa, Y., 2008. Preferential loss of serotonin markers in caudate versus putamen in Parkinson's disease. Brain : a journal of neurology. 131, 120-31.

Kostic, V.S., Lecic, D., Doder, M., Marinkovic, J., Filipovic, S., 1996. Prolactin and cortisol responses to fenfluramine in Parkinson's disease. Biological psychiatry. 40, 769-75.

Kurlan, R., Cummings, J., Raman, R., Thal, L., 2007. Quetiapine for agitation or psychosis in patients with dementia and parkinsonism. Neurology. 68, 1356-63.

Lauterbach, E.C.., Freeman, A., and Vogel, R.L. 2003. Correlates of generalized anxiety and panic attacks in dystonia and Parkinson's disease. Cognitive and behavioral neurology. 16, 225-233.

Lauterbach, E.C.., 2005. The neuropsychiatry of Parkinson's disease. Minerva medica. 96(3), 155-173.

Leentjens, A.F., Van den Akker, M., Metsemakers, J.F., Lousberg, R., Verhey, F.R., 2003. Higher incidence of depression preceding the onset of Parkinson's disease: a register study. Movement disorders : official journal of the Movement Disorder Society. 18, 414-8.

Leentjens, A.F., Scholtissen, B., Vreeling, F.W., Verhey, F.R., 2006. The serotonergic hypothesis for depression in Parkinson's disease: an experimental approach. Neuropsychopharmacology : official publication of the American College of Neuropsychopharmacology. 31, 1009-15.

Maker, H.S., Weiss, C., Brannan, T.S., 1986. Amine-mediated toxicity. The effects of dopamine, norepinephrine, 5-hydroxytryptamine, 6-hydroxydopamine, ascorbate, glutathione and peroxide on the in vitro activities of creatine and adenylate kinases in the brain of the rat. Neuropharmacology. 25, 25-32.

Mann, D.M., 1983. The locus coeruleus and its possible role in ageing and degenerative disease of the human central nervous system. Mechanisms of ageing and development. 23, 73-94.

Mann, D.M., Yates, P.O., 1983. Pathological basis for neurotransmitter changes in Parkinson's disease. Neuropathology and applied neurobiology. 9, 3-19.

Marien, M.R., Colpaert, F.C., Rosenquist, A.C., 2004. Noradrenergic mechanisms in neurodegenerative diseases: a theory. Brain research. Brain research reviews. 45, 38-78.

Marin, C., Aguilar, E., Rodriguez-Oroz, M.C., Bartoszyk, G.D., Obeso, J.A., 2009. Local administration of sarizotan into the subthalamic nucleus attenuates levodopa-induced dyskinesias in 6-OHDA-lesioned rats. Psychopharmacology. 204, 241-50.

Mavridis, M., Degryse, A.D., Lategan, A.J., Marien, M.R., Colpaert, F.C., 1991. Effects of locus coeruleus lesions on parkinsonian signs, striatal dopamine and substantia nigra cell loss after 1-methyl-4-phenyl-1,2,3,6-tetrahydropyridine in monkeys: a possible role for the locus coeruleus in the progression of Parkinson's disease. Neuroscience. 41, 507-23.

Mayeux, R., Williams, J.B., Stern, Y., Cote, L., 1984. Depression and Parkinson's disease. Advances in neurology. 40, 241-50.

Mayeux, R., Stern, Y., Williams, J.B., Cote, L., Frantz, A., Dyrenfurth, I., 1986. Clinical and biochemical features of depression in Parkinson's disease. The American journal of psychiatry. 143, 756-9.

McKinlay, A., Grace, R.C., Dalrymple-Alford, J.C., Anderson, T., Fink, J., Roger, D., 2008. A profile of neuropsychiatric problems and their relationship to quality of life for Parkinson's disease patients without dementia. Parkinsonism & related disorders. 14, 37-42.

McNaught, K.S., Jnobaptiste, R., Jackson, T., Jengelley, T.A., 2010. The pattern of neuronal loss and survival may reflect differential expression of proteasome activators in Parkinson's disease. Synapse. 64, 241-50.

Meltzer, H.Y., Mills, R., Revell, S., Williams, H., Johnson, A., Bahr, D., Friedman, J.H., 2010. Pimavanserin, a serotonin(2A) receptor inverse agonist, for the treatment of parkinson's disease psychosis. Neuropsychopharmacology : official publication of the American College of Neuropsychopharmacology. 35, 881-92.

Menza, M., Dobkin, R.D., Marin, H., Mark, M.H., Gara, M., Buyske, S., Bienfait, K., Dicke, A., 2009. A controlled trial of antidepressants in patients with Parkinson disease and depression. Neurology. 72, 886-92.

Meyer, J.S., Huang, J., Chowdhury, M.H., 2007. MRI confirms mild cognitive impairments prodromal for Alzheimer's, vascular and Parkinson-Lewy body dementias. Journal of the neurological sciences. 257, 97-104.

Michelsen, K.A., Prickaerts, J., Steinbusch, H.W., 2008. The dorsal raphe nucleus and serotonin: implications for neuroplasticity linked to major depression and Alzheimer's disease. Progress in brain research. 172, 233-64.

Miyawaki, E., Meah, Y., Koller, W.C., 1997. Serotonin, dopamine, and motor effects in Parkinson's disease. Clinical neuropharmacology. 20, 300-10.

Navailles, S., Bioulac, B., Gross, C., De Deurwaerdere, P., 2010. Serotonergic neurons mediate ectopic release of dopamine induced by L-DOPA in a rat model of Parkinson's disease. Neurobiology of disease. 38, 136-43.

Numan, S., Lundgren, K.H., Wright, D.E., Herman, J.P., Seroogy, K.B., 1995. Increased expression of 5HT2 receptor mRNA in rat striatum following 6-OHDA lesions of the adult nigrostriatal pathway. Brain research. Molecular brain research. 29, 391-6.

Parkkinen, L., Pirttila, T., Alafuzoff, I., 2008. Applicability of current staging/categorization of alpha-synuclein pathology and their clinical relevance. Acta neuropathologica. 115, 399-407.

Patt, S., Gerhard, L., 1993. A Golgi study of human locus coeruleus in normal brains and in Parkinson's disease. Neuropathology and applied neurobiology. 19, 519-23.

Paulus, W., Jellinger, K., 1991. The neuropathologic basis of different clinical subgroups of Parkinson's disease. Journal of neuropathology and experimental neurology. 50, 743-55.

Pintor, L., Bailles, E., Valldeoriola, F., Tolosa, E., Marti, M.J., de Pablo, J., 2006. Response to 4-month treatment with reboxetine in Parkinson's disease patients with a major depressive episode. General hospital psychiatry. 28, 59-64.

Politis, M., Wu, K., Loane, C., Turkheimer, F.E., Molloy, S., Brooks, D.J., Piccini, P., 2010. Depressive symptoms in PD correlate with higher 5-HTT binding in raphe and limbic structures. Neurology. 75, 1920-7.

Radja, F., Descarries, L., Dewar, K.M., Reader, T.A., 1993. Serotonin 5-HT1 and 5-HT2 receptors in adult rat brain after neonatal destruction of nigrostriatal dopamine neurons: a quantitative autoradiographic study. Brain research. 606, 273-85.

Ravina, B., Camicioli, R., Como, P.G., Marsh, L., Jankovic, J., Weintraub, D., Elm, J., 2007. The impact of depressive symptoms in early Parkinson disease. Neurology. 69, 342-7.

Remy, P., Doder, M., Lees, A., Turjanski, N., Brooks, D., 2005. Depression in Parkinson's disease: loss of dopamine and noradrenaline innervation in the limbic system. Brain : a journal of neurology. 128, 1314-22.

Richard, I.H., Schiffer, R.B., Kurlan, R., 1996. Anxiety and Parkinson's disease. The Journal of neuropsychiatry and clinical neurosciences. 8, 383-92.

Rommelfanger, K.S., Weinshenker, D., Miller, G.W., 2004. Reduced MPTP toxicity in noradrenaline transporter knockout mice. Journal of neurochemistry. 91, 1116-24.

Rommelfanger, K.S., Weinshenker, D., 2007. Norepinephrine: The redheaded stepchild of Parkinson's disease. Biochemical pharmacology. 74, 177-90.

Roselli, F., Pisciotta, N.M., Pennelli, M., Aniello, M.S., Gigante, A., De Caro, M.F., Ferrannini, E., Tartaglione, B., Niccoli-Asabella, A., Defazio, G., Livrea, P., Rubini, G., 2010. Midbrain SERT in degenerative parkinsonisms: a 123I-FP-CIT SPECT study. Movement disorders : official journal of the Movement Disorder Society. 25, 1853-9.

Scatton, B., Javoy-Agid, F., Rouquier, L., Dubois, B., Agid, Y., 1983. Reduction of cortical dopamine, noradrenaline, serotonin and their metabolites in Parkinson's disease. Brain research. 275, 321-8.

Schapira, A.H., Bezard, E., Brotchie, J., Calon, F., Collingridge, G.L., Ferger, B., Hengerer, B., Hirsch, E., Jenner, P., Le Novere, N., Obeso, J.A., Schwarzschild, M.A., Spampinato, U., Davidai, G., 2006. Novel pharmacological targets for the treatment of Parkinson's disease. Nature reviews. Drug discovery. 5, 845-54.

Schrag, A., Jahanshahi, M., Quinn, N., 2000. What contributes to quality of life in patients with Parkinson's disease? Journal of neurology, neurosurgery, and psychiatry. 69, 308-12.

Schrag, A., Morley, D., Quinn, N., Jahanshahi, M., 2004. Impact of Parkinson's disease on patients' adolescent and adult children. Parkinsonism & related disorders. 10, 391-7.

Schrag, A., 2006. Quality of life and depression in Parkinson's disease. Journal of the neurological sciences. 248, 151-7.

Schuurman, A.G., van den Akker, M., Ensinck, K.T., Metsemakers, J.F., Knottnerus, J.A., Leentjens, A.F., Buntinx, F., 2002. Increased risk of Parkinson's disease after depression: a retrospective cohort study. Neurology. 58, 1501-4.

Shiba, M., Bower, J.H., Maraganore, D.M., McDonnell, S.K., Peterson, B.J., Ahlskog, J.E., Schaid, D.J., Rocca, W.A., 2000. Anxiety disorders and depressive disorders preceding Parkinson's disease: a case-control study. Movement disorders : official journal of the Movement Disorder Society. 15, 669-77.

Stein,M.B., Heuser, I.J., Juncos, J.L., and Uhde, T.W. 1990. Anxiety disorders in patients with Parkinson's disease. American journal of pyschiatry. 41, 1086-1089.

Tadaiesky, M.T., Dombrowski, P.A., Figueiredo, C.P., Cargnin-Ferreira, E., Da Cunha, C., Takahashi, R.N., 2008. Emotional, cognitive and neurochemical alterations in a premotor stage model of Parkinson's disease. Neuroscience. 156, 830-40.

Taylor, T.N., Caudle, W.M., Shepherd, K.R., Noorian, A., Jackson, C.R., Iuvone, P.M., Weinshenker, D., Greene, J.G., Miller, G.W., 2009. Nonmotor symptoms of Parkinson's disease revealed in an animal model with reduced monoamine storage capacity. The Journal of neuroscience : the official journal of the Society for Neuroscience. 29, 8103-13.

Veazey, C., Aki, S.O., Cook, K.F., Lai, E.C., Kunik, M.E., 2005. Prevalence and treatment of depression in Parkinson's disease. The Journal of neuropsychiatry and clinical neurosciences. 17, 310-23.

Volpi, R., Caffarra, P., Boni, S., Scaglioni, A., Malvezzi, L., Saginario, A., Chiodera, P., Coiro, V., 1997. ACTH/cortisol involvement in the serotonergic disorder affecting the parkinsonian brain. Neuropsychobiology. 35, 73-8.

Von Coelln, R., Thomas, B., Savitt, J.M., Lim, K.L., Sasaki, M., Hess, E.J., Dawson, V.L., Dawson, T.M., 2004. Loss of locus coeruleus neurons and reduced startle in parkin null mice. Proceedings of the National Academy of Sciences of the United States of America. 101, 10744-9.

Walter, U., Dressler, D., Wolters, A., Wittstock, M., Benecke, R., 2007a. Transcranial brain sonography findings in clinical subgroups of idiopathic Parkinson's disease. Movement disorders : official journal of the Movement Disorder Society. 22, 48-54.

Walter, U., Hoeppner, J., Prudente-Morrissey, L., Horowski, S., Herpertz, S.C., Benecke, R., 2007b. Parkinson's disease-like midbrain sonography abnormalities are frequent in depressive disorders. Brain : a journal of neurology. 130, 1799-807.

Weintraub, D., Morales, K.H., Moberg, P.J., Bilker, W.B., Balderston, C., Duda, J.E., Katz, I.R., Stern, M.B., 2005. Antidepressant studies in Parkinson's disease: a review and meta-analysis. Movement disorders : official journal of the Movement Disorder Society. 20, 1161-9.

Zarow, C., Lyness, S.A., Mortimer, J.A., Chui, H.C., 2003. Neuronal loss is greater in the locus coeruleus than nucleus basalis and substantia nigra in Alzheimer and Parkinson diseases. Archives of neurology. 60, 337-41.

Zhang, X., Andren, P.E., Greengard, P., Svenningsson, P., 2008. Evidence for a role of the 5-HT1B receptor and its adaptor protein, p11, in L-DOPA treatment of an animal model of Parkinsonism. Proceedings of the National Academy of Sciences of the United States of America. 105, 2163-8.

10

Mesothalamic Dopaminergic Activity: Implications in Sleep Alterations in Parkinson's Disease

Daniele Q. M. Madureira
Laboratório Nacional de Computação Científica
Brazil

1. Introduction

Movement, sleep and cognition: three connected realms enriching to the human life. Three harmed realms limiting parkinsonian patients.

A degenerative process in dopaminergic neurons from the substantia nigra (SN) midbrain nucleus is the basic origin underlying a set of symptoms developed in patients with Parkinson's Disease (PD) (Andrade & Ferraz, 2003). The devastating motor difficulties usually do not appear isolated. Indeed, PD consists of distinct kinds of manifestations involving motor and mental rigidity as well as sleep alterations (Dubois & Pillon, 1996; Rye et al., 2000; De Cock et al., 2008; Arnulf & Leu-Semenescu, 2009).

Even though impairments in other brain nuclei also contribute to the symptoms present in PD (Braak et al., 2000), it is surprising how so distinct brain systems suffer influence of the degenerative alterations in the SN. This phenomenon may be regarded as a simple consequence of the connections between the SN and diverse brain areas. As a matter of fact, it also highlights that distinct behavioral aspects are achieved through the sharing of brain resources. Here, we examine - through a neurocomputational model - relationships between alterations in the mesothalamic dopaminergic activity (MDA) and sleep impairments in PD.

With origins in the SN, the mesothalamic pathway (MP) reaches the thalamic complex, in particular the thalamic reticular nucleus (TRN). Investigations on such dopaminergic pathway, evidenced by Freeman and colleagues (Freeman et al., 2001), have been contributing to a more global comprehension of cognitive processes in the brain. Based on experimental results (Florán et al., 2004), the mathematical model proposed in (Madureira et al., 2010) indicates a way by which the mesothalamic dopamine inhibits neurons in the TRN. And computational simulations of this model suggest that alterations in the MDA lead to inattention symptoms as observed in PD and Attention Deficit Hyperactivity Disorder (ADHD).

Thalamic neurons are able to spike under tonic and burst states (Steriade et al., 1993; Llinás & Steriade, 2006). Whenever in the tonic state, these neurons respond linearly to input stimuli. By this way, they propagate information reliably from perceptual systems to the cerebral cortex, where a more refined processing takes place. This mode of activity is crucial to the thalamocortical filtering of perceptual stimuli that allows attention focusing (Madureira et al., 2007, 2010; Carvalho, 1994).

Conversely, under the burst state thalamic neurons are no more reliable channels through which neural representations from sensorial inputs reach the cerebral cortex. As a matter of fact, this mode of activity underlies the thalamic behavior during sleep (Steriade et al., 1993; Pace-Schott & Hobson, 2002). In this case, the environmental stimuli are not perceived consciously as it occurs throughout wakefulness (Carvalho, 1994). The thalamic burst mode also permeates epileptic episodes during which environmental information is not processed reliably (Jeanmonod et al., 1996; Llinás et al., 1999). The dynamics of the ionic channels under the burst mode are different from the ones underlying the thalamic tonic state. That is why, under the burst mode, thalamic neurons spike quite autonomously, in such a way that their pattern of activity does not represent the input information.

Since the inattention symptoms addressed in (Madureira et al., 2010) concerned awakened people, the model considered the behavior of thalamic neurons under the tonic state. In the present work, we go further with the matter and scrutinize relationships between the MDA and the oscillatory state of neurons in the thalamic complex. Doing so, it becomes possible to widen the investigation to examine a possible MDA contribution to sleep alterations in PD and, to look at attention focusing aspects under a little more detailed point of view.

Clinical evidences indicating a variety of sleep alterations in PD suggest that this class of symptoms should not be considered as a secondary one: on the contrary, sleep problems certainly pertain to the core symptoms that define PD (De Cock et al., 2008; Arnulf & Leu-Semenescu, 2009). Such sleep alterations involve daytime sleepiness, inappropriate intrusion of REM sleep episodes throughout the day, and nocturne movement. In other words, parkinsonism disrupts the control of the sleep-wake cycle (Jancovic, 2002; Arnulf & Leu-Semenescu, 2009).

The question thus that naturally arises concerns the dopaminergic role in the sleep-wake cycle control. Given the clinical evidence from sleep impairments in PD, a disease whose basic neural origins is the dopaminergic neurons degeneration, we tend to conclude that dopamine does participate in the sleep regulation. Is it the case?

Up to recently, the above mentioned clinical observations have been quite disregarded. If, through PD, the dopaminergic participation in the control of the sleep cycle may be inferred (Rye, 2004), there is, on the other hand, a number of neuroscientific studies showing that the variation in the dopaminergic level throughout the sleep-wake cycle is too small to be taken into account (Jancovic, 2002).

A series of experiments undertaken by (Dzirasa et al., 2006), however, illuminated this controversy. They were capable of demonstrating that sleep-wake states are also controlled by dopamine. This seminal work shows the importance of the dopaminergic influence in the sleep regulation – even under small variations. In addition, they emphasize the relationship between dopaminergic alterations and sleep impairments in PD.

Here, we address – through a neurocomputational approach – the interference of SN neurons, particularly the degenerated ones, in the thalamocortical spiking modes. Our goal consists in investigating if the PD dopaminergic disruption alters the typical spiking patterns associated to sleep and wake states, thus compromising the normal sleep-wake cycle in PD.

We now outline the contents of this chapter. In Section 2 we introduce our hypothesis of dopaminergic influence on the control of the sleep-wake cycle, and describe the model. In Section 3, we explain how the computational simulations of the model are designed, and present the computational results. Finally, we conclude by discussing the consequences of our results in terms of sleep alterations in PD, in the context of the neuroscience of sleep.

2. The model

In (Madureira et al., 2010), we proposed a mathematical model indicating how the mesothalamic dopamine influences the thalamocortical loop, through the TRN, and thus modulates the attentional focus formation. In particular, we investigated relationships between alterations in this dopaminergic pathway and attention deficits in PD and ADHD.

Here, we extend this model to address how dopamine influences the emergence of distinct spiking modes in thalamic neurons. Since the thalamic modes of spiking are specifically related to sleep and wake neuron states, our modeling enables us to discuss if and how dopaminergic alterations in PD are related to the sleep problems observed in the disease.

Throughout the sleep-wake cycle, complex chemical and electrical networks of events occur in the thalamocortical neural circuit. They give rise to distinct patterns of neural behavior that underlies the different brain rhythms specifically associated to different sleep phases and also to the wake state (Pace-Schott & Hobson, 2002; Hobson & Pace-Schott, 2002; Diekelmann & Born, 2010).

The variety of brain rhythms extensively studied by the neuroscience of sleep (Steriade et al., 2003; De Gennaro & Ferrara, 2003; Llinás & Steriade, 2006; Steriade, 2006; Pace-Schott & Hobson, 2002; Hobson & Pace-Schott, 2002; Hobson, 2009; Diekelmann & Born, 2010) reflects the behavior of neural groups. Indeed, such brain rhythms, e.g. spindles, slow oscillation and theta activity, are measurements of field potential oscillations captured by EEGs experiments – not by single cell recordings. Therefore, they provide information from a scale above the cellular one.

Our model, on the other hand, addresses the dynamics of ionic and synaptic currents. It thus deals with information at the same level of single cell recordings, in particular, variations in the membrane electric potential.

Under this approach, it is reasonable to examine sleep issues by mathematically modeling neurons in the thalamocortical loop, and computationally simulating the action of neuromodulators throughout this brain area.

As an outcome of our neurocomputational model, we conjecture that the inhibitory action of mesothalamic dopamine in the thalamic reticular nucleus (TRN) (Florán et al., 2004) affects the spiking mode of thalamocortical neurons. This is possible whenever the dopaminergic action leads to a period of neuron hyperpolarization that activates the calcium conductance, thus changing the way by which the neuron behaves (Carvalho, 1994). Next, we present the model and develop such ideas more deeply.

2.1 The neural network

We model a thalamocortical circuit with a dopaminergic projection from SN to the TRN, according to Figure 1. We can note the excitatory and inhibitory connections in the modeled neural network. Thalamocortical and corticothalamic projections are excitatory, mediated by glutamate. Both areas send glutamatergic excitatory collateral axons to the TRN. Conversely, efferent projections from the TRN to thalamus are GABAergic inhibitory (Guillery & Harting, 2003).

With relation to the dopaminergic action, the architecture of the network incorporates results gathered together from Freeman et al. (2001) and Florán et al. (2004), which reveal the inhibitory dopaminergic projection from SN to the TRN, or the mesothalamic dopaminergic pathway. The explanation we suggest for the dopaminergic action in TRN is that dopamine acts on the calcium dependent potassium channels, possibly by increasing its conductance. By this way, the level of potassium that leaves the cell increases, which consequently inhibits neuron spiking. Thus, the GABA release becomes inhibited – for more details see (Madureira et al., 2010).

Given such a structure, external stimuli X and Y are projected through excitatory pathways to neighboring thalamic regions, T_x and T_y, respectively. Once stimulated, T_x activates TRN_x beyond collaterals of an ascending glutamatergic projection, whose final destiny is the PFC. Since our work does not model the PFC explicitly, such excitatory projection ends up in TRN in the model. Also, through an excitatory glutamatergic descending pathway, the cortical region enhances the activation of T_x, and also sends collateral axons to TRN_x. Thus, once activated, the TRN_x inhibits the thalamic region T_y through a GABAergic inhibitory projection. Summarizing, the thalamocortical circuit activation by an external stimulus X excites a central thalamic region T_x and inhibits its neighborhood, represented by the neuron T_y. As the mesothalamic dopamine inhibits neurons in TRN, a rise in the dopaminergic level contributes to deactivating such cells. This leads to a more active thalamic region T_y. Conversely, a reduction in the dopaminergic level activates TRN, and increases the inhibition of T_y. A symmetrical case involves the T_y and TRN_y neurons, as illustrated in Figure 1.

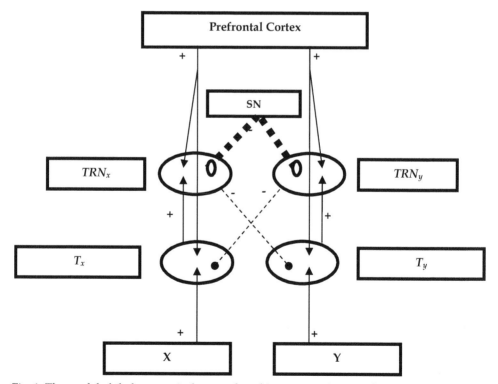

Fig. 1. The modeled thalamocortical network architecture: excitatory glutamatergic synapses (arrows), inhibitory GABAergic synapse (black sphere), inhibitory dopaminergic synapse (white sphere).

In the following, we describe the systems of equations that model the behaviors of T_x, T_y, TRN_x and TRN_y. The neural activities of the SN and the PFC, as well as the excitatory projections from X and Y are codified as temporal sequences representing their respective spiking times. As this work takes further the model presented in (Madureira et al., 2010), throughout the next section we examine specially the particular aspects of this extension.

2.2 Ionic currents

To better investigate alternate thalamic states, this model incorporates physiological features related to the tonic and the bursting modes of thalamic spikes. Thus, we address the neuron spike by considering the sodium, I_{Na}, and the calcium, I_{Ca}, currents, which depolarize the neuron, and the potassium current, I_K, which restores the cellular membrane potential (Kandel, 2000). With relation to the patterns of intervals between spikes, associated to different potassium currents (McCormick et al., 1995), our model incorporates the calcium dependent-potassium current, I_c, particularly, in the TRN neurons: it is a transient current, whose amplitude increases with intracellular calcium concentration, and it suffers dopaminergic influence (Florán et al., 2004; Madureira et al., 2010). Essentially associated to the bursting mode, the I_{ahp}, a current that underlies neural hyperpolarization, is modeled as described below.

The model deals with a network of ionic and synaptic events that leads to a specific mode of spiking. Particularly, under this approach we examine if dopamine is able to influence the spikes of thalamic neurons. In this model we assume that a high inhibitory dopamine action on D4 receptors in TRN neurons hyperpolarizes such cells, thus facilitating the activation of calcium currents. As a consequence, and according to thalamic properties (Carvalho, 1994), even a small membrane depolarization is capable of triggering an action potential, due to the low threshold calcium-currents. Whenever the inflow of Ca^{2+} in the cell, due to spikes, increases the Ca^{2+} concentration above a threshold, then the hyperpolarizing current I_{ahp}, becomes activated, hyperpolarizing the neuron. Therefore, the calcium currents become activate – or remain activated, depending on their previous state – and a cyclic or oscillatory behavior takes place in the TRN neuron. This is the burst thalamic mode of spiking, associated to sleep states (Steriade et al., 1993; Llinás & Steriade, 2006). It may be interrupted due to the calcium currents inactivation, which occurs whenever the neuron does not suffer hyperpolarization for around 100ms.

Based on this model, we speculate another possibility that is directly related to the PD origins: the generation of bursting in thalamic neurons, due to a strong inhibition imposed by TRN neurons. Such situation is plausible to occur in case of mesothalamic hypodopaminergy, which allows the inhibitory TRN neurons to become atypically over stimulated (Madureira et al., 2010, Florán et al., 2004).

Because of the dopaminergic modulation in the TRN, two types of neurons are modeled: the thalamic ones, T_x and T_y, and the TRN neurons. Both are single point spiking and are presented next.

2.2.1 Thalamic neurons

We define a simplified neuron model with a single compartment where dendrites, soma and axons are concentrated, and whose electric potential is V. The neural membrane is modeled according to the equation:

$$C_T \frac{dV}{dt} = I_k + I_{ahp} + I_{syn} + I_l ,$$

where we recall that I_k represents the potassium current, I_{ahp} the hyperpolarizing current, I_{syn} the dendritic current induced by synaptic action, and I_l the leak current, i.e., currents that are not modeled.

Considering the relation between membrane voltage and ionic currents, as

$$
\begin{aligned}
I_k &= g_k \left(E_k - V \right), \\
I_{ahp} &= g_{ahp} \left(E_k - V \right), \\
I_l &= g_l \left(E_l - V \right), \\
I_{syn} &= g_{syn} \left(E_{syn} - V \right)
\end{aligned}
\tag{1}
$$

where the constants E_k, E_{ahp}, E_l and E_{syn} are reversal potentials for the currents I_k, I_{ahp}, I_l and I_{syn}, respectively, and g_k, g_{ahp}, g_l and g_{syn} represent the conductances corresponding to these currents.

The occurrence of a spike is associated to a step function $s(V)$, whose unitary value indicates the action potential depolarizing phase, depending on the I_{Na} or I_{Ca} currents:

$$
s(V) = \begin{cases} 1, & \text{if } V \geq \theta_{spike} \\ 0, & \text{if } V < \theta_{spike}, \end{cases}
$$

where θ_{spike} is a voltage threshold for the channel opening. It is defined as:

$$
\theta_{spike} = \begin{cases} \theta_{Na}, & \text{if } I_{Ca} \text{ is inactivated} \\ \theta_{Ca}, & \text{if } I_{Ca} \text{ is activated}, \end{cases}
$$

where, θ_{Na} is the voltage threshold for the sodium channels opening, and θ_{Ca} for the calcium channels. We have $\theta_{Na} > \theta_{Ca}$, and the spikes triggered by the calcium ionic channels are the low threshold spikes (LTS).

During the network activity, the membrane potential, V, is monitored. When strong inhibitory events lead to periods of hyperpolarization, around 100ms, the I_{Ca} currents become activated (Carvalho, 1994). Once in activity, I_{Ca} currents cause the LTS.

Following a spike, the conductance g_k of the restoring current I_k increases rapidly, bringing the neuron back to a resting potential. Such a process is described by

$$\frac{dg_k}{dt} = \frac{s\beta_k - g_k}{\tau_k}$$

where the constant β_k represents a variation rate of g_k, and τ_k a time constant associated to the potassium channel.

According to the frequency of spikes, the calcium concentration increases – and decreases due to calcium buffers and pumps (Carvalho & Roitman, 1995). Then, we have:

$$\frac{d[Ca]}{dt} = \frac{s\beta_{Ca} - [Ca]}{\tau_{Ca}} \tag{2}$$

where β_{Ca} represents the rate of calcium concentration variation, and τ_{Ca} a time constant.
If the intracellular calcium concentration reaches a given threshold Θ_{Ca}, the potassium channels related to the hyperpolarizing current are opened. The step function $f([Ca])$ describes such event as:

$$f([Ca]) = \begin{cases} 1, \text{ if } [Ca] \geq \Theta_{Ca} \\ \\ 0, \text{ if } [Ca] < \Theta_{Ca}. \end{cases}$$

The following equation describes how its conductance, g_{ahp}, behaves with respect to the I_{ahp} current:

$$\frac{d\,g_{ahp}}{dt} = \frac{f\beta_{ahp} - g_{ahp}}{\tau_{ahp}}$$

where β_{ahp} represents a variation rate of g_{ahp}, and τ_{ahp} a time constant.
Once in the activated state, the I_{Ca} current facilitates the occurrence of LTS, and the consequent increase of the calcium concentration, $[Ca]$. As a result, the conductance g_{ahp} grows, and the neuron suffers a hyperpolarization.

2.2.2 TRN neurons

Since TRN and thalamic neurons main properties are similar, the equations for the TRN neuron are quite similar to the ones considered in 2.2.1, except for the inclusion of the calcium-dependent potassium current I_c.
We assume the final target of dopaminergic action is the calcium-dependent potassium channel, whose ionic current is I_c (Madureira et al., 2010; Florán et al., 2004). Thus, the membrane equation for the TRN neuron incorporates the ionic current I_c as:

$$C_{TRN}\frac{dV}{dt} = I_k + I_{ahp} + I_c + I_{syn} + I_l$$

Indeed, $I_c = g_c (E_k - V)$, where E_k represents the potassium reversal potential, and g_c the conductance of ionic current I_c.
The conductance g_c suffers dopaminergic influence, via D4 receptor, and depends on the intracellular calcium concentration. Thus, $g_c = \hat{g}_c\,D_4^*\,S(\,[Ca]\,)$, where $\hat{g}_c$ is a constant, D_4^* stands for the dopaminergic action on g_c, and $S(\,[Ca]\,)$ stands for a sigmoid function of the intracellular calcium concentration, which increases by virtue of a neural spiking. We set

$$S([Ca]) = \frac{1}{1 + \exp(-a[Ca])}$$

where the constant a controls the slope of S, and rhe calcium concentration behaves according to the equation (2). Indeed, in (2) the term s raises the calcium concentration whenever there is a neural spiking. Therefore g_c increases and inhibits the cell, if the cell is excited beyond a threshold.

The dopaminergic action on g_c is modeled by the summation of alpha functions (Carvalho, 1994) representing the rise and the decrease of the dopaminergic level, in each of the N presynaptic spikes that occurred at times t_i, before t, with $1 \leq i \leq N$:

$$D_4^* = \hat{g}_{d4} \sum_{i=1}^{N} (t - t_i) \exp[-(t - t_i) / t_{pd}]$$

Here, the constant t_{pd} stands for the peak time for the alpha function, and $\hat{g}_{d4}$ is the conductance constant of the dopaminergic projection. For further details, see ref. (Madureira et al., 2010).

2.3 Synaptic projections

Finally, we present the synaptic modeling (Carvalho, 1994). For the synaptic conductance g_{syn}, appearing in Equation (1), it follows that

$$g_{syn} = \hat{g}_{syn} \sum_{i=1}^{N} (t - t_i) \exp\left[-(t - t_i) / t_p\right]$$

where $\hat{g}_{syn}$ is the maximal conductance, which assumes different values for each particular synapse. In fact, each modeled synapse has a specific associated conductance, reflecting its influence: $\hat{g}_{c\text{-}trn}$ and $\hat{g}_{c\text{-}t}$ for synapses between the cortex and the TRN, and between the cortex and the thalamus, respectively; $\hat{g}_{t\text{-}trn}$ and $\hat{g}_{trn\text{-}t}$ for synapses between the thalamus and the TRN, and vice versa; and $\hat{g}_{e\text{-}t}$ for synapses between somatosensory projections and the thalamus.

The synaptic conductance g_{syn} is also represented by a summation of alpha functions, for each of the N presynaptic spikes that occurred at times t_i before t, for $1 \leq I \leq N$. We denote by t_p the peak time for the alpha function, and it assumes the values t_{pe} and t_{pi} for excitatory and inhibitory synapses respectively.

We used the ANSI C ® programming language to implement the model. The differential equations are integrated by the Euler's method. Ref. (Madureira et al., 2010) and Table 1 present glossaries with all necessary parameter values.

I_{ahp}	Hyperpolarizing potassium current	($\mu A.cm^{-2}$)
g_{ahp}	Conductance of I_{ahp}	($m.mhos.cm^{-2}$)
θ_{Ca}	Threshold for calcium channel's opening	(0 mV)
θ_{Na}	Threshold for sodium channel's opening	(1 mV)
Θ_{Ca}	Intracellular calcium concentration threshold for I_{ahp} activation	(mM)
β_{ahp}	Variation rate of g_{ahp}	(100)
τ_{ahp}	Time constant of g_{ahp}	(2 ms)

Table 1. Glossary of parameters.

3. Computational simulations

Due to a mechanism of inhibitory feedback between thalamic and TRN neurons in the thalamocortical circuit, when a projected stimulus on the central thalamic area T_x is propagated for posterior cortical processing, its neighboring thalamic area T_y suffers inhibition from TRN. This property was highly explored in (Madureira et al., 2010), because our major concern was the attentional focus formation.

Here, we explore such inhibitory feedback to inspect how the activity degree in the TRN influences the thalamic excitatory state. Summarizing, our simulations illustrate how dopamine modulates the activation of TRN neurons and, consequently, that of the thalamic cells.

With relation to the dopaminergic action in the TRN, we assume a relationship between the level of mesothalamic dopamine released in the TRN and the nigral spiking frequency. Consequently, we simulate variations in the level of dopamine released in the TRN by varying the SN spiking pattern. We also address the dopamine receptor D4 degree of activity, through the term $\hat{g}_{d4}$ in (3). Indeed, $\hat{g}_{d4}$ model the weight of the connection between the SN and TRN neurons. Then, $\hat{g}_{d4}$ tells us how much receptor D4, in the TRN, is affected by the dopamine release due to a nerve impulse from SN, or due to the action of exogenous factors as drugs that alter the dopamine level throughout synaptic clefts.

Overall, throughout these simulations our major concern is the dopaminergic effect on the thalamocortical dynamics. We do not intend to focus our exploration on the consequences of variations in external or cortical stimuli.

3.1 Asymmetrical architecture

In this section, we describe a series of simulations performed using an artificial neural network that presents the architecture illustrated in the Figure 2. Since such network is the one used in (Madureira et al., 2010), we set it as our departure point.

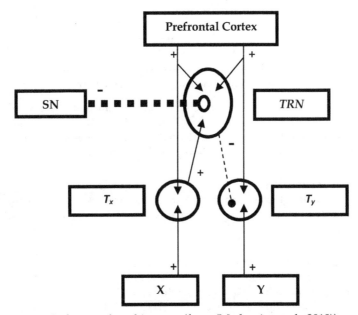

Fig. 2. The asymmetrical network architecture (from (Madureira et al., 2010)).

Here, we investigate if variations in the activity of receptor D4 in the TRN may influence the mode of spiking in neurons of the thalamic complex, along different SN spiking frequencies. We impose a drastic decrease in the nigral dopamine level, reflecting a disturbance in the mesothalamic system, and raise the dopaminergic level afterwards. Through the 500ms-simulations, variations in the dopaminergic receptor activation are modeled by altering the parameter $\hat{g}_{d4}$ after 250ms.

Table 2 describes all simulated variations in the SN spiking frequency, the imposed changes on receptor D4 activation, as well as the characteristic spike modes related to each situation. From these results, we gather that the bursting mode was elicited in two opposing situations: increase of D4 activation under mesothalamic hypoactivity (interval between spikes in SN equals 50 and above) and, decrease of D4 activation under mesothalamic hyperactivity (interval between spikes in SN equals 5).

In the first case, the mesothalamic hypoactivity turns the TRN_x neuron so highly excited, that T_y becomes strongly inhibited, thus activating the calcium current. The posterior increase of the D4 activity, plausibly representing the effect of some dopaminergic agonist, was able to elicit LTSs. Consequently, the calcium concentration reached a threshold value that activated the hyperpolarizing current, promoting the oscillatory pattern in the thalamic cell T_y.

Interval between Spikes in SN (ms)	Changes in the Activity of Dopamine Receptor D4 ($\hat{g}_{d4}$)	Neuron	Spike Mode
100, 150 and 200	1.0 to 1.2	T_y	Tonic to Bursting
50	1.0 to 1.2	T_y	Tonic to Bursting
10	1.0 to 1.2	-	Tonic
5	1.0 to 0.8	TRN	Tonic to Bursting

Table 2. Spiking modes examined through an asymmetrical network.

Conversely, in the second case, the mesothalamic hyperactivity generated the strong inhibition in the TRN neuron, which enabled the calcium currents activation. Then, the imposed decrease of D4 activity was sufficient to diminish the TRN inhibition, thus allowing LTSs and, finally, the bursting mode of spiking.

3.2 Symmetrical architecture
Following the first series of experiments, we extend the network architecture to incorporate the symmetry between neighboring thalamic areas. The symmetrical architecture is represented in the Figure 1.

3.2.1 SN spiking frequency and the attentional focus
We start exploring the extended architecture by addressing the dopaminergic action in neurons under the tonic mode of spiking. Therefore, as a first approximation, we apply the mathematical model developed in (Madureira et al., 2010). In this set of simulations, a weaker stimulus X is presented to the network before the a stronger one, Y. Again, we

initiate with a low SN spike frequency, characterizing the mesothalamic dopamine hypoactivity, and raise the SN activity in successive steps. Table 3 presents our simulations results. Overall, we gather that as the mesothalamic dopaminergic activity decreases, the TRN neurons become more excited. Also, T_x becomes be more inhibited than T_y, enlarging thus the difference between the activations of T_x and T_y, as showed in Table 4. Therefore the mesothalamic dopamine hypoactivity forces the attention to focus on the stimulus Y, implying in attentional shifting difficulty and mental rigidity. On the other hand, the almost identical neural activity of T_x and T_y, enhanced by the mesothalamic dopamine hyperactivity, lead to a no-winner competition between stimuli X and Y, which may represent distraction or lack of attentional focus. These results are compatible with the ones provided by our previous model.

Interval between Spikes in SN (ms)	Spikes in 100ms			
	T_x	T_y	TRN_x	TRN_y
	(100ms – 200ms)			
	(400ms – 500ms)			
50	11	0	25	14
	2	14	14	28
30	14	0	23	9
	4	14	16	25
20	12	0	21	10
	7	13	13	21
10	18	0	17	0
	10	15	5	10
5	18	0	0	0
	18	19	0	0

Table 3. SN spiking frequency and the thalamic tonic state.

3.2.2 Receptor D4 activity and the attentional focus

In the next series of experiments, we keep up our focus on the tonic mode of spiking. And, for each imposed SN spike frequency, we examine the effects of changes in the receptor D4 activation. Since the different degrees of D4 activation can be associated to not modeled exogenous or endogenous factors, that are not modeled, this approach makes it possible to speculate plausible outcomes of the dopaminergic agonists (or antagonists) action at the synaptic cleft. The simulations results are summarized in Table 4. First, we may note that the results presented in the column relative to $\hat{g}_{d4} = 1.0$ agree with the previous set of experiments. It is more interesting, however, to observe that as the receptor D4 activity diminishes, the thalamic neurons become less active, thus reaching a completely inhibited state. Conversely, as the receptor D4 activity increases, thalamic neurons become more active and tend to spike at the same frequency. Finally, we highlight that, except for the baseline case where the interval between spikes in SN equals 10, when $\hat{g}_{d4}$ assumes values lower than 1.0, the differences between T_x and T_y spiking frequencies disappear. So, the mesothalamic hypoactivity does not impose the attention to focus on the stimulus Y anymore.

	Spikes in 100ms					
Interval between Spikes in SN (ms)	Activity of Dopamine Receptor D4 $(\hat{g}_{d4})$					
	0.4	0.6	0.8	1.0	1.2	1.4
50	T_x -	0	2	2	11	14
	T_y -	0	2	14	16	19
	TRN_x -	46	32	14	9	4
	TRN_y -	46	32	28	15	6
30	T_x -	0	4	4	12	15
	T_y -	0	4	13	17	18
	TRN_x -	42	30	25	12	2
	TRN_y -	42	30	25	12	5
20	T_x -	0	5	7	12	18
	T_y -	0	5	13	15	18
	TRN_x -	40	30	13	10	5
	TRN_y -	40	30	21	12	2
10	T_x 0	0	0	10	16	18
	T_y 0	6	10	15	17	19
	TRN_x 52	30	20	5	5	0
	TRN_y 50	30	30	10	4	0
5	T_x 0	5	15	18	18	-
	T_y 0	5	15	19	19	-
	TRN_x 40	25	10	0	0	-
	TRN_y 40	20	5	0	0	-

Table 4. Receptor D4 activity and the thalamic tonic state.

3.2.3 Dopaminergic activity and the oscillatory state

Next, we simulate the mathematical model described in Section 2 through the extended symmetrical network illustrated in the Figure 1. In this set of experiments, two identical, external stimuli, X and Y, activate the network simultaneously. As in the previous experiments, we impose different SN spiking frequencies. We observe, in Table 5, that extreme and opposing situations lead to the bursting spiking mode in the thalamic complex: the drastic mesothalamic dopamine hypoactivity caused the oscillatory pattern in the T_x and T_y neurons, whereas the mesothalamic dopamine hyperactivity made the TRN neurons to spike through bursts. With relation to the T_x and T_y neurons, the appearance of the bursting mode comes from the strong inhibition they suffered through the GABAergic projection from the TRN neurons, which were over activated due to the low dopaminergic activity. Conversely, the oscillatory behavior of the TRN_x and TRN_y neurons originated from the inhibition suffered by the TRN due to the high dopaminergic level. The dynamics of the ionic currents involved in such processes are the same described in Subsection 2.2. Figure 3 illustrates the changes in the T_x behavior due to the diminishing of the receptor D4 activation, throughout the dopamine hypoactivity case, described in the first line of Table 5.

Interval between Spikes in SN (ms)	Activity of Dopamine Receptor D$_4^*$ ($\hat{g}_{d4}$)	Neurons	Spike Mode
100	0.8	T$_x$ and T$_y$	Bursting
	0.9	all	Tonic
	1.0	all	Tonic
50	0.8	all	Tonic
	0.9	all	Tonic
	1.0	all	Tonic
40, 30, 20, 10	1.0	all	Tonic
5	1.0	TRN$_x$ and TRN$_y$	Bursting

Table 5. Distinct dopaminergic activities in presence of similar stimuli.

3.2.4 Variations in the dopaminergic activity and the oscillatory state

In our last series of simulations, we deepen our investigations on the changes in the spiking mode. Now, we repeat the strategy undertaken in Subsection 3.2.1, where a stimulus X is presented to the asymmetrical network before a stronger one, Y. Through the extended mathematical model we propose in Section 2, here we look for situations where changes in the dopaminergic action lead to the burst mode in neurons of the thalamic complex. In this set of simulations, we examine only extreme cases of dopaminergic alterations. Such option was because all previous experiments indicated these extreme situations as the more plausible to initiate the ionic events that underlie the burst mode occurrence. Table 6 summarizes our results.

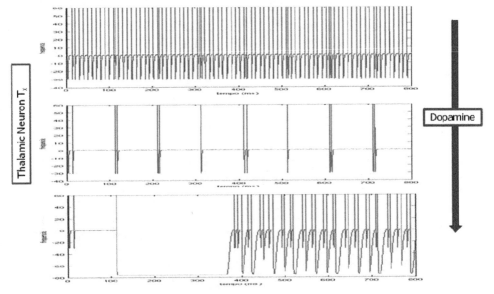

Fig. 3. Decreases in the receptor D4 activation, under mesothalamic dopaminergic hypoactivity, turned the tonic state into the burst one in T$_x$.

In the case of mesothalamic hypoactivity, where the SN neuron spikes every 150ms, the constant activation of D4 as $\hat{g}_{d4}$ = 0.9 made the T_y neuron to spike through bursts – not T_x one. This occurs because the T_y activation is greater than the T_x one by an amount enough to trigger the LTS - after the hyperpolarization due to the high activity in the TRN. In Figure 4, we can observe the T_x and T_y behaviors. The receptor D4 activations imposed by $\hat{g}_{d4}$ = 1.0 or $\hat{g}_{d4}$ = 1.1 did not allow the TRN neurons to spike highly enough to start the necessary hyperpolarization that activates the calcium currents.

Another case of mesothalamic hypoactivity we simulate by fixing the SN frequency in one spike each 100ms. Compared to the previous experiment, the SN is slightly more active. This time, it is the T_x neuron that presents an oscillatory pattern, when $\hat{g}_{d4}$ = 0.9. In this case, the inhibition from TRN_x was not strong enough to hyperpolarize T_y. However, the less stimulated T_x neuron suffered the necessary inhibition that activated calcium currents, thus facilitating the consolidation of the burst mode of spiking. Figure 5 illustrates the distinct spiking modes of T_x and T_y.

Interval between Spikes in SN (ms)	Activity of Dopamine Receptor D_4^* ($\hat{g}_{d4}$)	Neurons	Spike Mode
150	0.9	T_y	Bursting
	1.0	all	Tonic
	1.1	all	Tonic
100	0.8	all	Tonic
	0.9	T_x	Bursting
	0.9 to 1.0	T_x and T_y	Bursting
5	1.1 to 0.8	TRN_x and TRN_y	Bursting

Table 6. Distinct dopaminergic activities in presence of different stimuli.

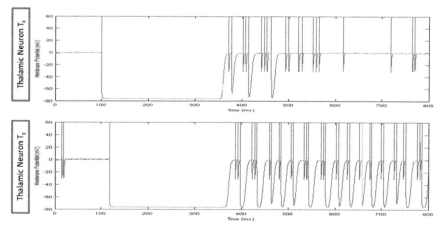

Fig. 4. Behaviors of T_x and T_y. Mesothalamic dopaminergic hypoactivity enables the oscillatory behavior of T_y. SN spikes every 150ms and $\hat{g}_{d4}$ = 0.9.

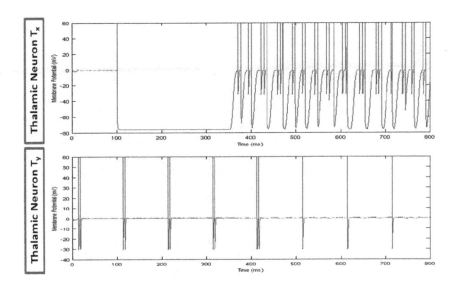

Fig. 5. The distinct spiking modes of T_x and T_y. When SN spikes every 100ms and $\hat{g}_{d4} = 0.9$, T_x presents the burst mode of spiking.

Also with the SN neuron set to spike each 100ms, we started a 800ms-experiment with the parameter $\hat{g}_{d4} = 0.9$. This time, however, we turned $\hat{g}_{d4}$ to 1.0 after 350ms. It is plausible to interpret such alteration in the $\hat{g}_{d4}$ value as a consequence of some increase in the dopaminergic level, due to an exogenous factor. In this case, both T_x and T_y start to oscillate. The last situation presented in Table 6 refers to the extreme case of mesothalamic hyperactivity. During a 800ms-experiment, the interval between spikes in the SN was set to 5ms. In addition, at the beginning we imposed a high activation in receptor D4 with $\hat{g}_{d4} = 1.1$. This dopaminergic context inhibited the TRN neurons, which suffer even a hyperpolarization. It was, however, the imposed decrease of $\hat{g}_{d4}$ to 0.8, after 350ms, that starts the burst mode in both *TRN* neurons. In this case, the lowering in the dopaminergic receptor activity enables the *TRNs* membrane potential to reach a threshold value that triggered LTS in such neurons. Figure 6 illustrates such situation.

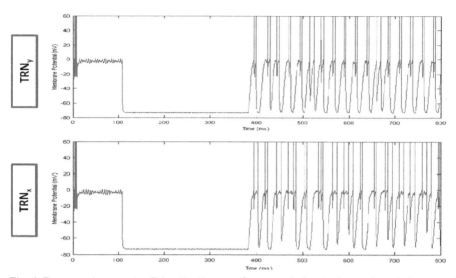

Fig. 6. Decrease in receptor D4 activation, under mesothalamic dopaminergic hyperactivity, originates the burst state in both TRN_x and TRN_y.

4. Discussion

Overall, the current knowledge in neuroscience conducts us through a multiscale world. The understanding of whatever peculiarity the human behavior exhibits requires us to travel throughout our brain's different levels of organization. In particular, this is the case with sleep neuroscience.

Here, we speculate the dopaminergic influence on neuron states associated to sleep and sleep alterations in PD. Our ideas, however, should be considered by keeping in mind the broad cascade of events that underlies the wake-sleep cycle.

Environmental as well as genetic factors trigger networks of intra and inter cellular signals, which promote the specific characteristics associated to wake or sleep states. For instance, due to the light impinging on the retina, signals from circadian oscillators reach specific hypothalamic regions. Such areas regulate the action of distinct brain systems associated to the different responses that an organism presents throughout the sleep-wake cycle. In this sense, the hypothalamus regulates wake-sleep switches through its suprachiasmatic, subparaventricular and dorsomedial nuclei; together with the basal forebrain, it controls ascending arousal systems, through its ventrolateral preopitic, lateral and tuberomammilary nuclei. The hypothalamus also regulates brainstem nuclei, as dorsal raphe and locus ceruleus, which control the cyclic transition between the rapid eye movement (REM) and non-REM (NREM) sleep phases. On the other hand, projections from such brainstem and diencephalon ascending arousal systems reach cortical and thalamic areas, known to be involved in the origin and maintenance of different brain rhythms that specifically underlie some sleep states (Pace-Schott & Hobson, 2002; Hobson & Pace-Schott, 2002).

Brain rhythms reflect the spike mode occurring in groups of neurons. And, as revealed by polysonographic recordings, the wake state as well as the NREM and REM sleep phases, are defined, each one, by characteristic field potential oscillations (Pace-Schott & Hobson, 2002;

Hobson & Pace-Schott, 2002). Accordingly, each behavioral state presents distinct cognitive activities and conscious experiences. Throughout the night, there is a cyclic occurrence of NREM and REM sleep phases, where the NREM stage is composed by the slow wave sleep (SWS) - that includes the sleep stages 3 and 4, besides the lighter sleep stages 1 and 2. In particular, the SWS is characterized by rhythms known as slow oscillations, spindles and sharp wave-ripples (Pace-Schott & Hobson, 2002; Hobson & Pace-Schott, 2002; Hobson, 2009; Diekelmann & Born, 2010).

Thalamocortical systems are highly involved in the achievement of oscillations associated to the SWS, in special, slow oscillations and spindles (Steriade et al., 1993; Steriade, 2006). Whereas slow oscillations originate at the cortex and propagate to the thalamus, the spindles have their origins in the thalamus and propagate to the cortex mediated by the TRN pacemaker (Steriade et al., 1993; Llinás & Steriade, 2006; Steriade, 2006). In both cases, however, the origin of the oscillatory pattern is associated to some strong inhibition leading to a consequent burst mode of spiking. More, according to (Steriade et al., 1993), different types of rhythms may appear depending on the magnitude of such inhibitory event.

Indeed, the cholinergic and noradrenergic neuromodulatory systems are known to regulate the neurophysiologic aspects underlying the brain rhythms in the NREM and REM sleep phases (Diekelmann & Born, 2010). However, the experiments revealing the existence of the mesothalamic dopaminergic pathway (Freeman et al., 2001) made it possible to hypothesize on the dopaminergic influence on neuron states associated to sleep (Pace-Schott & Hobson, 2002).

In this work, we propose that the mesothalamic dopamine action in the thalamocortical circuit is able of generating oscillatory patterns that are typical in sleep states, both in thalamic and TRN neurons, depending on the level of dopaminergic activity. In particular, we consider that the dopaminergic alteration in PD is an essential factor underlying the sleep problems observed in such disease. In this case, both the dopaminergic hypoactivity - due to the SN neurons degeneration -, and the increases in the dopaminergic activity due to the appliance of dopamine-related drugs, would contribute to the appearance of sleep alterations.

Basically, our computational simulations explore two ways by which mesothalamic dopamine may affect the thalamocortical dynamics: the SN activity and the dopamine receptor D4 activation. Overall, we conclude that an extreme dopaminergic mesothalamic hypoactivity favors the appearance of the burst mode in thalamic neurons. Conversely, a high degree of dopaminergic mesothalamic hyperactivity propitiates such an oscillatory rhythm in the TRN neurons. In addition, our simulations hint that, when the SN activity is markedly diminished, a slight factor inducing an increase in the receptor D4 activation triggers the bursting pattern in thalamic neurons. On the other hand, the application of some agent that lowers the D4 activation, under a situation of extreme mesothalamic dopamine hyperactivity, enables the burst mode in the TRN.

In the context of PD, such results point anomalous somnolence as a consequence of the lack of dopamine, due to the SN degeneration. More, neural sleep states may appear as a consequence of drugs administration to increase the dopamine action, when the SN activity is highly disrupted. Another situation we consider important to emphasize refers to the dopaminergic hyperactivity case. Due to the lifelong need of medication for equilibrating the nigral dopaminergic level, PD patients usually present symptoms related to excess of dopamine (March, 2005). We illustrate such situation by increasing the dopaminergic activity. We then observe that a slight diminishing in the receptor D4 activation induces the burst mode of spiking in the TRN. Since the TRN plays an essential role in the consolidation of brain rhythms associated to sleep states, it is plausible supposing that such unnatural dopaminergic hyperactivity underlies the emergence of some spurious sleep states, via TRN, in PD. On the other hand, with relation to the thalamic neurons, such dopaminergic hyperactivity prevents them from entering into an oscillatory state. It thus suggests that symptoms pointing to lack of sleep may have origins in the abnormal presence of high dopaminergic activity, due to drug administration. This situation would also contribute to the understanding of why, in PD, a night of sleep deprivation is commonly followed by a daytime of high alertness (Rye et al., 2000).

Our results agree with the striking ideas exposed in (Dzirasa et al., 2006), which shows that dopamine does play a role in the control of the sleep-wake cycle. Here, through a neurocomputational model, we indicate possible ways by which sleep-related states should emerge as a consequence of alterations in the mesothalamic dopamine activity.

Altogether, this work proposes a link between sleep neuroscience and PD. Through a mathematical and computational approach, we infer that the dopaminergic alterations in PD reach brain nuclei highly engaged in the control of rhythms that characterize different sleep states. Therefore, the presence of anomalous dopaminergic activities facilitate the appearance of spurious sleep states, not achieved in normal conditions through the brain systems directly associated to the circadian control of the sleep-wake cycle.

5. Acknowledgments

This work is kindly dedicated to the memory of Magdalena C. L. Madureira. The author thanks the Brazilian agency CNPq (PCI/LNCC, grants 560108/2010-9, 474218/2008) for the financial support.

6. References

Andrade LAF, Ferraz HB. Quadro clínico. In: Meneses MS, Teive HA (Eds). Doença de Parkinson. Rio de Janeiro: Guanabara Koogan, 2003:80-90.

Arnulf I and Leu-Semenescu S. Sleepiness in Parkinson's Disease. *Parkinsonism and Related Disorders* 1553, S101-S104 (2009).

Braak H, Rüb U, Sandmann-Keil D, Gai WP, de Vos RA, Jansen Steur EN, Arai K, Braak E. Parkinson's disease: affection of brain stem nuclei controlling premotor and motor neurons of the somatomotor system. *Acta Neuropathol* 99, 5:489-95 (2000).

Carvalho LAV. Modeling the Thalamocortical Loop. *International Journal of Bio-Medical Computing* 35, 267-296 (1994).

Carvalho LAV and Roitman VL. A Computational Model for the Neurobiological Substrates of Visual Attention. *International Journal of Bio-Medical Computing* 38, 33-45 (1995).

De Cock VC, Vidailhet M, Arnulf I. Sleep Disturbances in Patients with Parkinsonism. *Nature Clinical Practice Neurology* 4 (5), 254-266 (2008).

De Gennaro L and Ferrara M. Sleep Spindles: An Overview. *Sleep Medicine Reviews* 7, 5,432-440 (2003).

Diekelmann S and Born J. The Memory Function of Sleep. *Nature Reviews Neuroscience* 11, 114-126 (2010).

Dubois B, Pillon B. Cognitive deficits in Parkinson's disease. J Neurol. 1996;244:2–8.

Dzirasa K, Ribeiro S, Costa R, Santos LM, Lin S-C, Grosmark A, Sotnikova TD, Gainetdinov RR, Caron MG, Nicolelis MAL. Dopaminergic Control of Sleep-Wake States. *The Journal of Neuroscience* 26, 41, 10577-10589 (2006).

Florán B, Florán L, Erlij D, Aceves J. Activation of dopamine D4 receptors modulates [3H]GABA release in slices of the rat thalamic reticular nucleus. Neuropharmacology 2004;46:497-503.

Freeman A, Ciliax B, Bakay R, et al. Nigrostriatal collaterals to thalamus degenerate in parkinsonian animal models. Ann Neurol 2001;50:321-329.

Guillery RW, Harting JK. Structure and connections of the thalamic reticular nucleus: advancing views over half a century. J Comp Neurol 2003;463:360-371.

Hobson JA and Pace-Schott EF. The Cognitive Neuroscience of Sleep: Neuronal Systems, Consciousness and Learning. *Nature Reviews Neuroscience* 3, 679-693 (2002).

Hobson JA. REM Sleep and Dreaming: Towards a Theory of Protoconsciousness. *Nature Reviews Neuroscience* 10, 803-813 (2002).

Jankovic J. Emerging Views of Dopamine in Modulating Sleep/Wake State from an Unlikely Source: PD. *Neurology* 58 (3), 341-346 (2002).

Jeanmonod D, Magnin M, Morel A. Low-threshold Calcium Spike Bursts in the Human Thalamus: Common physiopatology for sensory, motor and limbic positive symptoms. *Brain* 119, 363-375 (1996).

Kandel, E.R., Schwartz, J.H. and Jessel, T.M., 2000, *Principals of neuroscience*. 4ed. International Edition: Mc-Graw Hill.

Llinás RR and Steriade M. Bursting of Thalamic Neurons and States of Vigilance. *Journal of Neurophysiology* 95, 3297-3308 (2006).

Llinás RR, Ribary U, Jeanmonod D, Kronberg E, Mitra PP. Thalamocortical Dysrhythmia: A Neurological and Neuropsychiatric Syndrome Characterized by Magnetoencephalography. *Proceedings of the National Academy of Science* 96, 26, 15222-15227 (1999).

Madureira DQM, Carvalho LAV, Cheniaux E. Attentional Focus Modulated by Mesothalamic Dopamine: Consequences in Parkinson's Disease and Attention Deficit Hyperactivity Disorder. *Cognitive Computation* 2, 1, 31-49. DOI 10.1007/s12559-009-9029-4 (2010).

Madureira DQM, Carvalho LAV, Cheniaux E. Modelagem Neurocomputacional do Circuito Tálamo-cortical: Implicações para Compreensão do Transtorno de Déficit de Atenção e Hiperatividade. *Arq. Neuro-Psiquiatr.* 65, 4a, 1043-1049 (2007).

March L. Psychosis in Parkinson's Disease. *Primary Psychiatry* 12, 7, 56-62 (2005).

McCormick, D.A., Connors, B.W., Lighthall, J.W. and Prince, D.A., 1985, Comparative electrophysiology of pyramidal and sparsely spiny stellate neurons of the neocortex. *Journal of Neurophysiology*, 54, 782-806.

Pace-Schott EF and Hobson JA. The Neurobiology of Sleep: Genetics, Cellular Physiology and Subcortical Networks. *Nature Reviews Neuroscience* 3, 591-605 (2002).

Rye DB, Bliwise DL, Dihenia B, Gurecki P. Daytime Sleepiness in Parkinson's Disease. *Journal of Sleep Research* 9, 63-69 (2000).

Rye DB. Parkinson's Disease and RLS: The Dopaminergic Bridge. *Sleep Medicine* 5, 317-328 (2004).

Steriade M, McCormick DA, Sejnowski TJ. Thalamocortical Oscillations in the Sleeping and Aroused Brain. *Science* 262, 679-685 (1993).

Steriade M. Grouping of Brain Rhythms in Corticothalamic Systems. *Neuroscience* 137, 1087-1106 (2006).

Permissions

The contributors of this book come from diverse backgrounds, making this book a truly international effort. This book will bring forth new frontiers with its revolutionizing research information and detailed analysis of the nascent developments around the world.

We would like to thank Dr. Abdul Qayyum Rana, for lending his expertise to make the book truly unique. He has played a crucial role in the development of this book. Without his invaluable contribution this book wouldn't have been possible. He has made vital efforts to compile up to date information on the varied aspects of this subject to make this book a valuable addition to the collection of many professionals and students.

This book was conceptualized with the vision of imparting up-to-date information and advanced data in this field. To ensure the same, a matchless editorial board was set up. Every individual on the board went through rigorous rounds of assessment to prove their worth. After which they invested a large part of their time researching and compiling the most relevant data for our readers. Conferences and sessions were held from time to time between the editorial board and the contributing authors to present the data in the most comprehensible form. The editorial team has worked tirelessly to provide valuable and valid information to help people across the globe.

Every chapter published in this book has been scrutinized by our experts. Their significance has been extensively debated. The topics covered herein carry significant findings which will fuel the growth of the discipline. They may even be implemented as practical applications or may be referred to as a beginning point for another development. Chapters in this book were first published by InTech; hereby published with permission under the Creative Commons Attribution License or equivalent.

The editorial board has been involved in producing this book since its inception. They have spent rigorous hours researching and exploring the diverse topics which have resulted in the successful publishing of this book. They have passed on their knowledge of decades through this book. To expedite this challenging task, the publisher supported the team at every step. A small team of assistant editors was also appointed to further simplify the editing procedure and attain best results for the readers.

Our editorial team has been hand-picked from every corner of the world. Their multi-ethnicity adds dynamic inputs to the discussions which result in innovative outcomes. These outcomes are then further discussed with the researchers and contributors who give their valuable feedback and opinion regarding the same. The feedback is then collaborated with the researches and they are edited in a comprehensive manner to aid the understanding of the subject.

Apart from the editorial board, the designing team has also invested a significant amount of their time in understanding the subject and creating the most relevant covers. They scrutinized every image to scout for the most suitable representation of the subject and create an appropriate cover for the book.

The publishing team has been involved in this book since its early stages. They were actively engaged in every process, be it collecting the data, connecting with the contributors or procuring relevant information. The team has been an ardent support to the editorial, designing and production team. Their endless efforts to recruit the best for this project, has resulted in the accomplishment of this book. They are a veteran in the field of academics and their pool of knowledge is as vast as their experience in printing. Their expertise and guidance has proved useful at every step. Their uncompromising quality standards have made this book an exceptional effort. Their encouragement from time to time has been an inspiration for everyone.

The publisher and the editorial board hope that this book will prove to be a valuable piece of knowledge for researchers, students, practitioners and scholars across the globe.

List of Contributors

Laura B. Valdez and Alberto Boveris
Laboratory of Free Radical Biology, School of Pharmacy and Biochemistry, University of Buenos Aires, Argentina

Manuel J. Bandez and Ana Navarro
Department of Biochemistry and Molecular Biology, School of Medicine, University of Cádiz, Spain

Dorszewska Jolanta and Kozubski Wojciech
Poznan University of Medical Sciences, Laboratory of Neurobiology Department of Neurology, Chair and Department of Neurology, Poland

Lynda J. Peterson and Patrick M. Flood
The University of North Carolina at Chapel Hill, U.S.A

Janet Best and Grant Oakley
Ohio State University, USA

Michael Reed and H. Frederik Nijhout
Duke University, USA

Ben Ampe, Anissa El Arfani, Yvette Michotte and Sophie Sarre
Vrije Universiteit Brussel, Belgium

Tommaso Beccari
Dipartimento di SEEA, Università di Perugia, Italy

Chiara Balducci, Silvia Paciotti and Emanuele Persichetti
Dipartimento di SEEA, Università di Perugia, Italy

Davide Chiasserini, Anna Castrioto, Nicola Tambasco, Aroldo Rossi, Paolo Calabresi and Lucilla Parnetti
Clinica Neurologica, Ospedale S. Maria della Misericordia, Università di Perugia, Italy

Veronica Pagliardini
Dipartimento di Pediatria, Università di Torino, Italy

Bruno Bembi
Centro Regionale per le malattie Rare, Ospedale Universitario 'Santa Maria della Misericordia', Italy

Kaoru Takakusaki and Kazuhiro Obara
Research Center for Brain Function and Medical Engineering, Japan

Toshikatsu Okumura
Department of General Medicine, Asahikawa Medical University, School of Medicine, Japan

Ruiping Xia
Department of Physical Therapy, Creighton University, Omaha, Nebraska, USA

Nirmal Bhide and Christopher Bishop
Department of Psychology, Binghamton University, Binghamton, NY, USA

Daniele Q. M. Madureira
Laboratório Nacional de Computação Científica, Brazil

Printed in the USA
CPSIA information can be obtained
at www.ICGtesting.com
JSHW011409221024
72173JS00003B/480

9 781632 411907